INTERNATIONAL CONGRESS AND SYMPOSIUM SERIES 213

Editor-in-Chief: Lord Walton of Detchant

Essays on the history of anaesthesia

D1476472

Selected and revised contributions by
members of the History of Anaesthesia Society Series 1:
1986–1989

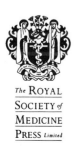

The ROYAL
SOCIETY *of*
MEDICINE
PRESS *Limited*

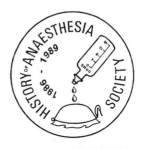

These proceedings are published by Royal Society of Medicine Services Ltd with financial support from the sponsor. The contributors are responsible for the scientific content and for the views expressed, which are not necessarily those of the sponsor, of the editor of the series or of the volume, of the Royal Society of Medicine or of the Royal Society of Medicine Press Ltd. Distribution has been in accordance with the wishes of the sponsor but a copy is available to any Fellow of the Society at a privileged price.

British Library Cataloguing in Publication Data
A catalogue record for this book is available from the British Library
ISBN 1-85315-293-5
ISSN 0142-2367

Phototypeset by Dobbie Typesetting Limited, Tavistock, Devon
Printed in Great Britain by Ebenezer Baylis, The Trinity Press, Worcester

List of illustrations

List of contributors

Aileen K Adams	*Hon Archivist, Royal College of Anaesthetists, Formerly Consultant Anaesthetist, Addenbrooke's Hospital, Cambridge*
RS Atkinson	*Honorary Consulting Anaesthetist, Southend Hospital, Essex*
A Marshall Barr	*Formerly Consultant Anaesthetist, Royal Berkshire Hospital, Reading*
R Colin Birt	*Consultant Anaesthetist, Southend*
TB Boulton	*Formerly Consultant Anaesthetist, Royal Berkshire Hospital, Reading and Nuffield Department of Anaesthetics, Oxford*
OP Dinnick*	*Formerly Consultant Anaesthetist, The Middlesex Hospital, London*
Barbara M Duncum	*Formerly Researcher in Nuffield Department of Anaesthetics, Oxford*
RH Ellis*	*Consultant Anaesthetist, St Bartholomew's Hospital, London*
CA Foster	*Formerly Consultant Anaesthetist, St Thomas's Hospital, London*
Phillida Frost	*Formerly Consultant Anaesthetist, Glan Clwyd Hospital, North Wales*
Sally E Garner	*Technician, Glenfield Hospital, Leicester. Formerly Chief Operating Department Assistant*
Elizabeth Gibbs	*Formerly Consultant Anaesthetist, Basildon and Thurrock Hospitals*
DDC Howat	*Formerly Consultant Anaesthetist, St George's Hospital, London*
J Alfred Lee*	*President of the History of Anaesthesia Society (1986–1989). Formerly Consultant Anaesthetist, Southend-on-Sea*
KG Lee	*Consultant Anaesthetist, Wythenshawe Hospital, Manchester*
ID Levack	*Consultant Anaesthetist, Western General Hospital, Edinburgh*
JM Lewis	*Formerly Consultant Anaesthetist, Morriston and Singleton Hospitals, Swansea*

JR Maltby	*Professor of Anaesthesia, The University of Calgary*
Ruth Mansfield*	*Formerly Consultant Anaesthetist, Royal Brompton Hospital, London and Christian Medical College, Vellore, India*
AHB Masson	*Honorary Archivist, Royal College of Surgeons of Edinburgh. Formerly Consultant Anaesthetist, Royal Infirmary, Edinburgh*
ET Mathews	*Formerly Consultant Anaesthetist, United Birmingham Hospitals*
SW McGowan	*Formerly Consultant Anaesthetist, Dundee Teaching Hospitals, Dundee, Tayside*
I McLellan	*Consultant Anaesthetist, Glenfield Hospital NHS Trust, Leicester*
RW Patterson	*Department of Anesthesiology, University of California, Los Angeles*
AW Raffan	*Retired, now Honorary Consultant Anaesthetist, Grampian Area Health Board*
J Rupreht	*Professor of Anaesthesiology and Resuscitation, University of Llubljana, Slovenia; Erasmus University, Rotterdam, The Netherlands*
CA Russell	*Clinical Research Manager, Portex Ltd, Hythe, Kent*
JF Searle	*Consultant Anaesthetist, The Royal Devon and Exeter Healthcare Trust*
WDA Smith	*Formerly Reader, Department of Anaesthesia, Leeds University*
JB Stetson*	*Formerly Professor of Anaesthesia, Rush Medical College, Chicago*
KA Stewart	*Emeritus Consultant Anaesthetist, The Leicester Royal Infirmary*
P Sykes	*Past President, Society for the Advancement of Anaesthesia in Dentistry*
JAW Wildsmith	*Professor of Anaesthesia, University of Dundee*
DJ Wilkinson	*Consultant Anaesthetist, St Bartholomew's Hospital, London.*
J Wilson	*Formerly Consultant Anaesthetist, Simpson Memorial Maternity Pavilion and Royal Infirmary, Edinburgh*
D Wright	*Consultant Anaesthetist, Western General Hospital, Edinburgh*
D Zuck	*Formerly Consultant Anaesthetist, Chase Farm Hospital, Enfield*

*Deceased

Contents

ORGANIZATION AND COMMUNICATIONS

Preface

A Marshall Barr, Thomas B Boulton,
David J Wilkinson

The papers presented at the first meeting of the History of Anaesthesia Society in June 1986 appeared in abridged form only. Booklets containing the full texts of the presentations at all subsequent meetings have been prepared and circulated to the members of the Society, thanks in large measure to the generosity of Abbott Laboratories Ltd, and the publishing skills of their Medical Adviser, Dr Frank Bennetts.

Council of the Society has felt for some time that the presentations are of a quality which merits a more permanent form of publication and a wider readership; to this end, the editors were asked to select a representative cross-section of essays, and to give their authors the opportunity to revise, update and provide new illustrations. Selection was perplexingly difficult. We have reluctantly omitted papers which have been published elsewhere, and listed these as an appendix. Even with this reduction, the excellence of the remaining material has meant that this volume of essays only covers the first four years of the meetings of the Society, from 1986 to the end of 1989. Much effort has gone into providing full presentations from the historic first meeting, reworking the later contributions to give a new freshness and vitality, and grouping the resultant essays into categories which offer interesting comparisons and contrasts.

The editors are most grateful for the cooperation of all the contributors and the literary executors of those now sadly deceased. We thank also the staff of the Royal Society of Medicine Press for much advice and help. This volume is intended to be first of an ongoing series, which we believe will be a valuable addition to the literature on anaesthesia.

The early history of the History of Anaesthesia Society

TB Boulton

The very successful First International Symposium on the History of Anaesthesia was organized by Joseph Rupreht and held in Rotterdam in 1982 [1,2]. It was followed by a world-wide revival of interest in the subject and a perceived need for the formation of specialist societies dedicated to its study. The Anesthesia History Association (AHA) was formed in the US in 1984, and the process leading to the inauguration of the History of Anaesthesia Society (HAS) in the United Kingdom began in 1985 [2].

The initiative which led to the formation of the History of Anaesthesia Society came from David J Wilkinson (Consultant Anaesthetist to St Bartholomew's Hospital, London) and Ian McLellan (Consultant Anaesthetist at Leicester). Both Wilkinson and McLellan were elected to Honorary appointments by Council of the Association of Anaesthetists of Great Britain and Ireland (AAGBI) about this time; Wilkinson was Honorary Curator of the Charles King Collection of Historical Anaesthetic Apparatus, and has later become Honorary Archivist and Honorary Secretary of the Association of Anaesthetists, and McLellan is Honorary Librarian.

Wilkinson and McLellan approached the then President of the AAGBI (Thomas B Boulton, 1984–1986, Consultant Anaesthetist Reading and Oxford) for support and assistance. An exploratory meeting was consequently held during the AAGBI Annual Scientific Meeting in Leicester on 12 September 1985 with the President of the AAGBI in the chair. The meeting was well attended and the proposal to form a specialist society devoted to the study of the history of anaesthesia was unanimously adopted. A Steering Committee was nominated and J Alfred Lee (Consultant Anaesthetist, Southend-on-Sea 1947–1971 and President of the AAGBI, 1971–1973) was elected to become the first President of the proposed society on its formation [3]. Adrian Padfield (Consultant Anaesthetist, Sheffield) having volunteered the use of his personal computer, was asked to collect names and addresses and £2 from each potential member.

The Steering Committee consisted of J Alfred Lee as Chairman, Boulton, Wilkinson, McLellan and Padfield. Some degree of nepotism can perhaps be detected! The four more junior members of the committee had all trained at St Bartholomew's, Lee (a graduate of Durham Medical School) was the odd man out; but Tom Boulton had been Lee's Senior Registrar at Southend-on-Sea, and both Southend Hospital and St Bartholomew's were in the North East Thames Region of the British National Health Service at that time.

The Inaugural Meeting was held at the Royal Berkshire Hospital, Reading, on 7 June 1986. The meeting included a scientific programme of invited papers and a general business meeting. The name of the Society was confirmed as The History of Anaesthesia Society (HAS). A national designation was avoided with the intention of attracting members from outside the UK, particularly from Europe. The AHA had similarly avoided a national label when it was formed in the US. A Constitution was proposed by the Steering Committee and was accepted with minor modifications. This constitution was based with permission on that drawn up by TM Young (Consultant Anaesthetist, Manchester) for the Association of Dental Anaesthetists formed in 1976. Membership is open to all those over 18 interested in the history of anaesthesia, whether medically qualified or not, subject only to proposal and formal election by Council. The Officers and Council of the HAS are elected by nomination of Council at the Annual General Meeting after counter nominations have been invited by post.

The members of the Steering Committee were elected *en bloc* to be Members of the First Council with the addition of Richard S Atkinson (Consultant Anaesthetist, Southend-on-Sea), A Marshall Barr (Consultant Anaesthetist, Reading) and JA (Tony) Wildsmith (Consultant Anaesthetist, Edinburgh, and now (1996) Professor at the University of Dundee). The Officers elected were: President: A Alfred Lee; Vice-President and President Elect: TB Boulton; Honorary Treasurer and Membership Secretary: A Padfield; Honorary Secretary: I McLellan.

Three Honorary Members were elected by acclamation, two of whom were present at the meeting. These were Professor Sir Robert Macintosh (the first Nuffield Professor of Anaesthetics in the University of Oxford [4] and Dr Barbara M Duncum author of the classic text *The Development of Inhalation Anaesthesia*, first published in 1947, which was subsequently reprinted by the Royal Society of Medicine for HAS in 1994 [5]. Mr Thomas E Keys (Librarian to the Mayo Clinic, Rochester, USA), author of several important texts on the history of anaesthesia was also elected as an Honorary Member [6,7].

The next meeting of the HAS was held at St Bartholomew's Hospital, London on 7 February 1987 at which the Constitution was confirmed. The offer by Abbott Laboratories, obtained through the good offices of Frank Bennetts (Consultant Anaesthetist at Maidstone, Abbott's Medical Adviser, and a member of HAS), for financial and practical support for the publication of a Proceedings booklet for each meeting was gratefully accepted and David Wilkinson was elected Editor.

The Second International Symposium on the History of Anaesthesia was held at the Royal College of Surgeons of England in London in July 1987. It was sponsored by the Association of Anaesthetists of Great Britain and Ireland, but the Organizing Committee was predominantly composed of Officers and Members of Council of the HAS [2].

The next meeting of the HAS was at Southend-on-Sea on 6 February 1988 when the Members of the First Council of the HAS presented the Society with a Presidential Medallion. This was worn for the first time by J Alfred Lee at the meeting.

In subsequent years meetings have been held twice each year: 1986: Reading; 1987: St Bartholomew's, London; 1988: Southend-on-Sea and Leicester; 1989: Croydon and Edinburgh; 1990: Epsom and Huddersfield; 1991: Rotterdam and Southampton; 1992: Cambridge and the Royal Society of Medicine, London; 1993: Llangollen and Birmingham; 1994: Guernsey and the Royal Society of Medicine, London; and in 1995: Glasgow and Poole.

There are now (in 1996) almost 500 members of the HAS.

REFERENCES

(1) Rupreht J, van Lieburg MJ, Lee JA, Erdman W. *Anaesthesia. Essays on its history.* Berlin: Springer Verlag, 1985.

(2) Rupreht J. Foreword. In: Atkinson RS, Boulton TB, eds. *The History of Anaesthesia. Proceedings of the Second International Symposium on the History of Anaesthesia 1987;* International Congress and Symposium Series 134. London: Royal Society of Medicine, 1989: xxiii.

(3) Lunn JN. John Alfred Lee (1906–1989). *Anaesthesia* 1989; **44**: 631.

(4) Beinart J. *A history of the Nuffield Department of Anaesthetics, Oxford 1937–1987*. Oxford: Oxford University Press, 1987.

(5) Duncum BM. *The development of inhalation anaesthesia*. Oxford: Oxford University Press, 1947. (Reprinted by the Royal Society of Medicine, London 1994).

(6) Faulconer A, Keys TE. *Foundations of anesthesiology*. Springfield: Illinois, USA, 1965.

(7) Keys TE. *The history of surgical anaesthesia*. New York: Dover Publications, 1963.

Officers and Council Members 1986–1989

President	J Alfred Lee	1986–88
	TB Boulton	1989
Vice-President	TB Boulton	1986–88
	Aileen K Adams	1989
Honorary Treasurer	A Padfield	
Honorary Secretary	I McLellan	
Honorary Editor	DJ Wilkinson	
Council Members	RS Atkinson	
	AM Barr	1986–88
	JA Wildsmith	
	DJ Wilkinson	
	CA Fuge	1988–89
	JA Bennett	1988–89
	DDC Howat	1988–89
	D Zuck	1988–89
	Buddug Owen	1989
	D Wright	1989
Honorary Members	Sir Robert Macintosh	
	Barbara Duncum	
	Thomas Keys	
	AR Hunter	1989
	Rex Marrett	1989

THERAPEUTICS AND SCIENCE BEFORE 1846

Benjamin Pugh and his air-pipe

DJ Wilkinson

Original presentation Reading 1986

Benjamin Pugh was born in Bishop's Castle, Shropshire in 1715 and was baptized on October 22 1715 in St Mary's Church, Shrewsbury. He was one of 10 children, the son of an excise officer. His uncle, John Wollaston, was a surgeon in Bishop's Castle and might well have influenced his choice of medicine as a career. Benjamin left Shropshire for London at some time in his teens. There is a semi-fictional account of him leaving London in the company of David Ogbourne, an itinerant limner and painter. Both of them settled in Essex, and their lives seemed interwoven from time to time.

In January 1738 Pugh married Amey Evans, a widow and the daughter of the local apothecary, Sherman Wall, who left him his house in Chelmsford when he died in 1743. Records show that in the same year that he married Benjamin was able to buy the Mansion House in Chelmsford, which over the next few years he extensively renovated and enlarged the gardens. By this time he was working as a surgeon, specializing in obstetrics. His father died in 1744 leaving Benjamin the sum of £40, while his elder brother inherited all his father's estate and money. In 1747 he tried to raise money for the printing of a *Treatise of Midwifery* by subscription, but this failed, as did an offer the following year in the *Ipswich Journal* for a set of his obstetric forceps for half a guinea, if the *Treatise of Midwifery* was bought at the same time.

In 1752 he published a letter [1] in the *Gentleman's Magazine* on the 'Success of the Peruvian Bark on the treatment of smallpox', and this was followed the next year by another letter on methods of inoculation [2]. In 1754 he finally published *A Treatise of Midwifery* [3] in which he described obstetric forceps with a pelvic curve as well as an 'air-pipe'. In 1760 he was awarded the MD by examination at St Andrew's University.

In 1772 he co-authored a paper about the Miller of Billericay, Thomas Wood [4] who had survived for the last 20 years of his life on a diet of sea biscuit pudding and water. Wood was the subject of an engraved portrait by Ogbourne, who otherwise seemed to have specialized in painting local scenes around Chelmsford and Great Baddow and the occasional strange creature such as a winged fish at Battle Bridge and a calf with six legs at Great Baddow.

Essays on the history of anaesthesia, edited by A Marshall Barr, Thomas B Boulton and David J Wilkinson. 1996: International Congress and Symposium Series No. 213, published by Royal Society of Medicine Press Limited.

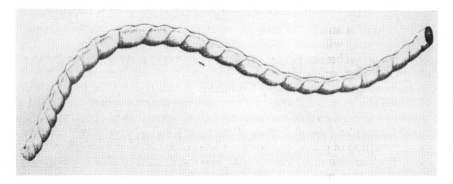

Figure 1   *The 'air-pipe'*

Pugh was obviously a very successful doctor, and through his marriage and his hard work he soon amassed a considerable fortune. He sold the Mansion House in 1773 for £3000 and bought farms in nearby villages, as well as a house in Great Baddow. Ogbourne settled in the same village having married the niece of the landowner who had sold Pugh his farm. Ogbourne taught drawing at Baddow School, died in 1801, and was buried in Chelmsford. Pugh continued to appear in the medical press; he was referred to in a paper on a case of retroverted uterus by his nephew William Bird [5] and wrote further letters on inoculation to the *Gentleman's Magazine* in 1779 [6,7], the year he retired from medical practice. His wife had died 2 years previously and was buried in St Mary's Church, Chelmsford.

For the next few years he seems to have travelled on the Continent. In 1784 he published a small book [8] entitled *Observations on the Climates of Naples, Rome, Nice etc.* and the following year a translation of the work of the French doctor M Pouzaire [9] *A Treatise on the Mineral Waters of Balaruc in the South of France* to which he added 'some additional cases and remarks on the city of Montpellier, its university, environs and the different routes from England to the said baths'. It is interesting to note that one of his companions/patients on this latter trip of several months was a Mr Wollaston, presumably a maternal relative.

In 1788 he bought Midford Castle, a large country house outside Bath where he spent the rest of his days. He had married again at some stage; his wife was Sarah Anne Page of Fillongley, Warwickshire. He died on February 14 1798 [10] at the age of 83 and was buried at Freshford Church where there is a memorial to his name above the entrance. His wife lived on at Midford Castle until 1808 when she moved to Landsdowne Terrace in Bath where she died on 29 March 1811, and was buried with her husband at Freshford.

Pugh's interest to anaesthetists can be found in his *Treatise of Midwifery* [3]. This book described some 14 years of obstetric experience. Pugh believed that 'every young surgeon now intends practising midwifery and so every help must be acceptable to these young practitioners and improvements are agreeable to older ones'. It is a very detailed obstetric work and is based on over 2000 personal cases. Pugh is believed to be the first to have described the pelvic curve of an obstetric forceps. His work was ready for publication in 1747 and indeed the forceps was advertised by the *Ipswich Gazette* for sale at this time. His book describes how the apparatus had been made by a cutler in Chelmsford, one Mr Archers, many years before and this definitely gives him precedence over the other two claimants of the pelvic curve forceps namely Smellie (1751) and the Frenchman André Levret (1747).

His air-pipe (Fig. 1) is described 'as big as a swans quill in the inside, ten inches long, is made of a small common wire, turned very close (in the manner wire springs are made) will turn anyway and covered with thin soft leather'. Pugh described its use in breech deliveries when the child's head could be trapped by a narrow pelvis and suffocate. He would introduce his fingers into the child's mouth trans-vaginally 'one end of the tube is introduced up the palm of the hand and between the fingers as far as the larynx—the other external'. The practitioner could then blow on the tube and maintain an airway. 'Every operator must know there is difficulty and great danger of losing the child by its stay in the passage, but by this method of giving the child air I have saved great numbers of children's lives which otherwise must have died.' Having described this elegant technique he then wrote that more recently he had abandoned it as he found that the presence of his hand and fingers afforded an adequate airway under these circumstances. 'You must then introduce the fingers of your left hand into the vagina, under the child's breast, and put the first and second fingers into the child's mouth pretty far, so far however that you are able to press down the child's tongue in such a manner that by keeping your hand hollow and pressing it upon the mother's rectum, the air may have access to the larynx you will soon perceive the thorax expand so the air gets into the lungs.'

He was also a believer in mouth to mouth resuscitation of neonates. 'If the child does not breathe immediately on delivery which sometimes it will not—wipe its mouth and press your mouth to the child's at the same time pinching the nose with your thumb and finger to prevent air escaping; inflate the lungs rubbing it before the fire by which method I have saved many.'

This is an amazing description of neonatal resuscitation from an age where such techniques were by no means commonplace. Although Fothergill and others were beginning to consider expired air ventilation for adult resuscitation in the early 1740s, it would be another 20–30 years before the Humane Societies were founded and these ideas could be fully developed.

Dr Benjamin Pugh was a man of many talents: a writer, traveller, obstetrician, physician and surgeon. He made numerous major medical contributions during his 84 years and should be remembered by anaesthetists for his air-pipe—a flexo-metallic paediatric airway and for his descriptions of neonatal resuscitation.

REFERENCES

(1) Pugh B. Success of the Peruvian Bark in a deplorable smallpox. *Gentleman's Magazine* 1752; **22**: 209–10.
(2) Pugh B. Methods of inoculation. *Gentleman's Magazine* 1753; **23**: 216–8.
(3) Pugh B. *A treatise of midwifery*. London: J Buckland, 1754.
(4) Baker G, Pugh B, Chaplyn R. The case of Mr Thomas Woods, a miller, of Billericay, in the county of Essex. *Med Trans Coll Physic Lond* 1772; **2**: 259–74.
(5) Bird W. An account of a retroverted uteri. *Med Obs Inq Soc Physic Lond* 1776; **5**: 110–12.
(6) Pugh B. General inoculation. *Gentleman's Magazine* 1779; **49**: 192–3.
(7) Pugh B. Inoculation. *Gentleman's Magazine* 1779; **49**: 247.
(8) Pugh B. *Observations on the climates of Naples, Rome, Nice etc*. London: G Robinson, 1784.
(9) Pugh B. *A treatise on the mineral waters of Balaruc*. Chelmsford: W Clacher & S Gray Co, 1785.
(10) Obituary. *Gentleman's Magazine* 1798; **68**: 177.

Sir Robert Christison and *A Treatise on Poisons*

JR Maltby

Original presentation Edinburgh 1989

Sir Robert Christison was one of the famous 19th century medical professors in Edinburgh, and a contemporary of Simpson and Syme. He was born in Edinburgh in 1797 and received his early education at the High School. At fourteen, he went to the University of Edinburgh for four years where he studied literature and natural and physical science. He then became a medical student and developed a special interest in botany and chemistry [1]. Having graduated as a Doctor of Medicine in 1819, he spent several months at St Bartholomew's Hospital in London and then went to Paris to take advantage of the exceptional facilities there to acquire theoretical and practical knowledge of chemistry. He studied chemistry under Vauquelin and Thenard, physics under Guy-Lussac, and toxicology under Orfila. He also visited the French Institute when discoveries were announced of the chemical composition of vegetable substances, in particular the separation and characters of the alkaloids. He received a thorough training in practical chemistry, and studied under the most distinguished toxicologist of the time.

In 1822, while he was still in Paris, the Chair of Medical Jurisprudence in Edinburgh became vacant. Although he was only 25 years old, Christison's friends proposed him for the appointment which he competed for and received. He held the chair from 1822 to 1832, during which time the number of students in his class rose from 12 to 90. He succeeded in producing order and precision in the teaching of medical jurisprudence, which had previously been confused and indeterminate. In addition, he conducted research and gained a national reputation as a medical jurist.

From 1832 until his retirement in 1877 at the age of 80, Christison had a distinguished career as Professor of Materia Medica and held numerous other appointments. He was Dean of his Faculty while still a junior professor, member of the University Court 1858–82, twice President of the Royal College of Physicians of Edinburgh, in 1838 and 1846, and President of the Royal Society of Edinburgh 1868–73. He was the Scottish representative on the General Medical Council from 1858 until 1873, and in 1875 he became President of the British Medical Association. For many years he was Physician in Ordinary to Queen Victoria in Scotland, and in 1871 a baronetcy was conferred on him.

Christison's reputation as Scotland's leading medical jurist was founded on his *Treatise On Poisons* which was first published in 1829. This book became the standard work of reference for 50 years. At the time of Christison's death, it was said that the book would always show the author's power of 'systematizing existing knowledge, of educing principles from judiciously considered facts, acquired with much industry from a wide range of literature and from laborious

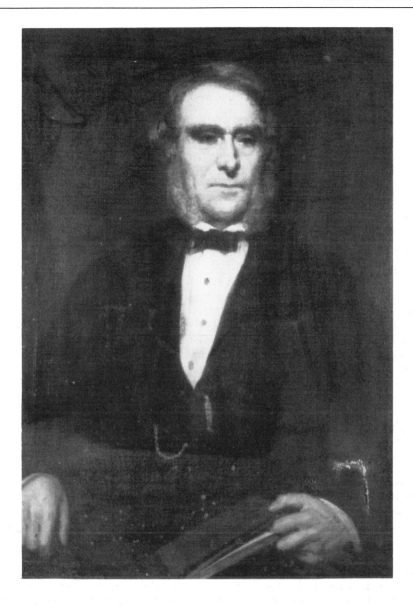

Figure 1 *Sir Robert Christison (1797–1882) (Reproduced with permission of the Royal College of Physicians of Edinburgh)*

personal observations, and of stating in terse and lucid language the results of original experiments and the details of chemical processes.'

A TREATISE ON POISONS

Four editions of this book were published, the last in 1845, just a year before Morton gave the first public demonstration of ether anaesthesia. The fourth edition [2] is of most interest to anaesthetists because it summarizes the extent of pharmacological and toxicological knowledge, immediately before anaesthesia was discovered.

The first part of the book runs for 100 pages and deals with general aspects of poisoning. These include the physiological action of poisons, their symptoms, morbid appearance, chemical analysis, and the results of animal experiments. More than half of the second part, which runs to nearly 900 pages, is devoted to inorganic poisons, and the remainder to organic poisons, mostly from plants, and poisonous gases. In the final section Christison described the effects of several of the drugs that were used in the first 100 years of anaesthesia: opium, morphine, atropine, hyoscyamine, nitrous oxide, ether and curare although, except for opium and morphine, their beneficial effects were not predicted. The importance and value of the book is enhanced by comprehensive footnote references to earlier publications on each drug.

OPIUM

In the years between 1825 and 1850 opium was one of the most important poisons for suicide or murder, or to induce stupor in victims before robbing them. Christison described several cases, including the tests for identifying morphia and its salts. It was known that opium was absorbed more quickly when applied to the surface of a wound than orally, and fastest of all when injected into a vein. Although it was generally believed that opium was carried through the bloodstream to the brain, there were some who thought it was carried along nerves.

The effect of a small dose taken orally was initially stimulating, however this effect varied among individuals and was usually insignificant. The symptoms of overdose began with giddiness, then rapidly increasing stupor until the person became motionless and insensible. At this stage, slow respiration and contracted pupils were observed. If recovery took place, it followed prolonged sleep of 24 to 36 hours and was accompanied by nausea, vomiting and giddiness. Survival for 6 hours following ingestion of opium signified a good prognosis. Christison observed that the sleep of opium overdose differed from that of true coma in that the patient could usually be roused, but would relapse as soon as the stimulus was withheld.

Opium, in the form of laudanum, was commonly used in poultices applied to the skin. Accidental overdoses were recorded when the skin was broken, although overdose could also occur through the unbroken skin.

The treatment of opium poisoning was by the use of a stomach-pump and emetics. However, Christison recommended that, in desperate circumstances, artificial respiration should be used. He observed that the heart continued to beat for some time after breathing had ceased. He felt that it was 'not improbable that the only ultimate cause of death from opium is suspension of the respiration and that if it could be maintained artificially so as to resemble exactly natural breathing, the poison in the blood would be at length decomposed and consciousness gradually restored'.

HYOSCYAMUS

Medicinal doses induced a pleasant sleep, and poisonous doses caused loss of speech, dilatation of the pupils, coma, and delirium commonly of the 'unmanageable and furious kind'. Poisoning usually occurred from confusion between poisonous and nonpoisonous leaves or roots. Treatment was similar to that for opium poisoning, and the claim by an Italian that a large dose of lemon juice was an immediate antidote was dismissed by Christison as 'improbable'.

ATROPINE

Atropine poisoning usually occurred in September from ingestion of the black berries of the deadly nightshade, *Atropa belladonna*. Christison described the properties of atropia crystals in detail, but did not record any medicinal use of this alkaloid. Dilatation of the pupil occurred after atropine application to the skin around the eye, the surface of a wound, or following ingestion. The main symptoms of overdose were dryness of the throat, then delirium with dilated pupils followed by coma. The delirium was sometimes accompanied by uncontrollable laughter and constant talking. Convulsions were rare. Recovery was common, although occasionally delirium lasted for up to 3 days.

NITROUS OXIDE

Christison quoted the writings of Davy and other researchers. However, he did not mention Davy's observation that nitrous oxide dulled the pain of an erupting wisdom tooth [3], or his suggestion that it might be used in small surgical operations, nor did he record Horace Wells' use of nitrous oxide in his dental practice in Hartford, Connecticut in 1844 [4].

ETHER

Sulphuric ether and nitric ether were considered poisons of the same nature as alcohol. Inhalation of ether vapour produced a strong sense of irritation in the throat, fullness in the head, and other symptoms similar to those produced by nitrous oxide. As a habitual treatment for asthma, gradually increasing doses were required, although there appeared to be no material injury with long-term use. Two cases of overdose were described in which breakage of large containers of ether occurred in confined spaces. In one case, a druggist's maid-servant died in her sleep after accidentally breaking a three gallon jar of ether in her apartment. In a similar case, a young man was found unconscious but recovered after several hours.

CURARE

Christison commented that poisons used by the American Indians were 'mere objects of curiosity' in Europe, and therefore scarcely merited discussion. Nevertheless, he quoted six authors and concluded that death occurred by suspension of respiration. He also referred to Waterton's successful use of artificial respiration in two curarized donkeys in 1839 [5], in one case for $7\frac{1}{2}$ hours, in the other for 2 hours.

DISCUSSION

Christison was a pharmacologist and toxicologist with a deep interest in research, and also a practising physician. He was not searching for analgesic or anaesthetic effects of drugs to relieve pain in dentistry, childbirth, or surgery. Although he described the effects of most of the drugs that would achieve importance in the first century of anaesthesia, he did not recognize their potential in that field. Many years later, in 1876, he became an enthusiastic advocate of chewing coca leaves to relieve exhaustion and increase energy [6], although again he did not appreciate the significance of numbness in his mouth for either anaesthesia or analgesia. The true pioneers of anaesthesia were those like Horace Wells [4] and William TG Morton [7] who, seeking pain relief for dental surgery, introduced nitrous oxide and ether, Sir James Y Simpson [8] who found chloroform to be a better agent than ether for pain relief in labour, Carl Koller [9] who recognized the local anaesthetic effect of cocaine in the eye, and Griffith [10] who used curare safely and effectively in anaesthetized patients.

Nevertheless, in *A Treatise on Poisons*, Christison has left us a wonderful legacy, providing a comprehensive review of pharmacology and toxicology of the available drugs at the time that general anaesthesia was discovered.

REFERENCES

(1) Anonymous. Sir Robert Christison, Bart, MD, LLD, DCL. *Edinburgh Med J* 1882; **XXVII (Part II)**: 852–62.
(2) Christison RA. *A treatise on poisons*. 4th ed. Edinburgh: Adam and Black 1845. (Reprinted 1988 for The Classics of Medicine Library, Division of Gryphon Editions, Inc., P.O. Box 76108, Birmingham, Alabama, 35253).
(3) Davy H. *Researches, chemical and philosophical; chiefly concerning nitrous oxide*. London: Johnson, 1800: 465.
(4) Colton GQ. *Anaesthesia. Who made and developed this great discovery?* New York: AG Sherwood and Co, 1886: 1–15.
(5) Waterton C. The wourali poison. *Lancet* 1838–39; II: 285–6.
(6) Christison R. Observations on the effects of cuca, or coca, the leaves of Erythroxylon coca. *Br Med J* 1876; I: 529.
(7) Warren JC. Inhalation of ethereal vapour for the prevention of pain in surgical operations. *Boston Med Surg J* 1846; **35**: 375–9.
(8) Simpson JY. On a new anaesthetic agent, more efficient than sulphuric ether. *Lancet* 1847; II: 549–50.
(9) Koller C. *Bericht ber die sechszehnte Versammlund der ophthalmolischen Gesellschaft*. Heidelberg 1884; Rostock, Universitts-Buchdruckerei von Adlers Erben 1884: 60–3.
(10) Griffith HR, Johnson GE. The use of curare in general anesthesia. *Anesthesiology* 1942; 3: 418–20.

Dependency of an American discovery on Edinburgh

RW Patterson

Original presentation Edinburgh 1989

On the martyr's monument in Greyfriars Churchyard, Edinburgh, is the inscription 'Which truths were Sealed by Famous Guthrie's Head'. It refers to a prominent Covenanter whose beheading prompted some of his relations to seek security in America. In 1830, one of his descendants, Samuel Guthrie, produced a novel chemical compound — chloroform. Prompt recognition of its incomparable boon was obscured by the teachings of the worldwide-prevailing Brunonian theory of medicine promoted in Edinburgh — the authoritative centre of medical education at the beginning of the 19th century. Perhaps Simpson's introduction of the drug into clinical practice was in some way a curious completion of a cycle that had ensured chloroform's links with Edinburgh at an earlier time.

Samuel Guthrie was essentially a product of a pioneer culture. He studied medicine as an apprentice under his father. During the winter of 1810–11 he attended a course of medical lectures in New York and again during January 1815 he attended lectures at the University of Pennsylvania, Philadelphia [1]. These studies together with his father's teaching indoctrinated him to believe that there were only two classes of disease: sthenic and asthenic. Treatment was equally straightforward: 'the indication for the cure of sthenic diathesis is to diminish, that for the cure of the asthenic diathesis is to increase the excitement, and to continue to increase it' [2]. His father's legacy underlined the importance of this tradition. He left his son one dollar, the five volumes of Rush's *Medical Inquiries and Observations*, and a set of silver catheters.

Dr Benjamin Rush of Philadelphia graduated from the University of Edinburgh in 1778. In a 1790 eulogy he summarized the teachings of the school and the accomplishments of the late Professor of Medicine, William Cullen. Referring to Cullen, 'He stripped Materia Medica of most of the errors that had been accumulating in it for two thousand years and reduced it to a simple and practical science' [3]. As though presaging the profound impact of his own teaching on American medical practice, Rush continued the eulogy: 'Dr Cullen is now no more. What a blank has been produced by this death in the great volume of Science! Behold! The genius of humanity weeping at his feet while the genius of medicine lifts up the key which fell from his hand with the last breath, and with inexpressible concern, cries out: to whom shall I give this instrument? Who will now unlock for me the treasures of universal nature?' [3].

Rush was not about to let the enlightening Scottish torch splutter out. Accepting the hypothetical abstraction 'The Principle of Excitability' as dogma and applying observable features common to the known fevers, he was able in a consistent and inexorable progression of reason to explain that all remote causes of disease (cause defined as the abstraction, or unusual application of stimuli) produced only differing 'states' of one disease. Treatment was accordingly simplified; if depleted of excitement, stimulants were added; if excited, drugs and procedures to exhaust the patient were required. Rush advocated uniformity of treatment. Rush believed that a multiplicity of treatments to fit the individual case was not only a mistake but a form of quackery. His explicit enlightenment of faith in the simplicity, predictability, and rationality of the universe and his Jeffersonian conviction that in real and important ways all men had been created equal, were reflected in his advocacy of a minimalist equating of one mankind, one disease, one therapy. During his long tenure as Professor of Medicine at the University of Pennsylvania, two-thirds of the physicians formally educated in America graduated from the University.

At another American Medical School, Columbia in New York City, the students were exposed to the teachings of John Brown, Alexander Monro, William Hunter and Joseph Black through the intermediary of their chemistry professor, Dr Samuel Latham Mitchell, who graduated from the University of Edinburgh in 1787. Mitchell's theory linking yellow fever contagion with exposure to nitrous oxide (published in 1795) stimulated Davy's research into nitrous oxide [4].

A mainstay of Brunonian therapy was the use of diffusible stimulants. Davy noted that 'the immediate effects of nitrous oxide upon the living system are analogous to those of diffusible stimuli' [5]. This prompted him to suggest combining CO_2, which he believed acted as a sedative, with N_2O to obtain; 'a regular series of exciting and depressing powers applicable to every deviation of the constitution from health'. Davy further suggested: 'The quickness of the operation of nitrous oxide will probably render it useful in cases of extreme debility produced by deficiency of common exciting powers. Perhaps it may be advantageously applied mingled with oxygen or common air, to the recovery of persons apparently dead from suffocation by drowning or hanging' [5]. By 1800, the use of N_2O [6] and ether [7] as diffusible stimuli was recommended for resuscitation. The occasional observation of temporary or permanent unconsciousness failed to call into question the principles of Brunonian dogma, being attributed to 'fainting' in the former case, and to severity of disease in the latter.

By 1817 Samuel Guthrie had settled in the town of Sackets Harbor on the eastern shore of Lake Ontario in upper New York State. He indulged his innate studiousness and curiosity by setting up a workshop for 'all sorts of tinkering', and a chemical laboratory for experiments. His chemical investigations were not those of a dilettante, but were designed to solve specific needs or problems and frequently led to commercial undertakings which for the time and place were extensive and profitable.

In Volume 2 of Benjamin Silliman's *Yale College of Chemistry* published in February 1831, Guthrie read that the 'alcoholic solution of chloric ether is a grateful diffusive stimulant and that as it admits of any degree of dilution it may probably be introduced into medicine'. He immediately set to work to produce this diffusive stimulant in cheap and easy way and by that spring a new compound dripped from the water-encased 'worm' of his still. In the summer of 1831 he sent a description of his method for publication in the *American Journal of Science and Arts* [8], the leading scientific journal in America at the time. Benjamin Silliman, the editor, as well as the first Professor of Chemistry at Yale College, considered the communication from this untutored chemist to be 'honorable to the rising chemical arts of this country'. Presumably no one suspected that such things were occurring in a remote region on the shore of Lake Ontario. In the fall of that year Silliman noted in his journal 'I have written to Mr Guthrie. Having been requested by some of our physicians to obtain a supply for regular use'. Numerous testimonials attested to its usefulness in various disease states without discovering its most useful attribute. This oversight may be attributed to yet another instance where the significance of a pivotal fact was obscured because there was a 'rational' explanation for its occurrence.

Guthrie's children were accustomed to playing in his laboratory when he was experimenting and an event which happened to his eight-year-old daughter, Cynthia, was described in a family letter: 'He had large tubs of liquid standing on the floor and she used to stick her fingers in the tub and taste the liquid; one tub she liked to taste, so did often, and he was watching her and one day she got too much and fell over and he ran to her and picked her up and then found that the liquid in this tub put her to sleep' [9].

It is remarkable that this astonishing event was not recognized there and then, for Guthrie was accustomed to capitalizing on his observations. According to the prevailing theory, unconsciousness could be expected as a side effect of 'too much stimulus'. His 'true' use of his new diffusive stimulus was also recounted in another family letter; writing to his eldest daughter he recalled her need to be resuscitated from carbon monoxide poisoning: 'Dear Harriot . . . sweet whiskey which you remember taking when suffocated with charcoal. You see it called chloroform and the newspapers are beginning to give me credit of discovering it. I made the first particle that was ever made and you are the first human being that ever used it in sickness' [9].

During the early 1800s Rush's legacy of authoritative pronouncements served as the standard of American professional health care. Although the single-minded attempt to bind mutually exclusive, individually unsolved, problems into a unified whole produced an unwieldy dogma which eventually led to confusion between cause and effect of disease processes, to therapeutic excesses, and to the nearly acute demise of orthodox US medicine [10]. Rush's 'diffusible stimulant' standby was mercury (in toxic doses, frequently transforming the patient's disease into a mercurial disease) combined with massive doses of Mexican jalap to be followed by the 'letting' of eight to ten ounces of blood for good measure. Additionally, 'whipping' and the 'hot iron' were part of his therapy. He believed a body could have only one disease at a time. Since he considered pain itself to be a disease, secondarily inflicting greater pain on a patient should drive the original disease from the body.

During the 1830s the public began to baulk at the harshness of standard therapy and at the pretension and power of a perceived elitist medical profession. This was the era of Jacksonian democracy; the intellectual aristocracy that had theorized about equalitarianism was now supplanted by a de facto social and political equalitarianism which combined a celebration of the common man and anti-intellectualism with hatred of authority and monopoly. It generated widespread distrust of professional medicine, distrust expressed most forcibly in the repeal of virtually all state medical licensing laws during the 1830s and 1840s.

Concurrent with the collapse of 'heroic practice' and the subsequent re-examination of disease cause and effect and re-evaluation of therapeutic measures, there was also a rethinking of the scientific implications of pain resulting in the antithetical view expressed by Hahnemann 'there is nothing to cure but the suffering of the patient'.

With these expansions of medical thought the way was prepared for acknowledgement of the usefulness of anaesthetic-induced reversible loss of consciousness, pain relief and Simpson's revelation from Edinburgh.

REFERENCES

(1) Guthrie O. *Memoirs of Dr Samuel Guthrie*. Chicago: GK Hazlitt Publishing Company, 1887.
(2) Brown J. *The elements of medicine, or a translation of the elementa Medicinae Brunonis, with large notes, illustrations and comments*. Philadelphia: Wm Spotswood, 1791; **1**: 32.
(3) Rush B. *An eulogium in honor of the late Dr Willliam Cullen. Professor of the Practice of Physics in the University of Edinburgh; delivered before the College of Physicians of Philadelphia*. Philadelphia: Thomas Dobson, 1790.
(4) Bergman NA. The earliest description of nitrous oxide narcosis. *Sem Anesth* 1987; **5**: 253.
(5) Davy H. *Researches, chemical and philosophical; chiefly concerning nitrous oxide or dephlogisticated nitrous air and its respiration*. London: J Johnson, 1800.
(6) Hancock J. *Observations on the origins and treatment of cholera and other pestilential diseases, and on the gaseous oxide of nitrogen as a remedy in such diseases, as also in cases of asphyxia from suffocation and drowning and against the effects of narcotic poisons*. London: J Wilson, 1831.
(7) Conner E. Anesthetics in the treatment of cholera. *Bull Hist Med* 1966; **40**: 52.
(8) Guthrie S. New mode of preparing a spiritous solution of chloric ether. *Am J Sci Arts* 1831; **21**: 64.
(9) Robinson V. Samuel Guthrie. *Medical Life* 1927; **34**: 102.
(10) Coulter HL. *Divided legacy. A history of the schism in medical thought*. Washington DC: McGrath Publishing Co, 1978: vol 3.

William Clayfield's mercurial airholder

WDA Smith

Original presentation Leicester 1988

Humphry Davy's early experiments of the measurement of nitrous oxide uptake and of lung volume used an apparatus called William Clayfield's Mercurial Airholder. Clayfield derived the idea from James Watt's gasometer, then called the hydraulic bellows, but Clayfield's airholder was made of glass and sealed by mercury instead of water [1,2].

Full excursion of the bell turned a pulley, from which it was suspended, through one revolution. The counterpoise weight was suspended from a spiral pulley, mounted on the same axle, to allow for change of upthrust with depth of immersion. The cavity at the top of the internal cylinder was intended 'to contain any liquid it may be thought proper to expose to the action of the gas'.

For respiratory experiments the subject breathed directly into the bell, allowing his head to follow. Davy emphasized that only after many experiments breathing air could he begin and end in the same posture.

A replica of this airholder was made in Leeds University, the glassware in the Department of Chemistry by Mr HS Butler, and the non-vitreous parts by Mr KD Horner in the Department of Anaesthesia.

THE PORTRAIT

In early 1988, Mr Horner visited the Antique Scientific Instrument Fair in London. There he saw an oil painting of a young gentleman behind whom was depicted Clayfield's mercurial airholder. The subject, apparatus and artist were unidentified (Fig. 1). The young subject might have been Davy because only he published results obtained using this unique airholder. The painting was about 14" × 11", and Clayfield's mercurial airholder was quite undeniable.

The face in the portrait possibly seemed young enough to be Davy at Bristol, but it looked older than in the Sharples likeness of Davy taken there and he looked a little older than the Howard portrait of Davy at the Royal Institution when he was 23. The face was not convincingly Davy's, but, knowing that two artists can sometimes make one subject look like two different people, the idea could not be rejected. Against the young face and the heavy dark eyebrows the hair looked inappropriately grey and unlike the hair in Davy's portraits.

The dealer asserted that the subject must have invented the apparatus but Clayfield was vague about the use of his airholder, as if it were an invention awaiting an application. Cartwright [3], referring to Clayfield, quoted Gregory Watt. 'Oh that I could hear of the reformation of that profligate Clayfield' and added that Clayfield seemed to have been a pupil of James Watt and was in general charge of the apparatus for producing gases. He further described

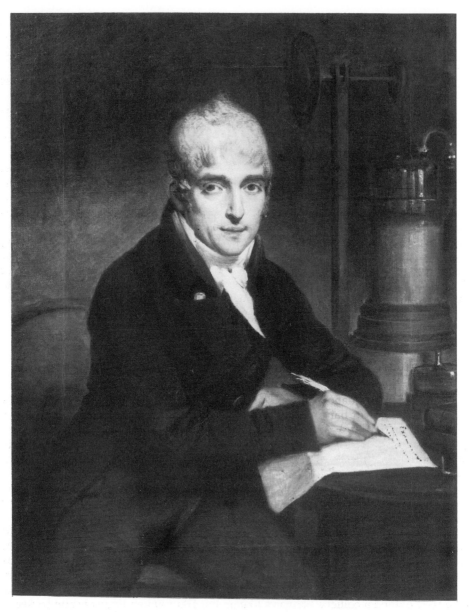

Figure 1 *Presumed portrait of William Clayfield painted by Singleton. Reproduced by kind permission of the Association of Anaesthetists of Great Britain and Ireland*

Clayfield as 'dissolute and lazy but still an eager chemist and a follower of the elder Watt'. That description did not seem to quite match the gentleman portrayed in the painting. Furthermore, heading the sheet of paper on the portrait is the word 'Experiments' and any experiments performed by Clayfield using the airholder were not well known.

It was likely that the presence of the airholder might point as much to the Pneumatic Institution as to Clayfield himself. A portrait of the founder of the

Medical Pneumatic Institution bears no resemblance, nor would James Watt be a likely candidate. Other people for consideration are: John King but that was ruled out in Bristol after comparison with known portraits and written descriptions; Dr Kingslake did not perform many experiments in the Pneumatic Institution although he was part of it; Mr Sadler, an interesting person, but not as likely as Clayfield; and Tobin and Cox who are probably very unlikely.

The Bristol art gallery's solution to the grey hair was the use of hair powder. The black trousers were said to date the portrait at about 1815 to 1820. The National Portrait Gallery has records of a portrait of W Clayfield, Esq by Henry Singleton, exhibited at the Royal Academy in 1805, but its location is unknown.

The Wood Library Museum of Anesthesiology in Chicago has manuscripts said to have been addressed to William Clayfield. They probably were for him but his name had been erased from most of them. The writers were Beddoes, Davy, Davies Gilbert, J and JW Tobin and JW Williams. They refer to analyses of metal ores and wastes, to an iron cement, to the marriage of JW Tobin, to current affairs and to fishing. They include an interesting note from Dr Beddoes to Dr Darwin, most probably referring to Clayfield, which reads: 'The bearer is my particular friend, the most ingenious philosopher in this part of the world and who nothing but money getting prevents from being among the most successful explorers of nature anywhere'.

EVIDENCE FROM THE UNIVERSITY OF KEELE

Much has been unearthed by Dr Hugh Torrens at the University of Keele whose files reveal that William Henry Clayfield died in 1837 aged 65, so he was about 29 when Gregory Watt bantered about his profligacy. Obituaries described Clayfield as a gentleman of high philosophic and scientific attainments, having from a very early period devoted all his leisure time to the acquisition of knowledge, chiefly in the departments of chemistry, botany, mineralogy and geology. Davies Gilbert, later President of the Royal Society noted in his diary that William Clayfield's father, Michael Clayfield, was 'a man of much science and knowledge, of very low origin, but he married Miss Morgan of rather high connections'. Directories recorded him as a tobacconist and distiller.

Michael had three sons, Edward, Charles and William. Davies Gilbert noted about William: 'well known as a chemist and philosopher', he ascended with Mr Sadler in a balloon and had the misfortune of descending in the Severn. He was unmarried in 1825. James Sadler was father of the Pneumatic Institution's Sadler.

Edward and William Clayfield were partners in a wine merchants' business, and they owned a colliery. Edward was on the original management committee of the Somerset Coal Canal. Trevithick visited them in 1802 to discuss the installation of a high pressure steam engine for pumping and winding at Clayfield Colliery. In 1799, James Sowerby and Dawson Turner recorded that at Bristol they had received kind attention from Dr Dyer and Mr William Clayfield, who pointed out the more remarkable local plants.

William Clayfield, was associated with the Medical Pneumatic Institution circle. In November 1798 Davy wrote to Davies Giddy (Davies Gilbert, who changed his name): 'I suppose you have not heard of the discovery of the native sulphate of strontium in England. We have it in large quantities, mistaken for sulphate of barytes till our friend Clayfield detected strontium. Clayfield has been working on it, we have persuaded him to publish his analysis.'

CLAYFIELD AND HUMPHRY DAVY

The friendly correspondence between Clayfield and Davy up till at least 1816, aired their common interest in fishing. When Davy published his *Elements of Chemistry* in 1812, he wrote to Clayfield: 'I have not sent you a copy of my book, for I have thought that the best mode of avoiding giving offence to some was by not making any presents at all. Had I not so determined, one of the first copies would have been sent to you'.

Did Davy learn from Clayfield in the early days? Did Clayfield conceive his air holder in the context of chemical analysis? Had respiratory experimentation been his main objective he might have produced something easier to use. The idea of using it for respiratory purposes may have been suggested by Davy or Beddoes, as Clayfield's previous lignum vitae versions of the air holder would have been quite impractical for respiratory experiments.

In his *Life of Sir Humphry Davy* [4], John Aryton Paris noted that 'Thomas Beddoes was occasionally assisted by Mr William Clayfield, a gentleman ardently attached to chemical pursuits and whose name is not unknown in the annals of science. Indeed, it appears that to him he was indebted to the invention of the mercurial air holder by which he was enabled to collect and measure the various gases submitted to examination'.

This portrait is most probably of Clayfield. It has its own charm, and one could wish for it to be bought by an institution where the association with Dr Beddoes, Sir Humphry Davy, the Medical Pneumatic Institution and nitrous oxide would be understood and appreciated.

Editors' Note: The portrait was subsequently purchased by the Association of Anaesthetists and can be seen at 9 Bedford Square. The portrait is still believed to be that of William Clayfield and was probably painted by Singleton.

ACKNOWLEDGEMENT

The author is most grateful to Dr Hugh Torrens, University of Keele for sight of his Clayfield file.

REFERENCES

(1) Clayfield W. Description of a mecurial apparatus in Beddoes T and Watt J. *Considerations on the medicinal use and production of factitious airs.* Bristol: Bulgin and Rosser, 1795.
(2) Clayfield W. Description of a mercurial airholder suggested by an inspection of Mr Watt's machine for containing factitious airs. *Phil Mag* 1800; **7**: 148.
(3) Cartwright FF. *The English pioneers of anaesthesia.* Bristol: John Wright and Sons Ltd, 1952.
(4) Paris JA. *The life of Sir Humphry Davy.* London: Henry Colburn and Richard Bentley, 1831.

EARLY DAYS OF ANAESTHESIA IN BRITAIN

Surgery and anaesthesia: the start of a tandem alliance

Barbara Duncum

Original presentation London 1987

John Snow was a professional anaesthetist from the last week of January 1847 until his death from apoplexy on June 16 1858, just three months after his 45th birthday. During those years Snow worked with most of the leading surgeons in London and kept a record of his cases. The list of operations could have been matched at almost any time during the quarter of a century preceding the discovery of anaesthesia. The difference after the discovery, was that whilst a surgeon was operating neither he, nor his patient, had pain to contend with. William Fergusson, Professor of Surgery at King's College, London, summed up the situation as it still was in 1864 'Although before the discovery of anaesthesia most if not all the great achievements of our art, had already been accomplished', he said, 'anaesthesia permits the surgeon to perform his duty with a security of thought and action quite unknown to his predecessors' [1]. All the same, a good many surgeons did not feel that security, until docile-seeming chloroform had superseded obstreperous ether in November 1847.

A week after Liston's famous amputation at University College Hospital, Snow saw for the first time a patient with a clip on his nose struggling to draw air through ether-drenched sponges in a glass container, along narrow tubing and into a mouthpiece. He realized at once that etherizing needed a firm physiological and practical basis; the etherist must know the appropriate strength for the ether/air mixture entering the patient's lungs and must be able to control it [2]. Before starting to experiment Snow already had two key pieces of information. He knew that at different temperatures 100 in^3 of air would take up different percentages of ether vapour and he knew of an inhaler, invented by Julius Jeffreys FRS in 1836, which would serve as a model for a dosimetric vaporizer. Jeffreys had used his inhaler for treating bronchitis with moist air. It was a round tin box about 5 ins across and 4 ins deep with warm water in the bottom. The lid had an air inlet and an inhaling tube, and inside the box was a spirally-coiled baffle plate which caused the drawn in air to pass several times over the liquid before reaching the

Essays on the history of anaesthesia, edited by A Marshall Barr, Thomas B Boulton and David J Wilkinson. 1996: International Congress and Symposium Series No. 213, published by Royal Society of Medicine Press Limited.

mouthpiece [3]. Essentially Snow's portable regulating ether inhaler was the same except that when in use, it stood in a basin of water at between 60° and 65 °F which produced an ether/air mixture containing around 47% ether vapour.

Snow introduced his inhaler at a meeting of the Westminster Medical Society on January 23, 1847 and it was well received [4]. He lost no time in offering his services as an etherist to the surgeons at St George's. His first operating session there was on January 23rd. Operating sessions in the London teaching hospitals were open occasions held weekly and they were normally attended by medical students and practitioners. However, since the beginning of 1847, they had been attracting crowds of casual spectators curious to see painless operating. After Snow's second session at St George's, the senior surgeon, Mr Caesar Hawkins, publicly thanked him and added that Dr Snow's instrument was very much superior to those he had previously used [5]. Snow later said that he believed St George's was the first institution in which the vapour of ether was constantly applied with uniform success in surgical operations [6].

During the spring of 1847 Snow improved his inhaler and tried out the facepiece invented and sent to him by Francis Sibson. He then evolved a facepiece of his own based on Sibson's prototype. It was nearly ready to go into production at the beginning of May when Snow began to work with Liston at University College Hospital, London and in Liston's private practice. Soon Liston was recommending him to other surgeons in private practice and between that help and the grapevine, Snow's own practice was beginning to build up. By September when he published his book on ether, much of the most important and interesting anaesthetic work in London was already being offered to him [7].

Liston died unexpectedly in December 1847. In the New Year, Snow began working with William Fergusson at King's College Hospital, and increasingly in Fergusson's very extensive private practice. Fergusson was only 5 years older than Snow and the two men evidently got on and worked well together since the association lasted until Snow's death 10 years later. Fergusson, apparently, never once referred to Snow or mentioned his skill as an anaesthetist; indeed, from the way Fergusson wrote about anaesthesia in his published work one might have thought he gave all the anaesthetics himself.

Snow's interests covered the whole field of anaesthesia, but his main concern was always the safety and comfort of his patients, and their individual responses within the five stages of anaesthesia he had earlier identified. Whilst still at St George's and afterwards at other hospitals, he occasionally took some preoperative responsibility for certain cases, notably when a leg about to be amputated could not be moved without intense pain. Snow would then anaesthetize in the ward, and at St George's at any rate, where the doorways and corridors were wide, he would accompany the patient still in his bed to the theatre, giving a last whiff of anaesthetic just before the transfer from the bed or the stretcher, to the table [8].

An account of Snow's postoperative care occurs in connection with piles, then treated by threading ligatures through the mucous membranes with a needle. A dose of opium was always given as soon as the patient came round from the anaesthetic, but postoperative pain was often severe. Many of these cases were Fergusson's private patients, operated on, of course, at home. Snow would remain at the bedside sometimes for an hour or two giving chloroform intermittently until the opium took full effect. He thought it would have been helpful if the opium could have been given 3 or 4 hours before the operation. Surgeons had used preoperative sedation before the discovery of anaesthesia but now thought it unnecessary.

Snow had a theory about piles. He noticed that they were much commoner in the upper classes of society than amongst working class and even middle class people, and had nothing to do with what they ate or drank. The disorder was purely related to when they had the main meal of the day. The lower classes had their dinner at midday while the upper classes took it in the evenings which had the unfortunate effect of leaving their liver and bowels congested overnight [9].

Fergusson was very emphatic in believing that 'all the horrors of our art', as he put it, 'should be concealed from common observation as much as possible', and he was ironically scathing about surgeons who seemed to delight in a show of blood. 'If the patient's clothes and bed coverings could be spotted all over or saturated,' they thought that was good; and if the operator and assistants were spattered from head to foot, so much the better. 'I have heard of a surgeon', he said, 'who, not content with using towels for his hands, actually seized the white bed curtains and wiped his bloody paws! And I have seen a man of fame proceed from one operation to another with his hands still covered with the first patient's blood.' In Fergusson's opinion, a good surgeon not only dealt promptly with haemorrhage, he did his best to remove all traces of it. Before he started to operate a sufficient supply of sponges and hot and cold water had to be ready at hand [10].

Contrasting sharply with the niceties of Fergusson's procedures, a macabre search for a strangulated hernia in the abdomen of an unanaesthetized patient was reported in *The Lancet* in July 1858, just a month after Snow's death. The patient was a youngish greengrocer, on the portly side, but usually in good health, who was taken acutely ill after eating rather a lot of veal for his dinner. A private doctor was sent for and he, in turn, sent for Mr Tatum from St George's. The greengrocer's surgeon, *The Lancet* said, did not consider him a suitable patient for taking chloroform and Tatum, apparently without more ado, slit open the man's belly and fished around first with one finger, then with three, until he could grasp the knot and pull it out to be dealt with. The real trouble started when Tatum tried to put the gut back; 'this I found extremely difficult to do', he said, 'for as fast as I returned a portion a greater volume escaped'. At last all was once more confined. 'Our patient', the two surgeons blandly remarked, 'felt very little fatigue or was the worse for the operation, though we considered him in great danger for a day or two' [11].

On the subject of operations without anaesthesia, Fergusson, lecturing at the Royal College of Surgeons in 1864, asserted that the question of giving chloroform in lithotrity was still a moot point in some quarters and he made a similar comment about excision of tumours of the upper jaw. He dismissed the suggestion that chloroform should not be given in these operations, particularly the jaw excisions which he described as frightful to behold. He himself had always given chloroform, he said, and had never seen any ill effects [12]. Snow, recording 11 excisions of the upper jaw he and Fergusson had done together, made some prefatory remarks. Mr Syme, Mr Lizars and some other surgeons expressed an opinion at one time that chloroform could not be safely used as the blood would be liable to flow into the lungs. 'This is not the case' Snow said, 'as the glottis retains its sensibility apparently unimpaired, if the influence of the chloroform is not too deep or long continued. It is only necessary to hold the head forward now and then, when the throat is very full of blood, in order to allow the patient the same opportunity of breathing that he would require if he were awake'.

Snow, in these cases, induced anaesthesia with his inhaler and then changed to a mixture of chloroform and alcohol on a hollow sponge, holding this as near as he could to the patient's face without getting in anybody's way, but he had to admit that he couldn't always keep the patient insensible [13].

He used a small sponge moistened with chloroform and alcohol when Fergusson was repairing hare-lips in infants. Most of these babies were aged between 3 and 6 weeks, some were younger, the youngest was only 8 days old. The success of the operation depended on Fergusson's dexterity and he was so quick that scarcely any blood was lost. A nurse sat opposite him supporting the baby with its head in his lap and between his thighs while an assistant compressed the labial artery. Twenty seconds from the start the pins were in and the cut edges of the lip were pressed together. Some of these babies were operated on at home, others at King's College Hospital. 'I have no doubt', said Snow, 'that many lives are saved by early operation especially amongst the poor, as a child with a bad hare-lip cannot take the breast and there is a very great mortality amongst infants brought up by hand' [14].

Out of nearly 100 cases of lithotomy anaesthetized for Fergusson, 34 were children, some of them as young as 4 years old. For them Snow used his inhaler fitted with a small version of his ordinary facepiece. While two assistants held down the child's legs it was the anaesthetist's job to steady the head and shoulders to prevent a reflex jerk as the first cut was made. Older patients were restrained with bandages as they had been in the past, for 'it would be an abuse of chloroform', Snow said, 'if merely to save the trouble of bandaging, its effects were carried so far that not the slightest contraction of the muscles could be excited by the use of the knife' [15].

Snow noted several cases in which ovaries were tapped but there were only three occasions when a cyst was actually removed. The first and third patients died from peritonitis 3 or 4 days postoperatively. On the second occasion, in August 1850, Snow gave chloroform whilst Fergusson and two other well-known surgeons assisted the operating surgeon, EW Duffin. The patient, a 38-year-old unmarried dressmaker, whose cysts made her appear 8 months pregnant, had begged Duffin to operate, saying she was confident it would be a success. She proved to be right and was able to go back to her dressmaking.

Duffin later described her case at a meeting of the Royal Medical and Chirurgical Society. In the discussion, several surgeons claimed they were removing ovarian cysts with success, but Caeser Hawkins spoke out against the operation. He himself had removed an ovarian cyst on a single occasion, and although he had been successful, he now thought that except in an emergency, the procedure was too dangerous to be justified [16,17].

Among Snow's most numerous, often distressing cases, were 222 mastectomies. The majority of them were for malignancy and in private practice. Snow wrote in his book on chloroform, published after his death, that 'there is no surgeon I am in the habit of assisting who does not occasionally have to remove a malignant, as well as a non-malignant tumour of the breast. I have not seen any case where the patient did not go through the operation and live, as far as I can remember, for two or three days, but the combination of a great haemorrhage and a great wound is apt to be fatal' [18].

An instance of what Fergusson meant by the security of thought and action conferred by anaesthesia, showed up as a trend in Snow's records of amputations before and after the introduction of chloroform. In 9 months in 1847, 32 arms and legs were cut off; but in a 3-year period ending in March 1858, the total number of cases was only 16. One of Fergusson's great interests was the excision of joints and he acknowledged the influence of James Syme who, in 1823 in Edinburgh, had excised his first elbow and left his patient with a still usable arm. It was an aphorism of Fergusson's that there had never been a time when conservative surgery, a term he himself coined in 1852, had not been the true aim of all good surgeons [19,20].

Other kinds of surgery appearing in Snow's casebooks included a variety of eye operations, such as the correction of squint in children; a vast number of dental extractions by dentists working in Snow's own neighbourhood, Soho, and obstetric cases. One of Snow's first administrations of chloroform, on the 25 November 1847, was for Edward Murphy, the Professor of Midwifery at University College. Murphy, who had an exceptionally difficult delivery in prospect, wanted to try the powerful new agent, and there was nobody but Snow he would trust to give it for him. The occasion did indeed prove formidable; the baby, mercifully dead, had to be hooked out piecemeal. The mother survived. She had been in labour for 39 hours [21].

Benjamin Ward Richardson, who piloted Snow's book on chloroform through the press soon after his friend's death, prefaced it with a memoir. In it he said that on average over the past decade, Snow had anaesthetized some 450 times a year, and latterly had been earning about £1000 a year, but never more because so often Snow would not take a fee from the patient [22]; £1000 a year was not a bad income in those days.

Today it seems strange to find that neither the *British Medical Journal* nor *The Lancet* marked Snow's death with an obituary. When they received a copy of Snow's book, however, both journals, particularly the *BMJ*, reviewed his work appreciatively and at some length, and each added a few comments on the kind of man they thought Snow had been. The *BMJ* said 'Richardson's memoir was entertaining, and not uninstructive as exhibiting the struggles of a poor man of sterling integrity and merit, but destitute of the popular talents by which early success is sometimes attained'. The editor of *The Lancet* first rebuked Richardson for not alluding to the active part taken by that journal in bringing Dr Snow's merits before the profession, at a time when such an encouragement was all important to him at the start of an arduous career. 'We have nothing but good to say of Dr Snow, alive or dead', the editor went on. 'He was a patient and earnest worker for the good of his fellow men, one of those practical philanthropists whose efforts were none the less meritorious because they were exerted for his own advancement, as well as for the benefit of others. It was from his hand that the sufferer, whether alone in the curtained bedroom or publicly on the hospital table, could best obtain the full advantage of this greatest and most beneficial discovery of modern medical science' [23,24]. A little patronizing, perhaps, those two journals.

REFERENCES

(1) Fergusson W. *Lectures on the progress of anatomy and surgery*. London: 1867; 22–3.

(2) Snow J. *On the inhalation of the vapour of ether in surgical operations*. London: John Churchill, 1847: 15.

(3) Jeffries J. On the atmospheric treatment of the lungs. *London Med Gazette* 1842; **6**: 5–7.

(4) Snow J. Apparatus for inhaling the vapour of ether. *Lancet* 1847; **1**: 120–1.

(5) Anon. Operations without pain. St. George's Hospital. *Lancet* 1847; **1**: 184

(6) Snow J. *On the inhalation of the vapour of ether in surgical operations*. London: John Churchill, 1847: 16.

(7) Richardson BW. Memoir. In Snow J. *On chloroform and other anaesthetics*. London: John Churchill, 1858: xiv.

(8) Snow J. *On chloroform and other anaesthetics*. London: John Churchill, 1858: 276.

(9) Snow J. *On chloroform and other anaesthetics*. London: John Churchill, 1858: 307.

(10) Fergusson W. *Lectures on the progress of anatomy and surgery*. London: J Churchill & Sons, 1867: 283–5.

(11) Tatum T. Hernia strangulated within the abdomen, successfully operated on. *Lancet* 1858; **2**: 58–9

(12) Fergusson W. *Lectures on the progress of anatomy and surgery*. London: J Churchill & Sons, 1867: 197, 237, 24.

(13) Snow J. *On chloroform and other anaesthetics*. London: John Churchill, 1858: 281.

(14) Snow J. *On chloroform and other anaesthetics*. London: John Churchill, 1858: 291.

(15) Snow J. *On chloroform and other anaesthetics*. London: John Churchill, 1858: 271.

(16) Anon. Royal Medical Chirurgical Society. *Lancet* 1850; **ii**: 583–7.

(17) Snow J. *On chloroform and other anaesthetics*. London: John Churchill, 1858: 308–309.

(18) Snow J. *On chloroform and other anaesthetics*. London: John Churchill, 1858: 285–6.

(19) Fergusson W. On resection of bone. *Medical Times and Gazette* 1852; **4**: 8–11.

(20) Snow J. *On chloroform and other anaesthetics*. 1858. London: John Churchill, 1858: 277–8.

(21) Murphy EW. Administration of chloroform in cases of difficult parturition. *Lancet* 1847; **2**: 653

(22) Richardson B W In Snow J. *On chloroform and other anaesthetics*. London: John Churchill, 1858: xi.

(23) Anon. Reviews and notices. *Br Med J* 1858; **2**: 1047–9.

(24) Anon. Reviews–notices of books. *Lancet* 1858; **2**: 555–6.

Early ether anaesthesia—the enigma of Robert Liston

RH Ellis

Original presentation Reading 1986

Ether anaesthesia was first publicly and successfully used in Boston Massachusetts in October 1846 [1,2]. Within a few weeks a long and detailed medical article on the subject by Henry Bigelow, a Boston surgeon had been sent across the Atlantic to Dr Francis Boott, an expatriate American physician living in London [1–7]. Within a few days Boott had not only organized the first anaesthetic ever to be given in England [1,2], but had also stimulated the train of events which was to lead to the first, and much publicized, use of ether for major surgery in England [5,7].

THE FIRST USE OF ANAESTHESIA IN ENGLAND

Anaesthesia was first used in England on Saturday 19 December 1846 at Dr Boott's home in London. It was given by a leading London dentist, James Robinson, who then extracted a young lady's molar tooth [1–3,5]. During the rest of the weekend of 19–20 December, Boott and Robinson made several other attempts to produce the state of insensibility with ether, but only their first administration was a success [3,5].

THE FIRST USE IN ENGLAND OF ANAESTHESIA FOR MAJOR SURGERY

Anaesthesia was first used for major surgery in England by Robert Liston, on Monday 21 December 1846, two days after its use by Boott and Robinson [1–3,5,7]. This was at the North London Hospital, now known as University College Hospital (UCH). Liston operated before an invited audience made up largely of influential doctors. He performed two operations, the first a mid-thigh amputation and the second the removal of a toenail. The patients were etherized by William Squire—a young medical student. The demonstration was judged a success and Liston himself was clearly very pleased, and enthused about it to his audience [7]. The whole event attracted a great deal of comment. The most effective publicity was that generated by Dr Francis Boott in a letter in *The Lancet* of 2 January 1847 quoting a private letter he had received from Liston enthusiastically reporting the success of these first two cases [5].

Boott's letter to *The Lancet* ended with the optimistic words, 'I hope Mr Liston will report of these cases more fully'. But Liston never reported these or any other of his ether cases. Indeed he did not write a single word intended for publication about ether; nor did he speak at (or seemingly even attend) any of the medical meetings held in London at the time to discuss the new and exciting discovery. The few comments of his that were published, appeared solely as the result of being reported by others. This at first sight may seem surprising. Liston in 1846 was London's leading surgeon, and at the height of his career. He was a Vice President of the fore-runner of the Royal Society of Medicine and had spoken at its recent meetings. In addition he had numerous recent publications in the leading medical journals, and had written two successful textbooks, the fourth edition of one having appeared only a short while before his first use of ether.

THE ENIGMA

Thus if Liston had wished to promote ether he could have commanded a large and attentive audience or readership. And this is the enigma of Robert Liston as far as anaesthesia is concerned. Why, with his reported enthusiasm for ether, and with more opportunities than anyone else involved to promote its use, did he not do so? In public, why did he of all people remain so silent?

The solution to this enigma is to be found in still surviving primary sources. A study of hitherto overlooked material shows that Liston's views about ether changed markedly soon after his dramatic and successful demonstration. His initial reaction of enthusiasm gave way, almost within hours, to one of qualified endorsement, and then within days to near abandonment of the process. Some months were then to pass before his eventual acceptance of ether anaesthesia. This paper explores in more detail these four separate phases of Liston's thinking about ether.

INITIAL ENTHUSIASM

Liston's enthusiasm for ether began as soon as he heard of its successful use in Boston, Massachusetts; but it lasted only for a few days, until just a matter of hours after his successful demonstration at the North London Hospital. This enthusiasm was generated, and until that demonstration sustained—despite setbacks—almost entirely because of the ways in which Liston heard the news from Boston.

He heard the news in two ways, only one of which has previously been recognized. Firstly, he heard about ether in a private letter from Dr Francis Boott on either 17, 18 or 19 December 1846. This is well documented [1–3]. But he also heard about it directly from Boston, almost certainly on 17 December, from Edward Everett. This fact has not hitherto been recorded, but the evidence for it was found in 1985 in Boston, when I had the chance to study Edward Everett's papers. Everett was an eminent non-medical Bostonian, a scientifically-aware man of letters. He was at the time President of Harvard University, and had in 1845 completed a highly successful four-year term as the United States Ambassador in London. He was therefore well-known in influential academic and scientific circles in both the United States and in Britian [8].

Interestingly enough, my researches in Boston also revealed that by the time Liston had heard about ether from Boott and Everett, several other leading medical men in London had also learned from Everett about the introduction of ether anaesthesia in Boston. For a variety of reasons, none of these other leading doctors responded positively to the news. Liston, however, did so and his initial enthusiastic reaction may, in part at least, be explained by his having received the news from not one, but two, independent reliable sources. Boott's letter conveyed the approval of the eminent doctors of Boston, and Everett's the approbation of the community's considerable lay intelligentsia. As a result of these two letters Liston would not really have been left in any doubt that ether anaesthesia was worth trying. We can well understand his immediate acceptance of the invitation from Boott and Robinson to see one of their early trials of ether for dental extraction.

And so, sometime on Saturday 19 December, taking with him the young medical student William Squire (who over 40 years later wrote an account of Liston's actions) [9], Liston went to Boott's house to see James Robinson give ether for dental extraction [6,9]. They did not see the first, and only successful, case of the day, but saw one or possibly more of the later unsuccessful ones. Undeterred by this lack of success Liston, his confidence apparently undiminished, left to pursue the matter further. He did so in three ways. Firstly he sought, in vain, a better inhaler, secondly he attempted, again vainly, his own trial of ether for dentistry, and thirdly he opted to demonstrate ether in public for major surgery. All these tasks were attempted within the next 48 hours of that brief, initial time when Liston was enthusiastic about ether [7,9].

In seeking a better inhaler Liston and Squire went off to Squire's uncle, Peter Squire, who was a London chemist. He designed an inhaler for them. This new inhaler was a modification of Nooth's apparatus which was originally designed to produce carbon dioxide to impregnate water. This was precisely the same device on which Boott and Robinson had already based their own inhaler, and which Liston and the younger Squire had seen in use a few hours earlier [1–3, 7, 9]. This identical choice of the relatively rare Nooth's apparatus could not possibly have been a coincidence; Liston and his group undoubtedly borrowed Boott and Robinson's ideas but this plagiarism was never acknowledged.

Liston's much overlooked unsuccessful trial of ether for dentistry also occurred in this initially enthusiastic period—on the following day, Sunday 20 December 1846. Peter Squire's inhaler was used, and to help him, Liston sought the aid of Edwin Saunders, another London dentist. The trial was unsuccessful because Liston and Saunders, unlike Boott and Robinson, had arranged for only one patient, and that patient refused to continue with the experiment after he had taken just a few breaths of ether [7,9]. Liston himself never referred to this episode.

By now, Liston had seen at least one of Boott and Robinson's unsuccessful cases and had failed in his own attempt to use ether for dental extraction. These failures would have discouraged most people, but clearly the reliance Liston placed on what he had learnt about ether's use in Boston from Francis Boott and Edward Everett was undiminished. He decided to go ahead on the next day with his plans for a public demonstration of the use of ether for major surgery. This took place in the operating theatre of the old UCH building in London, on Monday 21 December 1846. He operated on two of his patients, and he chose to do so in front of an invited audience, amongst whom were eminent physicians, surgeons and medical editors. Everyone present judged the demonstration a success and it established Liston's deservedly important place in the history of British anaesthesia. At the time he dominated the London surgical scene. Had the demonstration been made by a lesser surgeon, it would probably not have carried the same weight with medical, surgical and lay opinions.

The success of this demonstration confirmed Liston's enthusiasm, and this initial reaction to what happened was important because it was so widely reported, and referred to by the many others who then tried the process for themselves [5]. Liston's remark 'Gentleman! This Yankee dodge beats mesmerism hollow!' is, unfortunately apocryphal. Nonetheless, his initial reaction to ether was undoubtedly and unreservedly enthusiastic. At the end of this demonstration he praised ether in glowing terms. Within hours he held a dinner party at which he horrified the ladies present by trying ether on a guest, his surgical assistant, whom he rendered insensible (exactly as Simpson did after first using chloroform one year later) [10]. Furthermore, within hours he wrote at least two personal letters describing his operations and praising ether anaesthesia. The recipients of these two letters fortunately thought the contents to be so important that they sent them off to reputable journals for wider, more enduring publication.

One was the letter to Francis Boott, who sent it for publication in the *Lancet* of 2 January [5]. Thus was published Liston's famous comment: 'It is a very great matter to be able thus to destroy sensibility to such an extent, and without, apparently, any bad result. It is a fine thing for operating surgeons . . .' The second letter was written by Liston to a surgical friend in Edinburgh, Professor James Miller, who arranged for its publication in the *North British Review*. To Miller Liston wrote: 'Hurrah! Rejoice! Mesmerism and its professors have met with "a heavy blow and great discouragement" . . . In six months no operation will be performed without this prior preparation . . . Rejoice!'

FROM ENTHUSIASM TO QUALIFIED ENDORSEMENT

Soon after these eulogistic pronouncements, at the most within a few days, Liston qualified his opinion about ether's usefulness. This phase of his opinion lasted from around Christmas 1846 until early in the New Year. We know of this phase because in the memoirs of Sir James Young Simpson we can read how Simpson came down from Edinburgh to visit Liston during the Christmas holiday of 1846. The two men discussed ether anaesthesia and Simpson later recalled: 'When I saw Mr Liston in London during the following Christmas holidays he expressed to me the opinion that the new anaesthetic would be of special use to him—who was so swift an operator—as he thought that it could only be used for a brief time.' This was a commonly held misconception at that time, but it may have weighed more heavily with Liston than with other surgeons because Liston's great claims to fame as a surgeon were his physical strength and the speed with which he could operate. These were the only two attributes by which any surgeon in the pre-anaesthetic era could minimize the horror suffered by a patient having to endure an operation while fully awake. But the advent of anaesthesia was to change things, and quite predictably it would soon no longer be necessary for a surgeon to be either marvellously quick or wonderfully strong. Although there is no firm evidence for his having done so, it would have been quite understandable if Liston had had the disquieting thought that, when widely adopted, ether anaesthesia could diminish the importance of the two attributes, speed and strength, on which so much of his own considerable reputation had been built.

NEAR ABANDONMENT

Liston's phase of near abandonment of ether began early in the New Year, and was certainly established by 4 January 1847, which was just two weeks after his first, enthusiastic use. Liston seems to have lost faith in anaesthesia at this point, and was quite prepared to abandon its use altogether. It was unfortunate for the fledgling specialty of anaesthesia that these dispiriting occasions were publicized in the medical journals. Just as his initial enthusiasm helped the launching of anaesthesia in Britain so this later about turn by such an involved and eminent man may well have retarded its progess. In early January 1847 the *Medical Times* recorded that on Friday 1 January: 'At University College Hospital Mr Liston attempted the operation of amputation of the forearm with the assistance of Mr Squire's apparatus; but after endeavouring to produce insensibility for 10 minutes without success the arm was amputated with the usual amount of pain' [11]. And on Monday 4 January: 'A woman was to have a breast tumour removed by Mr Liston. After inhaling the vapour of ether for upwards of 20 minutes without any sensible effect the operation was performed with the usual amount of pain' [11]. Liston's reasons for nearly abandoning ether at this stage were complex, but his immediate reaction was probably the result of three factors. Firstly, his impatience at the prospect of having to wait for 20 minutes or so while anaesthesia was induced; secondly, the inefficiency of Squire's inhaler which clearly did not always produce satisfactory anaesthesia; thirdly, and I believe most importantly, genuine and growing doubts in Liston's mind about ether's usefulness.

Because of his silence on the subject we can only infer these doubts from the comments made by other surgeons, but there is every reason to believe that they would have occurred to Liston just as they did to his surgical colleagues. Without doubt some leading surgeons did oppose ether most strongly. In March 1847, an article in *The Lancet* stated: 'Amongst English surgeons, there are some, whom all of us have been accustomed to regard with immense admiration for their brilliant talents, who have steadily set their faces against the use of ether, and who are exerting all the influence their reputation gives them to discourage its employment.' We do not know whether Liston was one of the surgeons referred to, but he clearly must at least have been aware that some of his eminent colleagues opposed ether most strongly, and apparently with good reasons. Firstly, many surgeons insisted that the pain of awake surgery was the most important stimulus of the processes of healing and survival, and that the mortality rate of surgery, already in the order of 30%, would increase dramatically if ether was used to abolish this vital stimulus. Secondly, there was certainly a problem, then identified as the 'unpredictability' of ether, the essence of which was summarized in *The Lancet* in mid-January 1847: 'In some cases there is perfect insensibility to pain . . . (but) . . . there are cases in which ether does not act at all or appears to act as a violent stimulus' [13]. So at this early stage, in some instances ether worked well, and in others it did nothing; but the most dramatic, serious and worrying cases were those in which ether was reported to act as a 'violent stimulus'. This was of course the stage of excitement on induction or emergence, but at the time it was not at all understood. If, as often happened, the surgery coincided with this stage, an unmanageable shambles resulted, and the ether appeared to make the surgeon's task, which was already difficult, virtually impossible.

The third problem was that of indiscriminate administration. This arose because in the first few months of British anaesthesia, anyone so inclined, be he doctor, dentist, chemist or whoever, felt free to devise his own unique inhaler for ether, and then to try it out whenever he could. More often than not these episodes also resulted in a shambles, with the ether failing to work because of the hopeless inhalers and hapless administrators. But of course the ether was blamed for the deficiencies of both.

This certainly was a problem, as many inhalers must have been designed and used. Twenty-four different inhalers were illustrated in just three British journals within a few weeks of ether's first use in England. Presumably these were reasonably satisfactory and worth writing up, but hundreds more must have been invented, tried, found to be useless and never published or illustrated [1].

James Robinson's inhaler, developed from the one with which he had given England's first anaesthetic, was considered to be effective. The *Medical Times* of 9 January 1847 declared: 'That Mr Robinson has succeeded in inventing a most perfect apparatus cannot be questioned. . .' [14]. The editor's next and reassuring remarks make it clear that at the time some people in Britain thought that ether did not really produce anaesthesia, and that the Bostonian experience was not repeatable on this side of the Atlantic: 'The results have now been witnessed by hundreds of the medical profession, and they have acknowledged that it really exerts the influence attributed to it by our American brethren, and that it may be employed without danger or difficulty' [14]. James Robinson was sent for immediately following the second of those two horrendous cases at UCH, in which the surgery had gone ahead on fully conscious patients after the ether had seemingly failed. Already by that time (4 January), Robinson had obviously acquired a reputation as a skilled and effective ether administrator. Thereafter the cases were anaesthetized most satisfactorily. The same *Medical Times* reported: 'After this a woman was operated on for partial closure of the mouth. Mr Robinson superintended the inhalation of the vapour using his own apparatus. The patient became insensible in two minutes and the operation was completed before she was aware that it had begun' [11].

LISTON'S INTEREST IN ANAESTHESIA REVIVES

Following this success Robinson was asked to anaesthetize more of Liston's cases. This he did, competently, using his own inhaler. No further instances of awake surgery by Liston were recorded, and it appears that Liston's flagging interest in ether was revived by James Robinson's skill. For a while—a matter of several weeks—Robinson became Britain's premier anaesthetist, and at the end of January 1847 the *Medical Times* described him as 'a gentleman who has had more experience of ether than any other in the Kingdom' [15].

Despite Robinson's success, the problems created by inept etherizers and inadequate apparatus persisted, as John Snow later recalled: 'Mr Robinson, dentist, gave much time and attention to the exhibition of ether in London on its first introduction, and was on the whole very successful. This was not generally the case, however, with other operators during the first six weeks of the new practice. Owing to imperfections in the inhalers employed and in the method of using them, the ether often failed altogether or only made the patient partly insensible: and Mr Liston, and some other surgeons were inclined to discountenance the use of it, in consequence of the struggles and cries of the patients to whom it had been administered' [16]. By April 1847, however, John Snow had established his anaesthetic practice [17], and with his medical background and scientific approach he soon supplanted Robinson as Liston's regular anaesthetist [18]. Snow's efforts completely restored Liston's confidence in ether. Thus, in *The Lancet* of 22 May 1847, referring to operations by Liston on 3 May, it is noted: 'He had, at one time, doubts about the utility of ether but he had lately performed several operations in which the ether had been given by Dr Snow with perfect success, and he was inclined to modify his opinion' [19].

By the spring of 1847, when Liston eventually accepted ether anaesthesia, its use had been validated and established beyond all doubt by Robinson and Snow. Henceforth Liston's views, be they for ether or against it, were irrelevant and none of his opinions on the subject were publicized. Had he made any pronouncements about ether at this stage of things, he could well have been accused of merely following the leads already given by others, and that, most certainly, was not Liston's style. After May 1847, if for no other reason than this, Robert Liston remained silent on the subject of ether anaesthesia.

CONCLUSION

The next references to Liston in most medical journals recorded his unexpected death at the age of 53, in December 1847 [20–22]. This was less than a year after his original and short-lived exhortation to rejoice in the discovery of anaesthesia. That we can and do rejoice in the discovery of ether anaesthesia today is in no small part due to Liston's initial enthusiasm for the subject. His later attitudes to ether were adopted for reasons which seemed to him at the time to be quite sound, however it must be said that these later opinions did nothing whatsoever to help promote ether anaesthesia in this country. Quite the reverse, in fact! During its earliest weeks, the wellbeing of anaesthesia in Britain rested in the hands, not of Robert Liston, but initially James Robinson, and then of John Snow.

REFERENCES

(1) Duncum BM. *The development in inhalation anaesthesia*. London: Oxford University Press, 1947: 130–65. (Reproduced on behalf of the History of Anaesthesia Society. London: Royal Society of Medicine, 1994).

(2) Robinson JA. *A treatise on the inhalation of ether vapour for the prevention of pain in surgical operation*. London: Webster, 1847: 1–24.

(3) Ellis RH. *James Robinson on the inhalation of ether vapour*. London: Baillière Tindall, 1983: vii–xi.

(4) Ellis RH. The introduction of ether anaesthesia to Great Britain. 1: How the news was carried from Boston, Massachusetts to Gower Street, London. *Anaesthesia* 1976; **31**: 766–77.

(5) Boott F. Surgical operations performed during insensibility produced by the inhalation of sulphuric ether. *Lancet* 1847; **1**: 5–8.

(6) Ellis RH. The introdcution of ether anaesthesia to Great Britain. 2. A biographical sketch of Dr Francis Boott. *Anaesthesia* 1977; **32**: 197–208.

(7) Dawkins CJM. The first public operation carried out under an anaesthetic in Europe. *Anaesthesia* 1947; **2**: 51–61.

(8) Ellis RH. Early anaesthesia. The news of anaesthesia spreads to the United Kingdom. In: Atkinson RS, Boulton TB. *The history of anaesthesia: Proceedings of the 2nd international symposium on the history of anaesthesia 1987*. London: Royal Society of Medicine International Congress Series 134, 1989: 69–76.

(9) Squire W. On the introduction of ether inhalation as an anaesthetic in London. *Lancet* 1888; **2**: 1220.

(10) Sykes WS. *Essays on the first hundred years of anaesthesia*. Vol 1. Edinburgh: Livingstone, 1960: 117–36.

(11) Editorial. Painless operations. *Medical Times* 1847: **15**: 289–90.

(12) Gardner J. On ether vapour. Its medical and surgical uses. *Lancet* 1847; **1**: 349–55.

(13) Editorial. *Lancet* 1847; **1**: 74–5.

(14) Editorial. Painless surgical operations. Description of Robinson's inhaler. *Medical Times* 1847; **15**: 290–1.

(15) Editorial. Painless operations. *Medical Times* 1847; **15**: 328.

(16) Snow J. *On chloroform and anaesthetics. Their action and administration*. London: Churchill, 1858: 18–19.

(17) Snow J. A lecture on the inhalation of ether in surgical operations. *Lancet* 1847; **1**: 551–4.

(18) Hospital reports. University College Hospital. *Lancet* 1847; **1**: 639.

(19) Editorial. Operations without pain. University College Hospital. *Lancet* 1847; **1**: 546.
(20) Editorial. Robert Liston FRS. *Medical Times* 1847; **17**: 162.
(21) Post mortem examination of the body of the late Robert Liston, Esq, FRS. *Medical Times* 1847; **17**: 182.
(22) Death of Robert Liston, Esq, FRS. *Lancet* 1847; **2**: 633–4.

Early history of ether and chloroform anaesthesia from Welsh newspapers

JM Lewis

Original presentation Edinburgh 1989

Weekly Welsh newspapers printed in the 1847–1848 period are a fruitful source of information on the introduction of ether and chloroform. Another local source is the very detailed minutes of the Management Committee meetings of the old Swansea Infirmary and the old Swansea General & Eye Hospital. These were kept from 1817 to 1948, with practically no clinical material recorded — not even the introduction of ether in 1846 is mentioned. The major concern of these committees was always the lack of funds.

It is of some local interest that one of the medical men present when Liston used ether for the first time on 19 December 1846 was Dr James Couch. Dr Couch was later in medical practice in Swansea for 34 years and his son, Dr J Kynaston Couch in 1889 became the first pathologist and chloroformist appointed in Swansea.

EARLY REPORTS FROM DIVERSE PLACES

The newspapers of January, February and March 1847 record the use of ether at a number of places outside Wales. At Bristol on 31 December 1846, the second ether anaesthetic in Britain was given by Dr Fairbrother, the senior physician, it is significant that '. . . he kept his finger on the pulse' and watched the breathing. The failure of ether in three operations at University College Hospital, two of which were undertaken by Liston, was noted, as was the case of the lady at King's College Hospital who after two or three breaths preferred to be awake. Operations under anaesthesia at Guy's, the London and Westminster Hospitals are also recorded.

The first use in Ireland was in Dublin, by a Mr McDonnell who submitted himself to the influence of ether five or six times before using it on his patients. Its use in Birmingham, Boston in Lincolnshire, Doncaster, Dumfries, Shrewsbury and Stroud are recorded. In Edinburgh an un-united fracture of the left leg was operated upon by Professor Miller, using a Squire's apparatus for anaesthesia which had been sent to him by Liston, '. . . a very suitable gift from that eminent surgeon to his old pupil'. This original apparatus is thought to be the one that can now be seen in the museum housed at the Royal College of Surgeons, Edinburgh, having been rediscovered by the museum's curator Dr A Masson. Deaths at the Essex and Colchester Hospital and Grantham in Lincolnshire are recorded.

The first use of ether in Wales was at Swansea and is recorded in a letter dated 13 January 1847, to the editor of *The Cambrian* newspaper, from Mr Henry

Wiglesworth, once a pupil of Liston and now a surgeon to the Swansea Infirmary. The inhalation was for a tooth extraction at Mr Wiglesworth's residence. In his letter he used Liston's words: 'I feel sir, with Liston, that this remedy is indeed a great thing for operating surgeons,' and he added: ' I cannot but believe that it will considerably alleviate the suffering of thousands — that it will be the salvation of many lives — and one of the greatest boons which the public will receive from the medical profession'.

The first major operation under ether in Wales was at Wrexham on 5 February 1847. It was an amputation at the thigh and is of interest in that there was vomiting, '. . . the stomach during its administration having several times ejected its contents'. A fortnight later, the first capital operation in Swansea under ether anaesthesia — again amputation — was performed by Henry Wiglesworth at the Swansea Infirmary. On the same day, 19 February, 'etherism at Aberystwyth' was described. The operation was for the removal of a large breast tumour at the lady's residence. The surgeon first submitted his two pupils and his coachman to ether, 'to test the power of the ether and the soundness of his apparatus'. The inhaler was Mr Smee's, manufactured by Horne of Newgate Street, London. At Blaenavon, ether had been used on 13 February for surgery on a diseased bone of the foot. Other reports were from Abergavenny, Bala, Bangor (on a patient from Llanfair in Anglesey), Llanelli, Monmouth and from Llangefni in North Wales.

Of particular note is a case in late March 1847 at Bangor. A man suffered multiple comminuted compound fractures of both legs and one thigh. Due to shock, the surgeon of the week and the senior surgeon decided to postpone operation until the next morning. At 9am a double operation was performed, and the patient died after 15 minutes. This could possibly be the first anaesthetic 'death on the table'.

CHLOROFORM

Professor Simpson's use of chloroform in November 1847 is well documented in four Welsh newspapers. Later reports include a mastectomy in Liverpool, using a sponge; release of burns contractures in Gloucester, using a handkerchief; and removal of a tumour in Somerset, where writing paper and a handkerchief were used. Also recorded, under the headline 'Doctor caught napping', is a dental extraction on board a ship, where the surgeon sniffed the handkerchief afterwards and became unconscious. Two deaths associated with dental extraction were recorded. The son of the West Riding coroner died during the removal of six teeth, and Dr Anderson of Birkenhead died 48 hours after his extraction.

In Wales, the first chloroform anaesthetic was given in Swansea, recorded in another letter to *The Cambrian*. This was dated 17 December 1847 and written by Dr Edward Howell, Physician to the Swansea Infirmary. Dr Howell had read medicine at the Universities of London, Paris and Edinburgh. At the age of 22 he was awarded the Edinburgh MD for a thesis on *'De asthmate spasmodico'*. In private practice he undertook obstetrics, and it was for a midwifery case that the chloroform was given. Also in December, chloroform was used for a boy with severe injuries, the operation 'only made possible after the use of the most active stimulants'. At Blackwood in the same month, a patient with compound fractures had both legs amputated. He was so shocked that operation was only possible 24 hours after the accident, and the anaesthetic was given by Dr Young 'with such care'. In January 1848 at Monmouth a large tumour of the back was removed, the chloroformist being Dr Andrews. The report notes, 'we had the pleasure of inspecting Dr Andrews's apparatus and were particularly struck with its exceeding simplicity'. In June, an amputation at the thigh was performed in Swansea, ether having been previously tried unsuccessfully. Removal of a cancerous breast at Caernarvon is recorded in July.

The famous Hannah Greener case was reported as the death of a young girl of 15 in the practice of Dr Meggison of Winlanton, near Newcastle. Professor Simpson's objection in *The Lancet* of 12 February [1] was noted. He believed the verdict of death 'from the effects of chloroform' should have been 'from the means to revive her', water and brandy having been poured into her mouth. A few weeks later, Henry Wiglesworth, London trained and the first user of ether in Wales, addressed Simpson through *The Lancet* [2]. 'I will state my opinion that Simpson's reasons are not in accordance with sound physiological doctrines . . . I believe with the jury, with Drs Meggison and Glover, Sir John Fife and all those being immediately concerned with the case, that the poor girl died from the effects of chloroform and nothing else'. A few weeks earlier Wiglesworth had gained the MB degree of the University of London, with a scholarship, a gold medal in physiology and comparative anatomy, and another in midwifery and diseases of women.

OTHER USES OF ETHER AND CHLOROFORM

The improper use of ether or chloroform is mentioned on three occasions — by a nurse in June 1847, with the chemist saying 'ether is all the go now', by a sultan who ordered a quarter cask of chloroform for use by the ladies of his harem, and by a respected medical practitioner. This latter instance was reported in February 1848 with the headline, 'A form of mania in Edinburgh'. Instead of music and dancing, the learned doctor provided a flask of chloroform and a sponge, and every guest seems to have had a trip. One lovely lady said, 'Oh, my beloved Charles come to my arms', while some of the gentlemen 'committed slight breaches of etiquette'.

As therapy, repeated inhalation was used for two cases of tetanus and one of typhus. Veterinary use of chloroform was recorded for a dog, a horse and a rabid tigress. Local application of chloroform was used in delayed labour and in the removal of a tumour from the sole of the foot!

A final news item from *The Cambrian* is of more general interest. In March 1849, the sinking is recorded of an ex-passenger vessel which had been bought by the central German government, and equipped in Liverpool as a war steamer. This was the 500 horsepower *Acadia*, which had brought the news of ether across the Atlantic. Her last voyage ended in the North Sea.

REFERENCES

(1) Simpson JY. The alleged case of death from the action of chloroform. *Lancet* 1848; i: 175.
(2) Wiglesworth H. A letter to Professor Simpson on the fatal case of inhalation of chloroform that occurred at Newcastle. *Lancet* 1848; ii: 181.

Welsh newspapers reviewed 1847–1848
The Cardiff and Merthyr Guardian (Merthyr Tydfil)
The Monmouthshire Merlin (Newport)
The Monmouthshire Beacon (Monmouth)

The Cambrian (Swansea)
The Carmarthen Journal (Carmarthen)
The Welshman (Carmarthen)
The Caernarfon and Denbigh Herald (Caernarfon)
The North Wales Chronicle (Bangor)
Y Protestant (Mold)
The Salurian (Tenby)
The Pembrokeshire Herald (Haverfordwest)
The Tenby and Pembroke (Tenby)

Anaesthetizing: the early years of a growth industry

Barbara Duncum

Original presentation Southend 1988

In England, in the late winter of 1846–7, the quickest way for a medical man and indeed anybody else, to find out about painless surgery was to watch it being done in the nearest hospital. Operating sessions were open to the public and the first surgeons to follow Liston's lead held hospital appointments either in London or in towns and cities up and down the country. In those hospitals whenever word got round that a patient was to be made insensible, local physicians and surgeons eager to learn and laymen full of curiosity, crowded into the operating room [1]. That sometimes led to strange gatherings. At the Maidstone Ophthalmic Institution on January 16 1847, for instance, although only two adults for minor operations and a boy with a squint were on the list, the spectators included the mayor and other members of the corporation and the officers of the cavalry depot with their two army surgeons [2,3].

In early reports of painless surgery in London, each of the small number of self appointed etherists was given prominence. In reports from the provinces it was usually only the surgeon who stood in the limelight and the etherist, if he happened to be mentioned, was likely to be either one of the hospital's regular physicians or a particular medical crony of the surgeon. In private practice which catered for everyone not sufficiently poor to be eligible for hospital treatment, the role of etherist was virtually ready-made for the patient's physician. Long before etherizing was thought of, most general practitioners had a link with some surgeon to whom they referred cases needing more than fairly minor surgery. The GP attended the operation—done in the patient's bedroom no matter how unsuitable—his part being to support and encourage the sufferer during the surgical ordeal. The surgeon himself usually brought one or more colleagues with him to assist. When etherizing was adopted, the customary duties of the patient's physician made him the obvious person to act as anaesthetist and to monitor the patient's general condition until consciousness fully returned.

During January and February of 1847 professional enthusiasm for painless surgery was shared more soberly by patients. Those operated on were thankful, and a good many others previously too terrified to agree to surgery plucked up courage and asked to be etherized and treated. Although anaesthesia often went wrong, the difficulties were generally regarded as useful experience and were described along with the successes in letters to the press. 'Our office is literally inundated with details of new operations performed on patients under the influence of sulphuric ether', the editor of the *Medical Times* wrote in a leader on February 27 [4].

A shock was in store for everybody on March 19 1847. *The Times* reported an inquest on Ann Parkinson, the 23-year-old wife of a Grantham hairdresser. On March 9, at her own request, she had inhaled ether for the removal of a tumour on her thigh. She failed to rally after her operation and about 36 hours later she died. At the inquest it was said that six people had been present during the operation — her sister-in-law, her GP who operated (he was also the surgeon to the Grantham Workhouse Union), the etherist, two other medical men, and a nurse. After hearing their evidence, the coroner's jury returned a verdict that the sole cause of death had been the inhalation of ether vapour [5]. In fact, Ann Parkinson was the second patient in England to die some hours after inhaling ether. The first, a 52-year-old man, had died on February 12 after lithotomy at the Essex and Colchester Hospital. His death was not directly attributed to ether and there had not been an inquest, but Mr RR Nunn the surgeon in the case, reconsidering it in March, suggested that inhaling ether had so depressed the patient's nervous system that his powers of recovery were lost. Nunn was now inclined to believe, he said, 'that pain was a healthy indication and an essential concomitant of surgical operations which perhaps ought not to be artificially suppressed' [6]. A similar argument was already persuading obstetricians that the pangs of childbirth were salutary and so should continue to be bravely borne [7].

Apropos of the Colchester and Grantham deaths, the editor of the *Medical Times* drew his readers attention to several deaths on the Continent, and asked rhetorically whether ether inhalation should now be considered too hazardous for further use. Answering his own question he concluded that in careful, experienced hands the advantages of etherization decidedly outweighed the drawbacks [8]. Most people seemed to have agreed with him; nevertheless, the number of letters from tyro-etherists to the press sharply decreased and the remarkable speed and completeness of the switch to chloroform when Simpson announced its virtues in mid-November 1847 showed how greatly confidence in ether had been shaken. Once again a shock was in store.

On January 28 1848, young Hannah Greener, inexplicably as it seemed, died inhaling chloroform for the removal of a toenail [9]. Her death was only the first of many. That summer, for example, the meticulous and very experienced proto-etherist, James Robinson, acting as his own anaesthetist in his private dental practice in Gower Street, lost a patient — a solicitor named Mr Badger. The evidence at the inquest provides a glimpse as to how things were managed in a top-level dental surgery. Mr Robinson's maid servant said she was always present when ladies were being treated. When the patient was a man the footman attended, though the maid deputized for him if he was otherwise occupied. One of the footman's duties, should the occasion arise, was to run along Gower Street for medical help, but when Mr Badger collapsed it was too late [10].

In private medical practice, except when a leading surgeon brought his own anaesthetist — as Professor William Fergusson would bring Dr Snow — the patient's GP continued to act, generally becoming not only proficient but also interested in what he was doing. In English hospital practice however, there was a growing tendency to think like the Scots, that the chloroformist needed little special training and need not be a fully qualified medical man.

By March 1852 the number of chloroform deaths reported from London hospitals was becoming alarming and John Snow wrote to the *Medical Times and Gazette*. His letter followed a death at St Bartholomew's where the anaesthetist had been one of the dressers. Snow wrote 'The office of administering chloroform should no more be delegated to a dresser than the important operations of surgery'. Nor did he think house surgeons any more suitable. Their tenure of office was too brief for adequate experience, and understandably they were more interested in watching the surgeon than the patient. In Snow's opinion, as there must always be someone on the spot to administer in an emergency, the most appropriate person was the resident medical officer. That plan had been found to be perfect where it had been acted on. He used St George's Hospital as an example, where Mr Potter 'was appointed to the duty of giving chloroform between two and three years ago', and University College Hospital where, as he said, 'Mr Clover had, I believe, performed this duty since the early part of 1848, with equally satisfactory results' [11].

Just a year later, in March 1853, a patient died at University College Hospital, while being given chloroform by a house surgeon. The Medical Committee then announced that although the resident medical officer should continue to act as chloroformist whenever conveniently practicable, since he could not always be available they were appointing deputies: two specially assigned house surgeons — one of whom, as it happened was Joseph Lister [12].

At the turn of the year 1853–4 the UCH Medical Committee accepted a suggestion made to them by SF Statham, the junior assistant surgeon. Statham proposed that all the hospital's medical students, as part of their course of studies, should receive some practical instructions from the resident medical officer on how to administer chloroform, and that a certificate to that effect should be among the requirements for final qualification [13]. A notable advance along the meandering trail to professionalism in anaesthesia, one might think. Whether or not the scheme was put into practice is unclear.

REFERENCES

(1) Anon. Painless operations. *Med Times* 1846–7; **15**: 289–90.
(2) Plomley F. Operations upon the eye. *Lancet* 1847; **1**: 134–5.
(3) Plomley F. Maidstone Ophthalmic Institution. *Lancet* 1847; **1**: 159–60.
(4) Anon. Ether. *Med Times* 1847; **16**: 24.
(5) Anon. Fatal operation under the influence of ether. *Lancet* 1847; **1**: 340–2.
(6) Nunn RS. Essex and Colchester Hospital. Operation for stone in the bladder. *Lancet* 1847; **1**: 343.
(7) Smith WT. A lecture on the utility and safety of the inhalation of ether in obstetric practice. *Lancet* 1847; **1**: 321–3.
(8) Anon. Ether inhalation. *Med Times* 1847; **16**: 101–2.
(9) Anon. Fatal application of chloroform. *Lancet* 1848; **1**: 161–2.
(10) Coroners' Inquest. Death during the inhalation of the vapour of chloroform. *Lancet* 1848; **ii**: 46–8.
(11) Snow J. On the administration of chloroform in the public hospitals. *Med Times* 1852; **4**: 349–50.
(12) Merrington WR. *University College Hospital and its Medical School.* London: Heinemann, 1976: 38.
(13) Jewsbury ECO. *The Royal Northern Hospital 1856–1956.* London: HK Lewis, 1956: 5.

A busy week for John Snow (16–22 December 1850)

RH Ellis

Original presentation Croydon 1989

Dr John Snow recorded details of much of his clinical work in what are referred to as his *Casebooks*. Several years after Snow's death the *Casebooks* were presented to the Library of the Royal College of Physicians of London [1]. There are three Volumes. They cover the period from mid-July 1848 until a few days before his death almost 10 years later. They are in poor condition and in need of preservation and careful restoration. I am currently just over one-third of the way through the task of transcribing the whole of John Snow's *Casebook* material, hopefully for publication. This publication will mean that those wishing to study Snow's case material will no longer need to refer to the fragile, original volumes.*

It is often thought that Snow recorded details in his *Casebooks* of almost every case to which he gave anaesthesia to, during the period that they cover. However, I am sure that this is not true; Snow certainly gave anaesthesia on other occasions although no details of these appear in his records.

When the call for Free Papers came for the Meeting of the History of Anaesthesia Society in February 1989, I was working on Snow's entries for the week of Monday 16 to Sunday 22 December, 1850. I thought that it might be of interest to describe one of Snow's working weeks, and chose this one virtually by chance—although it does coincide with the fourth anniversary of anaesthesia's first use in Britain.

Information about the pattern of John Snow's work is to be found principally, but not only, in his *Casebooks*. Other sources include Benjamin Ward Richardson's *Memoir* of Snow [2], published Case Reports, and the proceedings of various medical meetings held in London.

It is instructive to learn what we can of Snow's work during this week as it tells us about John Snow as a family doctor, as an anaesthetist, and as a scientific researcher. He had suspended his interest in the epidemiology of cholera at this time. However, it should be emphasized that it would be quite wrong to assume that this week was a typical one for him. During the week in question Snow was involved with his medical work every day. In his capacity as a family doctor, he made no less than 26 separate domiciliary visits. He gave nine anaesthetics, and performed two animal experiments. He may also have attended a medical meeting. That Snow made so many visits unconnected with anaesthesia emphasizes that the oft-quoted notion that he was the first full-time physician

---

*Dr Ellis's monumental work, *The Case Books of Dr John Snow*, (1848–1858), was published by the Wellcome Institute for the History of Medicine, London, as *Medical History*, Supplement 14, 1994, shortly before his tragically early death. Conservation work on the original case books was sponsored by the History of Anaesthesia Society. Completion of this restoration was marked in April 1996 by a ceremony at the Royal College of Physicians.

anaesthetist [3] is clearly not correct. During the rest of his life he continued his work as a family doctor, researcher and epidemiologist in addition to his involvement with anaesthesia.

CASEBOOK ENTRIES—MONDAY—OPERATIVE HAEMORRHAGE

The first of Snow's *Casebook* entries for the week shows that on Monday 16 December 1850 he made three visits in his capacity as a family doctor, and gave one anaesthetic. He made two visits to a baby. The mother, a Mrs Bent, had been a patient of Snow's for at least two and a quarter years. The family lived in Castle Street, near Leicester Square. The baby whom he saw on this occasion was five months old and had been delivered by him in July 1850 (without the aid of chloroform). On the same day, he also saw a Mrs Hillier, whom he had first attended at least seven months earlier in May 1850. Mrs Hillier lived in Cecil Court, also near Leicester Square.

Snow rarely recorded further details of his domiciliary visits unless he prescribed for his patients, but he did make notes about the patients to whom he gave anaesthesia. Although he did not refer to it specifically in this section of his *Casebooks* there can be little doubt that the apparatus used for the anaesthetics during the week was Snow's usual chloroform inhaler with Sibson's face-piece [4].

Snow's anaesthetic note for Monday 16 December 1850 reads as follows: 'Administered chloroform to Mr Little, 28 Middleton Square (Snow misspelt the name of the Square, it should be spelt Myddleton), whilst Mr Bransby Cooper removed the right testicle on account of fungoid disease. The patient who did not appear more than 35 years of age is very fat.' Nothing is known of the patient, Mr Little, apart from his address but the house to which Snow was called to give his anaesthetic is still standing, although it appears to have undergone recent modifications. It is near the Angel, Islington. Mr Bransby Cooper, the surgeon, was a senior surgeon at Guy's Hospital [5]. In an article which he had written shortly before this episode Cooper had equated 'fungoid disease' with what was then called 'sarcoma of the testis' [6]. Snow's patient was in his mid-thirties, and this particular tumour was almost certainly a seminoma. Snow's narrative continues: 'There was great difficulty in arresting the haemorrhage; the patient consequently lost a great quantity of blood and was very faint, being at one time without pulse'. It is possible to discover how Snow and Cooper would have reacted to this situation. The treatment of surgical haemorrhage in the 1850s is well documented in contemporary textbooks—of which that by John Lizars of Edinburgh (published in 1847) is typical [7]. From this it is clear that the usual management was for the surgeon to try to arrest the haemorrhage with ligatures or direct pressure. If this proved ineffective then it was enough to await the signs of fainting, at which time the flow of blood would be so reduced that local coagulation and haemostasis would follow. In these circumstances the patient rested, with nothing active being done in case the slow-forming clot should be disturbed. Further intervention was discouraged and the patient was merely observed, and fortified with stimulants. Snow, himself, recommended that this course of action should be followed in similar situations [8]. He ended this case note by remarking that 'Brandy was given to him and he rallied in a satisfactory manner. No sickness'. (Snow was always very careful to note whether or not sickness had occurred after his anaesthetics.)

TUESDAY—LITHOTRITY

On the following day, Tuesday 17 December, Snow again made three visits—two to Mrs Bent's baby, and one to Mrs Hillier. In addition, he gave one anaesthetic—this time to an army officer. 'Administered chloroform today to Major Fawcett, apparently near 60, whilst Mr Coulson performed lithotrity. Dr Rowe being present'. Nothing is known of Major Fawcett, although various military records have been consulted. The surgeon was Mr William Coulson who lived near the Guildhall in the City of London. He was surgeon to The German Hospital and to the City of London Lying-in Hospital. Later, in 1851, he was also appointed Senior Surgeon at the newly-opened St Mary's Hospital, Paddington [9]. A few years earlier he had written a textbook on disease of the bladder and prostate [10].

Coulson was one of those who had recently introduced the operation of lithotrity to this country, claiming that it carried far less risk than the severe and open alternative of lithotomy. He gave a contemporary account of lithotrity in his textbook. The patient would have been held securely in the lithotomy position by attendants, who would also have restrained him had Snow's anaesthesia been less than perfect. Snow always insisted that whenever patients were operated on in the lithotomy position they should—on each side—have their hands and the soles of their feet, bound firmly together by restraining bandages [8]. Before the operation began the pelvis would have been raised on cushions and the bladder distended with warm water. Snow recorded elsewhere that the usual time for this operation was about 20 minutes.

Dr Rowe was almost certainly Dr George Rowe, who had been a surgeon in the army [11]. This probably explains his connection with Major Fawcett. By 1850 he had left the army and was in practice in Cavendish Square. The patient, Major Fawcett, must have been quite pleased to see John Snow, for Snow records, 'the stone had been crushed twice before without the chloroform' and he continued 'No excitement, very little rigidity, but after becoming unconscious but not yet insensible the breathing was very deep and rapid'. Coulson would probably have used two lithotrites (one for crushing the stone, the other for scooping up the debris) which he himself had designed and described in his textbook a few years earlier [10]. At the end of the operation Snow records 'No sickness although he had dined on a chop two hours previously'. Snow did not stipulate that patients should starve before anaesthesia, although he knew of the connection between post-operative (and intra-operative) vomiting and the recent taking of food [12]. The fact that the Major had 'dined' may imply that this procedure was carried out in the evening.

WEDNESDAY—RESEARCH

On Wednesday, Snow made six visits—two of which were to Mrs Bent's baby, and one to Mrs Hillier. He made no less than three visits during the day to a George Hogarth whose family (according to his *Casebook* entries) Snow had first attended some two and a half years earlier. He also administered one chloroform anaesthetic, and—in addition—found time to perform a lengthy and sophisticated animal experiment on a rabbit. Snow's account of the anaesthetic case reads 'Administered Chloroform . . . to a gentleman apparently about 30, lodging in Down Street, Piccadilly whilst Mr Avery removed the left testicle on account of fungoid disease. Very little excitement or rigidity. No sickness'. (This was, presumably, another seminoma). Down Street was, and still is, just off Piccadilly near Hyde Park Corner. Mr John Avery, lived in Mayfair [11], and was a surgeon at Charing Cross Hospital. He had qualified in both London and Paris, had invented a very ingenious endoscope, and had written on the surgery of cleft-palate [13].

The experiment which Snow performed was one of a lengthy series on carbon dioxide excretion and chloroform anaesthesia in various animals; on this occasion he used a rabbit. The series began earlier in 1850 and ended in 1851. Each experiment must have occupied him for at least 3 hours. Some of them may have been performed with Dr Benjamin Ward Richardson, although where they were performed is unknown. Snow's experiment consisted of placing an animal in a large, sealed jar. He measured the carbon dioxide which it breathed out in half an hour, and then anaesthetized the animal with chloroform and again measured the carbon dioxide produced. He also repeated his measurements during recovery. His results were remarkably consistent, and his deductions about the effect of anaesthesia on what we now know as the metabolic rate were reasoned and perceptive [14].

THURSDAY—DENTAL EXTRACTION

On Thursay 19 December Snow made five domiciliary visits. He made one visit each to Mrs Bent's baby and Mrs Hillier, and was still sufficiently concerned about George Hogarth to see him on three separate occasions during the day. He gave two anaesthetics. Firstly, he returned to Down Street, Piccadilly to give an anaesthetic to another of Mr Avery's patients. 'Administered Chloroform to a gentleman, about 30, lodging in Down Street whilst Mr Avery removed some cicatrices caused by a burn from the root and side of the penis. No sickness'. After this he travelled several miles to Upper Holloway (now in North London, but then some distance from the metropolis) to give a dental anaesthetic. 'Administered Chloroform to a son of Mrs Jourdain, aged 20, at Upper Holloway whilst Mr Catlin (Snow misspelt this surname; it should have been spelt 'Cattlin') extracted a lower molar tooth'.

The relevant *Kelly's London Directories* [15] show that the Jourdain family lived at 2 Lansdowne Place in Holloway which is, presumably, where Snow gave this anaesthetic. Lansdowne Place no longer exists. The surgeon was Mr William Cattlin, who was a Fellow of the Royal College of Surgeons, and a Licentiate of Dental Surgery. He lived in Islington, and was Surgeon-Dentist to the Islington and Holloway Dispensary and to the Royal Caledonian Asylum [11]. There was an onlooker at this operation, for Snow's record continues 'Mr Kesteven was present. No sickness or other sequalae'. Mr Kesteven seemed, then, not to have a hospital appointment and was a surgeon in private practice. He lived nearby in Upper Holloway [11]. He had written in the medical journals on diverse subjects, including croup and some aspects of anaesthesia [16].

FRIDAY—FISTULA IN ST JOHN'S WOOD

On the following day, Friday 20 December, Snow made a total of five visits—one each to Mrs Bent's baby and to Mrs Hillier, and three to George Hogarth. During the day he also went to give an anaesthetic. 'Administered Chloroform to a lady at St John's Wood whilst Mr Fergusson operated for fistula. No excitement, rigidity, or sickness. (A spare lady, about 45)'. Mr (and later Sir) William Fergusson was the colleague with whom Snow worked most frequently. He was the senior surgeon at King's College Hospital [17] and was London's most celebrated surgeon, having inherited that mantle on the death of Robert Liston.

SATURDAY—A DEAD BABY, OPERATIVE HAEMORRHAGE AND DEATH

Saturday 21 December was the longest and busiest day of the week for Snow. He attended a confinement, saw George Hogarth twice and Mrs Bent's baby and Mrs Hillier once. He also administered two anaesthetics, and performed another experiment on carbon dioxide production during anaesthesia—this time on a dog. He may also have gone to a medical meeting for Snow was a regular attender and speaker at the weekly meetings of the Medical Society of London. He was later its President. The reports of the meeting which was held at 8.00 pm on this Saturday do not mention his having taken part [18–21]. He may have decided to miss this particular meeting since I doubt that the subjects discussed would have been of special interest to him, and he had had a very early start to his day.

Very early in the morning Snow was sent for to attend a confinement. His *Casebook* entry begins 'Saturday 21 December. Mrs Desmajieu, 63 King Street, Westminster. Delivery. Mas. (presumably Masculine) DC (presumably 'dead child') First labour. Pains commenced 4.00 am. I was sent for soon afterwards, and found the liq. amnii evacuated and the os uteri rather larger than a shilling. Between six and seven the os was quite obliterated and soon afterwards the head began to bear on the perineum. The child was not born till between 10 and 11 owing to resistance of the perineum, the patient being over 30. Within the last hour before the birth of the child some meconium was discharged. The child was still-born, and its limbs were in a state of post mortem rigidity, both the superior and inferior extremities being semi-flexed. The head was elongated and compressed. The mother said that she had not felt the child for a day or two, and that the day before the labour her abdomen felt cold. She had not mentioned this before'. The patient's rooms, incidentally, were above the premises of either a hairdresser or a tailor [15].

Space does not permit a detailed discussion of the many points raised by this case note of Snow's. While his conduct of this labour would nowadays be criticized severely, it was in accordance with the practice of midwifery in 1850. He decided not to intervene actively to deliver the child, nor—surprisingly—did he give chloroform which he must have known had been used when progress was held up at the perineum, since it was said to relax the tissues and ease delivery [22]. During most of the time he spent with the mother, Snow it seems, had no reason to think that the baby had succumbed *in utero*. Even so, he did not attempt resuscitation of the child, despite his long-standing and published expertise in the technique [23].

On each Saturday Snow had a regular appointment to give anaesthesia at King's College Hospital, which was then close behind the Royal College of Surgeons. On this occasion there was just one case waiting for him. 'Administered Chloroform at King's College Hospital to a muscular, thin man, about 40, whilst Mr Luxton—the house surgeon—amputated the thumb and the first phalanx'. The house surgeon was William Luxton who had qualified at King's a short time before. He later became a GP in Wiltshire [24]. This administration of chloroform was somewhat eventful and, as frequently happened 'The patient struggled violently after losing his consciousness. No sickness'.

After this, Snow left King's College Hospital and travelled once more to meet Mr Coulson who wished to repeat the lithotrity which he had carried out on Major Fawcett 4 days earlier. This was quite usual, and Major Fawcett's operation was repeated several more times in the next few weeks. 'Administered Chloroform again to Major Fawcett whilst Mr Coulson repeated the lithotrity. He breathed deeply and quickly before losing his consciousness and becoming insensible; exactly as before. No sickness'. At some time on this Saturday Snow performed another, similar, 3 or 4 hour long experiment with his apparatus, this time on a dog.

Snow seemed to take little, if any, notice of weekends as far as his professional work was concerned, and his notes for Sunday 22 December record that while he made no visits to the Hilliers, Bents or Hogarths he did anaesthetize another of Mr Coulson's patients. 'Administered Chloroform to Mr MacKenzie (Snow may have misspelt this surname; elsewhere it has been spelt McKenzie [15]) at 10, Lower Calthorpe Street whilst Mr Coulson performed lithotomy'.

The house in which this drama occurred is still standing, and despite changes in the naming of the road and numbering of the houses, it can still be identified from Local Authority records [25,26]. It is now 44 Calthorpe Street, just off Gray's Inn Road. The relevant *Kelly's Directories*, incidentally, tell us that the patient was a Mr John McKenzie and that he worked as a diamond setter [15], possibly, I suppose, in nearby Hatton Garden. The house is now decrepit but, with a little imagination, one can picture that Sunday morning and the horse-drawn carriages arriving outside the door, Snow being admitted with his bag containing the inhaler and the chloroform, Coulson arriving with his instruments, and several assistants carrying in such ominous things as restraining bandages and sawdust to mop up the blood. Perhaps Mr McKenzie's neighbours watched as the drama began, some in the street itself and others from their windows nearby.

Snow's record tells us that Mr McKenzie was far from fit. 'The patient was an elderly man, very fat and asthmatic, having to rest himself for 2 or 3 minutes in order to recover his breath after walking upstairs'. Despite this, and even though the patient must have been held securely in the lithotomy position by two of the assistants and had his hands tied to the soles of his feet with Snow's obligatory restraining bandages, the anaesthetic proceeded uneventfully. The surgery, however, was far from straightforward. 'He became insensible without struggling or rigidity. The first calculus which was removed was imbedded in the prostate; two others afterwards removed from the bladder after some difficulty and delay'.

Snow's next comments will hardly surprise us. 'There was a great deal of blood lost during the operation, very large coagula being found on the sawdust afterwards. The patient became very faint from haemorrhage before the end of the operation'. Coulson would have been familiar with the problem. A few years earlier he had written in his textbook 'If any haemorrhage occur we must endeavour to compress the bleeding vessel with the finger. It is always a most untoward circumstance when it happens' [10]. Clearly, having operated to remove a stone from the prostate there must have been a huge loss of blood. Snow and Coulson seem to have followed the usual plan by trying to stop the bleeding directly, but as this failed they relied on fainting to reduce the haemorrhage and permit haemostasis, and were content to give routine stimulants.

Snow's record continues 'A good deal of sherry and some hot brandy and water were given to him, although he made great objection to swallowing, and in the course of 15 or 20 minutes after the operation he rallied in a great measure'. I am not surprised that Mr McKenzie made great objection to swallowing the sherry and hot brandy and water. He was not only elderly, wheezy and hypoxic, but was still partly under the influence of Snow's chloroform, may well still have been trussed up like a turkey, and in a state of haemorrhagic shock.

It was not Snow's normal custom to remain with his patient for long after his anaesthetic had worn off; whatever subsequent care was needed was the province of the surgeon, or of the patient's relatives. Nonetheless, he learnt of the outcome, and the last note in his *Casebooks* for this particular week records 'He died suddenly about 3 o' clock on the morning of the 24th whilst being lifted up in bed'. This was 2 days post-operatively. The most likely cause of death was—in the circumstances of late 1850—the effects of continuing post-operative haemorrhage superimposed on the major blood loss which occurred at the time of the procedure itself. Coulson, the surgeon, would not have been surprised at this, and had written in his book on the bladder and prostate '. . . it is rare that patients die immediately from loss of blood . . . but the draining sometimes continues for hours . . . and gradually exhausts the power of the patient'. [10] Nor, I think, would Snow have been surprised at this sad outcome for, elsewhere, he records that 75% of his private patients undergoing lithotomy had died as a result of the surgery [8].

I hope that this brief study of just one, busy and eventful week in John Snow's busy and eventful professional life is of interest. The *Memoir* of Snow, written by his great friend Benjamin Ward Richardson [2], is of great importance to us, having served as the main biographical source for some 130 years. However, I feel certain that by studying John Snow's *Casebooks* in detail, and reconciling their contents with other material which is still available, a more detailed and informative account of his life will emerge.

I am equally certain that such an account will lead us to realize that John Snow deserves even more admiration and even more respect than we now accord him.

ACKNOWLEDGEMENT

I am most grateful to Mr Geoffrey Davenport, the Librarian at the Royal College of Physicians, for his advice and encouragement and for allowing me to transcribe John Snow's *Casebooks*.

REFERENCES

(1) Snow J. *Three manuscript volumes of casebooks (1848–1858)*. Royal College of Physicians, London.
(2) Richardson BW. The Life of John Snow, MD In: Snow J. *On Chloroform and other anaesthetics*. London: Churchill, 1858.
(3) Owen D. The 1988 John Snow Lecture (summary). *Anaesthesia News* 1988; **17**: 4.
(4) Snow J. On narcotism by the inhalation of vapours—part 7. *London Med Gazette* 1848; **7**: 840–4.
(5) Cameron HC. *Mr. Guy's Hospital 1726–1948*. 1st ed. London: Longman Green, 1954.
(6) Cooper BB. Diseases of the organs of generation. *Lond Med Gazette* 1849; **8**: 265–72.
(7) Lizars JA. *System of practical surgery, including all the recent discoveries and operations*. 2nd ed. Edinburgh: Lizars, 1847.
(8) Snow J. *On chloroform and other anaesthetics*. 1st ed. London: Churchill: 1858.
(9) Cope Z. *The History of St. Mary's Hospital Medical School*. 1st ed. London: Heinemann, 1954.
(10) Coulson W. *On disease of the bladder and prostate gland*. 3rd ed. London: Longman, Brown, Green and Longmans, 1842.
(11) *The London and provincial medical directory*. London: Churchill, 1851.

(12) Snow J. *On the inhalation of the vapour of ether in surgical operations*. 1st ed. London: Churchill, 1847.
(13) Yearsley M. John Avery. *Charing Cross Hospital Gazette* 1913; **15**: 45–7.
(14) Snow J. On narcotism by the inhalation of vapours—Part 16. *London Med Gazette* 1851; **7**: 622–7.
(15) *The Post Office London Directories*. London: Kelly, 1850, 1851.
(16) Kesteven WB. Action of chloroform. *London Med Gazette* 1848; **7**: 245–6.
(17) Lyle HW. *King's and some King's men*. 1st ed. London: Oxford University Press, 1935.
(18) Annotation. Medical Society of London. *London J Med* 1851; **3**: 93.
(19) Annotation. Medical Society of London. *London Med Gazette* 1851; **11**: 1104.
(20) Annotation. Medical Society of London. *Medical Times and Gazette* 1851; **2**(N.S.): 21–2.
(21) Annotation. Medical Society of London. *Lancet* 1851; **1**: 45–6.
(22) Murphy EW. *Chloroform in the practice of midwifery*. 1st ed. London: Taylor and Walton, 1848.
(23) Snow J. On asphyxia and on the resuscitation of still-born children. *London Med Gazette* 1841; **1**: 222–7.
(24) *The London and provincial medical directory*. London: Churchill, 1855.
(25) *Names of streets and places in the administrative county of London, (1856–1955)*. 1st ed. London: London County Council, 1955.
(26) The Greater London Council Record Office and Library. *Plan 1732, Film X 91/8. Reference AR/BA/S/149/1726–1750*.

Chloroform for Mrs Dickens

Barbara Duncum

Original presentation Croydon 1989

In March 1847, before the birth of his seventh child, Charles Dickens brought his family back to London from Paris. Their house, just south of Regent's Park, was still let, so Dickens took a furnished house in Chester Place, looking into the park on one side and Albany Street on the other. There on a Sunday in mid-April, Kate Dickens suddenly found herself in labour of a most alarming nature. Dickens, as he described events to his actor friend William Macready, rushed off to fetch Kate's obstetrician, Dr Henry Davis, and at the same time got hold of the top London man, the Queen's accoucheur, Dr Charles Locock. Locock and Davis evidently coped effectively with the emergency, whatever it was, for Dickens reported that 'next day Kate, thank God, was as well as ever she had been at such a time, though Davis', Dickens said, 'had seen only one other case of the kind; and of course my dear Kate suffered terribly' [1]. Had Dickens not been living abroad during the previous few months he might well have heard of Dr Protheroe Smith who could have prevented Kate's ordeal. In the spring of 1847, Smith was one of the few London obstetricians resolutely following James Young Simpson in believing that since women could now safely be spared the pain and anxiety of childbirth by inhaling ether vapour, they should be offered the opportunity to do so.

Besides being in private practice, Smith taught midwifery at St Bartholomew's Hospital. If he had had any doubts about the safety of ether, there was at St Bartholomew's the notable pioneer anaesthetist Mr Samuel John Tracy, the hospital's surgeon-dentist. Since the end of December 1846, Tracy had quietly, resourcefully, and very successfully, been acting as etherist for various colleagues in and out of hospital, including Protheroe Smith. Smith's first account of his own etherized patients appeared in *The Lancet* on May 1 — just too late to enlighten Dickens. In his article he acknowledged the valuable services of Mr Tracy. He was one of the first obstetricians to suggest that in natural childbirth it would be sufficient and safer not to carry etherization beyond the second stage, keeping the patient conscious, although insensible to pain [2].

By the autumn of 1847, Kate Dickens was pregnant again. Charles had not forgotten the alarms of that dreadful Sunday in April, nevertheless he took Kate with him when he travelled north by train on December 27 to preside at the opening of a Workingmen's College, the Glasgow Athenaeum. At that time neither of the main lines from London to Scotland was fully open. On the western route the track was incomplete between Carlisle and Glasgow, and on the east coast route to Edinburgh the railway bridges over the Tyne and Tweed were still under construction. Though his destination was Glasgow, Dickens chose the eastern route, possibly because in bleak mid-winter it would be a little less gruelling than the long cold haul over Shap Fell, but chiefly so that he could spend a few days in Edinburgh with his friend Lord Jeffrey and break the homeward journey at York to meet his brother Alfred, a railway engineer working in the locality.

Charles and Kate spent what remained of the night of December 27 at the Royal Hotel in Edinburgh and next day caught a train to Glasgow. Some of the most popular music-hall jokes then in circulation suggested that pregnant women might precipitate labour by being jolted about on the railway. Dickens himself had thought the idea funny enough to rough out a sketch featuring Mrs Gamp in a train, on the look out for business. Between Edinburgh and Glasgow it ceased to be funny: poor Kate began to miscarry. Fortunately, their sympathetic Glasgow hosts lived in a warm and comfortable house and Kate was put to bed and cosseted. Dickens went off to be acclaimed at the Athenaeum but not before, as he put it in a letter to Alfred, he had been obliged to call in a famous doctor—who that doctor was Dickens didn't say.

After two days in bed Kate felt better and they caught the train back to Edinburgh and Lord Jeffrey's house. On New Year's Day they went out shopping to look for a little present for Alfred's wife, but Kate was taken violently ill in the street and had to be hustled into bed once more, to be attended by famous doctor number two [3]. This time however there can be no doubt about the doctor's identity. Famous doctor number two must have been Professor James Young Simpson. Jeffrey would certainly have recommended him; and it later became evident that Dickens had already heard a good deal about Simpson's much publicized use of the new wonder—anaesthetic chloroform—in childbirth, and was eager to learn all he could about it at first hand.

When a year later, on January 16 1849, Kate was brought to bed with their eighth child, everything had been carefully pre-arranged. Reporting again to Macready, then on tour in the United States, Dickens wrote at some length as follows: 'You have heard, perhaps, how that I now stand seised and possessed of six sons and two daughters. . . . Kate is wonderfully well—eating mutton chops in the drawing room—and sends you her dear love. The boy is . . .a "moon faced" monster. He did not, however, come into the world as he ought to have done (I don't know in what we have offended Nature, but she seems to have taken something in us amiss) and we had to call in extra counsel and assistance. Foreseeing the possibility of such a repetition of last time, I had made myself thoroughly acquainted in Edinburgh with the facts of Chloroform—in contradistinction to the talk about it—and had insisted on the attendence of a gentleman from Bartholomew's Hospital who administers it in the operations there, and has given it four or five thousand times. I had also promised her that she should have it . . . the doctors were dead against it: but I stood my ground, and (thank God) triumphantly. It spared her all pain (she had no sensation, but of a great display of sky rockets) and saved the child all mutilation. It enabled the doctors to do, as they afterwards very readily said, in ten minutes, what might otherwise have taken them an hour and a half; the shock to her nervous system was reduced to nothing; and she was, to all intents and purposes, well, next day. Administered by someone who has nothing else to do, who knows its symptoms thoroughly, who keeps his hand upon the pulse, and his eyes upon the face, and uses nothing but a handkerchief, and that lightly, I am convinced that it is as safe in its administration, as it is miraculous and merciful in its effects. This the Edinburgh Professors assured me, and certainly our experience thoroughly comfirms them' [4]. This was Dickens's first mention of more than one professor. Who else then had he encountered in Edinburgh? In all probability it was James Miller, Liston's former pupil and Simpson's friend and colleague and the first general surgeon to test chloroform for him, at the Royal Infirmary on November 12 1847. A more important speculation concerns the identity of the 'gentleman from Bartholomew's Hospital'. The editors of the fifth volume of the Pilgrim Edition of Dickens's letters, usually impeccable in their annotations, suggest that he was Protheroe Smith, on the grounds that he was one of Simpson's earliest converts and connected with Barts; but this may not be true. Had Smith been present on January 16 Dickens surely would not have written as he did that 'the doctors were dead against it' and Smith himself would have been most unlikely to affront his colleagues by chloroforming their patient against their expressed wishes. It seems that all those particulars about the chloroformist and his methods described by Dickens add up to the unmistakeble likeness of SJ Tracy.

As to the dissenting but defeated doctors, my guess is that once again they were Locock and Davis who had certainly done very well by Kate in April 1847 — apart from her suffering. But if it was Locock who had been browbeaten into letting Kate have a little chloroform, the success of that venture did not persuade him to alter his original stance. When in the following year he attended the Queen during the birth of Prince Arthur, he safely delivered Her Majesty, but let her suffer as usual.

REFERENCES

(1) Story G, Fielding KJ, eds. *The letters of Charles Dickens*. Pilgrim Edition 5. Oxford: Clarendon Press, 1981: 1847–9.
(2) Smith P. On the employment of ether by inhalation in obstetric practice. *Lancet* 1847; **1**: 452–7.
(3) Story G, Fielding KJ, eds. *The letters of Charles Dickens*. Pilgrim Edition 5. Oxford: Clarendon Press, 1981: 217–21.
(4) Story G, Fielding KJ, eds. *The letters of Charles Dickens*. Pilgrim Edition 5. Oxford: Clarendon Press, 1981: 486–7.

THE SCOTTISH TRADITION

Edinburgh threads in the tapestry of early British anaesthesia

RH Ellis

Original presentation Edinburgh 1989

In the latter half of the last century, although Edinburgh was just one of several schools of medicine in Britain, it occupied a disproportionately important place in the early history of anaesthesia. This was mainly in relation to chloroform. However, I suggest that, initially at least, Edinburgh can claim more than a passing interest in early ether anaesthesia, and that it upheld chloroform anaesthesia in ways that were not always direct.

FOUR PIONEERS IN EDINBURGH

At the end of the eighteenth century four men were born, each of whom, having studied medicine in Edinburgh, went on to be closely involved with early anaesthesia in Britain. These were Henry Hill Hickman, Francis Boott, Robert Liston and James Syme.

Hickman studied medicine in Edinburgh and, by 1821, had qualified and returned to England as a family doctor [1]. He was, in 1824, the first person to prove that insensibility during surgery could be induced by inhalation. He died prematurely with his pioneering work almost unacknowledged. Virtually as Hickman left Edinburgh so Francis Boott arrived to begin his formal medical education [2]. Boott was born in Boston, Massachusetts but settled in London and soon after came to Edinburgh to study medicine. He was there from 1821 to 1824, when he qualified and returned to medical practice in London. Robert Liston emerged from his Edinburgh medical studies in 1816 with a bias towards teaching anatomy and surgery — for which he had an excellent reputation [3]. Indeed, it is quite likely that both Hickman and Boott were taught in Edinburgh by the young Robert Liston. James Syme began his studies in 1817 and qualified a few years later [4]. Like Liston he had a strong bias towards surgery and its teaching.

When anaesthesia was discovered in 1846 it was not long before Boott, Liston and Syme became involved.

Francis Boott lived in central London. By 1846 he had given up his formal medical practice but still maintained close contacts with medical friends and

Essays on the history of anaesthesia, edited by A Marshall Barr, Thomas B Boulton and David J Wilkinson. 1996: International Congress and Symposium Series No. 213, published by Royal Society of Medicine Press Limited.

colleagues. As a result he was amongst the first to receive, from Boston, the news of ether's invention, and it was he who did more than anyone else to publicize and establish ether anaesthesia in the United Kingdom [5]. Boott, together with James Robinson (a leading London dentist) conducted the first trial of ether anaesthesia in England on Saturday 19 December 1846 [6]. He sent the news he had received from Boston to the leading medical journals of the day and wrote private letters to medical colleagues in Edinburgh and elsewhere in the United Kingdom. He also told London's leading surgeon about ether's invention. This was none other than Robert Liston, Boott's erstwhile Edinburgh contemporary and possible teacher who, by 1846, was Professor of Surgery at University College, London, of which college Boott was, by then, a Governor.

On 21 December, at University College Hospital, Liston performed his first operations under ether anaesthesia. Their success was publicized — mainly by Francis Boott and, to a lesser extent, by Liston himself.

EDINBURGH'S SURGEONS LEARN OF ETHER:
THEIR MUTED REACTION

Within a few days of the news of anaesthesia first arriving in Britain, several leading doctors in Edinburgh learnt of its invention from a number of different, but entirely reliable, sources. James Miller, the Professor of Clinical Surgery, heard in a most enthusiastic letter from Robert Liston [7]. Professor William Alison, the Professor of Medicine, heard in a letter from his London friend Dr Francis Boott. Without delay he passed Boott's letter on to James Syme, the Professor of Systematic Surgery [8]. James Simpson learnt all that he could from Robert Liston, with whom he went to stay in London a few days after Liston's first use of ether [9]. Since Simpson and Professor Miller were next door neighbours in Queen Street [10] it is likely that the 2 men discussed ether's invention together. Indeed, such discussion might have provided the stimulus for Simpson to meet Liston in London. In addition, the Edinburgh men would have been able to read about ether in the London and American journals. There is also evidence that one other, unknown informant travelled directly from London to Edinburgh with the news.

So, had they wished to adopt ether anaesthesia energetically, the Edinburgh surgeons had more than enough information on which to act. Nonetheless, their initial reaction to anaesthesia was surprisingly unenthusiastic, and ether was not used in Edinburgh until 9 January 1847 [11], 2 weeks after its use in London, by which time it had been used in several other, far less prestigious, hospitals [12,13]. This is a paradox which has yet to be explained.

At this point it is important to note that anaesthesia was an entirely American invention, and that its initial propagation throughout Britain came about solely because of events which took place in, and were reported from, London. Those in Scotland had no opportunity to play a significant part in the establishment of ether anaesthesia for general surgery, and the best they could do at this stage was to follow along behind their London colleagues. Bearing in mind the enormous rivalry which then existed between London and Edinburgh this would have hardly been to their liking. Whether or not the surprising delay was a result of chauvinist pique I cannot say but, patently, anaesthesia did not really inspire the men of Edinburgh until one month after its first use in Britain when James Simpson first described its use for obstetrics [14]. His use of ether for obstetrics was widely publicized, and the controversy surrounding it, and Simpson's spirited defence of his practice, helped to redress the imbalance between London and Edinburgh as did, later in 1847, Simpson's introduction of chloroform [15].

EARLIER EDINBURGH INTEREST IN CHLOROFORM — WALDIE AND GLOVER

It is interesting to note that two other Edinburgh-trained doctors had investigated the properties of chloroform before Simpson had his attention drawn to it as a possible anaesthetic. In 1842, Dr Robert Glover (in Newcastle) investigated the physiological effects of a whole series of halides, including chloroform [16], but did not deal of course with anaesthesia. Glover had qualified in Edinburgh in 1837 [17]. In 1847, yet another Edinburgh-trained doctor, David Waldie (in Liverpool) investigated the anaesthetic properties of chloroform. Early in 1847 reports appeared that 'Chloric Ether' had been used with partial success as an anaesthetic in London [18]. These reports came to the attention of Waldie [19] who had grown up in Scotland, where he and Simpson had become friends during their medical studies together at Edinburgh. After qualification their paths diverged and Waldie — eventually — gave up medicine to pursue a long and distinguished career in pharmaceutical chemistry.

Waldie had read of the Londoner's use of chloric ether to produce anaesthesia whilst working at the Apothecaries Hall in Liverpool. Aware that the chloric ether used in London was a mixture of chloroform and alcohol [20], Waldie reasoned that the chloroform must have been the active ingredient. Accordingly, in Liverpool, he prepared a sample of pure chloroform but, significantly, did not use it or publicize his work. Soon afterwards, he and Simpson met in Edinburgh and Waldie explained his theory about chloroform. Simpson tried chloroform and introduced it into clinical practice. Later, Waldie resigned from Liverpool and emigrated to India where he lived and worked until he died in 1889. We will return to the same year and the same sub-continent a little later.

THE SCHISM BETWEEN EDINBURGH AND LONDON

By 1848, the rivalry between Edinburgh and London was focused on anaesthesia. At first the debate was on the relative merits of ether and chloroform; this soon developed into a lengthy dispute over whether or not chloroform was inherently safe, and finally it settled into an argument over whether chloroform killed by its action on the respiration or by its action on the heart: this also bore on the safest method of its administration.

Initially, the disagreement was not extreme; but reasoned and professional. However, within a few weeks of first using chloroform, Simpson felt confident enough to lay down the law on its use. His starting point was that chloroform was an extremely powerful agent. His view was that the stage of excitement (so often troublesome with ether) could be eliminated if chloroform was used, and if it was given, as he said 'In a large and overpowering dose' [21]; given 'as rapidly and in as full strength as possible so powerfully and speedily as to apathize the patient at once' [22]. He gave chloroform in this way on a simple handkerchief or towel, and cautioned against using inhalers which, he said 'merely exhibited it by the mouth and not by the nostrils, in small and imperfect, instead of full and complete doses' [22]. He took pride in recording that 'I have seen a strong person rendered completely insensible by six or seven breaths . . . of the liquid' [23]. Simpson's belief that chloroform was entirely safe was supported unequivocally by his Edinburgh colleagues.

In London these views were countered by the intuitive and cautious John Snow. Starting with the same argument as Simpson — that chloroform was indeed extremely powerful — Snow reasoned that this potency made it essential to administer the agent gradually and to know what concentration was being breathed by the patient lest overdose should occur [24]. He emphasized the importance of a gradual induction, lasting 2 minutes or more, so that one could look for signs of impending trouble (by feeling the pulse) and could decrease the chloroform should alarming signs appear. All this, he argued, could only be achieved by using a well-designed, accurate inhaler. Snow's usual practice was to use his own chloroform inhaler, and he rarely used a handkerchief alone. Indeed he wrote 'Those who have but a handkerchief or a sponge had better use ether which . . . .has not yet been known to cause death' [23] — a suggestion which was hardly likely to appeal to the Edinburgh doctors.

It would be quite wrong to criticize Simpson and his Edinburgh colleagues for their initial beliefs — that chloroform was superior to ether, that it was safer, and that an inhaler was unnecessary or dangerous. By the standards of the time these points were quite defensible. But what was indefensible was the Edinburgh school's continued insistence on chloroform's safety when early in 1848, reports of chloroform deaths began to appear. Possibly, the ever-diplomatic Snow recognized this when he wrote, after the death of Hannah Greener: 'Dr Simpson cannot be blamed if in conferring on us the benefit of chloroform, his instructions did not issue, like Minerva from the head of Jupiter, perfect and incapable of improvement' [23]. Simpson ignored this olive branch.

By coincidence, one of the earliest chloroform deaths was reported from Hyderabad, in India [25]. Soon afterwards, similar reports appeared with ominous regularity from many parts of the world. By and large those with Edinburgh affiliations reacted by maintaining that chloroform was safe, and attributed the deaths to other causes. Those without Edinburgh affiliations asserted that the chloroform was, or could be, to blame, and particularly dwelt on the method of its safe administration. (Revealingly, Hannah Greener's surgeon was Edinburgh-trained, and he was one of the very few such men to dismiss, out of hand, Simpson's argument about chloroform's safety [26]).

Nonetheless, Simpson and the vast majority of his Edinburgh-trained colleagues refused to consider any view other than their own, even when faced with a relentlessly increasing number of deaths under chloroform. Indeed, it became — as one historian of Edinburgh medicine has suggested — that support for chloroform was, for many years, a test of loyalty to Edinburgh and its traditions [27]. In this connection it is noteworthy that few — if any — of the many attempts which were made to discover a safer alternative to chloroform originated in Edinburgh.

Eventually, when it was acknowledged that chloroform might indeed cause deaths, the argument between Edinburgh and London changed. The Edinburgh view became that chloroform deaths were due only to respiratory depression, and were therefore predictable; the London view was that they were due to sudden stoppage of the heart, and therefore unheralded.

JAMES SYME'S LECTURE ON CHLOROFORM

By the mid-1850s the Edinburgh position was clearly set out in a lecture by James Syme [28]. The lecture was remarkable for two features — Syme's fierce criticisms of those in London, and his certainty that the Edinburgh school of chloroformists was right and the Londoners' hopelessly, and dangerously wrong. Syme's teaching was that no special apparatus or training was required to give chloroform, the amount of chloroform should not be stinted, and the only worthwhile guide was the patient's respiration. It was important to prevent the tongue from falling back, but the circulation should be ignored completely. 'You never' he said, 'see anybody here with his finger on the pulse while chloroform is given'. These views were championed by the Edinburgh school for the next 60 years or more.

Snow replied to Syme's critical lecture [29], and, by and large, the London school was adherent to Snow's views, which were encapsulated in the later classical picture showing Clover giving an accurately metered dose of chloroform in air, with his finger on the pulse.

CHLOROFORM 'A LA REINE': SNOW USES SIMPSON'S METHOD

In 1853 and 1857, events at Buckingham Palace provided unintentional support (from London) for the Edinburgh school from a most high and unexpected quarter, namely Queen Victoria. During her eighth and ninth labours, she received chloroform — given to her by John Snow — and was delighted by the results [30,31]. However, on each occasion that Snow gave chloroform to the Queen he did not (as he might so easily have done) use the opportunity to pour scorn on the Scots and their methods but instead poured chloroform on a handkerchief. In short, he followed Simpson's method rather than his own, which usually involved the use of his inhaler. Snow's strange inconsistency over Queen Victoria's chloroform in the 1850s was a boost for the agent, and for the Edinburgh method of giving it.

There was yet another Edinburgh dimension to this episode. Just as the Queen's Accoucheur in Scotland was the Edinburgh-trained James Simpson so her Accoucheur in England was also Edinburgh-trained. This was Dr (later Sir) Charles Locock [32], an Englishman, who had qualified from Edinburgh in 1821 having, incidentally, been a contemporary of Hickman.

How Snow came to be selected for the honour of chloroforming his sovereign is uncertain, for Snow's *Casebooks* reveal that he and Locock had rarely worked together. However, it is unlikely that Locock and the Queen's other advisers would have omitted to ask the opinion of the one person who knew most about Snow's skills at first hand — the then leading London surgeon (later Sir) William Fergusson [33]. Fergusson, then in charge of surgery at King's College Hospital, was the surgeon with whom Snow had worked most closely. He was also surgeon to Prince Albert and had his confidence. He was yet another graduate from Edinburgh from where he qualified in 1828, and where he worked until coming to London in 1840.

LISTER, THE ENGLISH DEVOTEE OF THE EDINBURGH METHOD

Joseph (later Lord) Lister, upheld the Edinburgh view of chloroform before, during and after his 8 years as Professor of Surgery in Edinburgh from 1869 to 1877 [34]. He had been trained in London — and might have been expected to hold views somewhere between those espoused by Edinburgh and those by London. However, Lister endorsed Syme's views in every detail and wrote emphatically of their correctness over a period of at least 21 years between 1861 and 1882 [35,36].

Why such a brilliant and original man as Lister obdurately refused to consider any other view than his own and Syme's is difficult to comprehend, although the fact that he was Syme's son-in-law may have been a factor.

Lister's views on chloroform were opposed from London by Joseph Clover who, predictably, stressed the importance of watching the pulse and giving a known, controlled, and not excessive amount of chloroform [37]. But Clover was merely preaching to the converted and the distance between the two schools of thought, north and south of the Border, remained as wide as ever. What I have described so far is a tale of two cities, now it becomes a tale of two continents as well.

EDWARD LAWRIE AND THE HYDERABAD MEDICAL SCHOOL

In 1846, three remarkable things happened, entirely by coincidence. Firstly, anaesthesia was discovered in America [6]. Secondly, Edward Lawrie was born in Manchester [38]. Thirdly, in far-off India, a Medical School was opened in Hyderabad [39].

Twenty-one years later, in 1867, Edward Lawrie qualified in medicine in Edinburgh [38] (at the same time, incidentally, as Thomas Lauder Brunton, of whom more shortly). Lawrie became Syme's house surgeon, but was headstrong and outspoken and was soon in trouble with the surgical authorities in Edinburgh. He was summarily dismissed from the Royal Infirmary [40] even though he had the strong support and absolute confidence of his chief, James Syme, who was then enduring his last, lingering illness. For this support, Syme earnt the undying respect and gratitude of Edward Lawrie who thereafter hero-worshipped Syme and his teachings.

Soon after his dismissal from Edinburgh, Lawrie joined the Indian Medical Service, and was promoted to increasingly senior posts over the next few years. He continued to support Syme's views about chloroform. In 1879 he was stationed in Calcutta where, by chance, David Waldie was also living, although there is no evidence that the two men ever met. While in Calcutta, Lawrie delivered a lecture on chloroform which was, as he said, 'a repetition, almost word for word, of an old lecture by the wisest man I have ever known — the late Mr Syme' [41].

Lawrie was eventually appointed as the Residency Surgeon to the princely and independent State of Hyderabad where he was also in charge of the Medical School, the students of which were trained at the Afzul Gunj Hospital. Here, far away from Britain, he developed a huge and successful chloroform practice, and taught his students to give it by Syme's method [42]. He viewed with amazement and disbelief the reports of chloroform deaths in Europe, and with horror the criticism of the agent itself. For Lawrie the answer was simple. The chloroform was not being given correctly and if everyone would change to Syme's method — especially those in London who were creating such a fuss — the problem would no longer exist.

In 1889 (the year in which David Waldie died in India) an important anaesthetic event was about to happen which was to foster chloroform's use for decades to come. Lawrie decided to promote his views on chloroform in Britain, and he chose to begin his campaign at a royal occasion in Hyderabad when there was every chance that his remarks would be reported in far-off, misguided London.

In January 1889 the Duke of Connaught (one of Queen Victoria's sons) arrived to view the Hospital and Medical School in Hyderabad [43]. The Duke and Duchess were welcomed by an impressive group. This included, amongst others, the British Ambassador to Hyderabad, the young Nizam of Hyderabad, and Edward Lawrie himself.

Within minutes of a photograph being taken of the group, Lawrie launched into a scathing attack on the London method of giving chloroform, and emphasized its absolute safety if used, as he taught in Hyderabad, in the Edinburgh fashion as recommended by Syme. Lawrie announced that he had organized an investigation of chloroform's safety which had already been carried out by some of his junior military colleagues in Hyderabad. Under the leadership of Patrick Hehir, himself an Edinburgh graduate, they had formed what came to be known as the First Hyderabad Chloroform Commission. Its conclusions were published in 1888 and were entirely in support of Lawrie's (and therefore Syme's) views [44]. *The Lancet* published details of the episode and affirmed that the conclusions were wrong [45]. As a result Lawrie inveigled *The Lancet* to send an independent expert out to Hyderabad to repeat the experiments in order to settle the matter of chloroform's safety, or lack of it, once and for all. Significantly *The Lancet* chose as its independent expert Dr Thomas Lauder Brunton [46]. Brunton [47] had been a medical student at Edinburgh with Lawrie. Later he became a renowned researcher and physician at St Bartholomew's Hospital, London. He was chosen by *The Lancet* because — even though he was an Edinburgh man — he had already written that chloroform could kill suddenly by a direct action on the heart [48], the exact reverse of Lawrie's and Syme's beliefs.

Within a few weeks of arriving in Hyderabad, Brunton, out-manoeuvred by Lawrie, had changed his views about chloroform completely and subscribed to those of Lawrie and Syme. He informed *The Lancet* that chloroform could not possibly kill by a direct action on the heart and that its only danger was from respiratory depression [49]. This view was published in 1890 in the *Report of the Second Hyderabad Chloroform Commission* [50]. The essential conclusion was couched in terms which could have been — and probably were — taken from the text of Lawrie's oft-repeated version of Syme's lecture which had been delivered in Edinburgh 37 years previously.

Syme's thesis in 1854 had been that 'chloroform may be used judiciously so as to do good without exposing the patient to the risk of evil' [28]. Thirty-seven years later the conclusion of Lawrie, Brunton and the rest of the Second Hyderabad Chloroform Commission was that 'The administrator should be guided as to the effect entirely by the respiration....chloroform may be given in any case requiring an operation with perfect ease and absolute safety so as to do good without the risk of evil' [50].

In 1901 Lawrie retired from the Indian Medical Service — initially to London and then to Brighton — but, as an extremely persistent and forceful man, he continued to sweep aside all criticism of chloroform until his death in 1915 [51,52].

20TH CENTURY SUPPORT FOR CHLOROFORM

World War I and World War II perpetuated chloroform's use. Thus, in 1947, Edinburgh celebrated the centenary of chloroform, in the knowledge that Simpson's agent was still commonly used and, in keeping with Simpson's doctrine, a survey in 1948 showed that no less than 94% of family doctors in Scotland said that chloroform was their preferred anaesthetic for obstetrics [53]. Indeed, in the even more recent past, in 1963, an even more distinguished graduate of Edinburgh suggested that chloroform could be safely used and was reluctant to condemn it [54]. Eventually, chloroform was superseded only when a similar but safer alternative—halothane—appeared on the scene [55].

CONCLUSION

Without Syme and Lawrie and their followers, Simpson's chloroform would have been discarded many decades before its actual demise. That it continued so long can be attributed to the zeal with which the Edinburgh school supported their agent. They not only held their views sincerely but were also determined to see them prevail. With hindsight it is surprising that the compelling work of Embley in 1902 in Australia [56], and of Goodman Levy in 1911 in Britain [57] (each of whom showed the nature of sudden death under chloroform) should be so widely acclaimed and yet be so ineffective in eliminating chloroform from clinical practice. Similarly, the damning recommendations of many other investigations and commissions into chloroform's safety [58] were, over the decades, published, accepted and then ignored.

Earlier, I described the Edinburgh school's perpetuation of chloroform by refusing to accept criticism of it, as being 'indefensible'. I hold to that, but it is only one half of the story. For the London school was equally culpable. The evidence of chloroform's danger was, over the years amassed and assessed by an impressive body of experts, who were mainly in London. The evidence was convincing and the lessons were clear to see. The London school railed against chloroform for no less than 100 years, and its inability to force its well-based and overwhelming arguments into general acceptance is, surely, the greatest enigma of the whole chloroform story.

REFERENCES

(1) Cartwright F. *The English pioneers of anaesthesia*. Bristol: Wright, 1952: 272.
(2) Ellis RH. The introduction of ether anaesthesia to Great Britain—2. A biographical sketch of Dr. Francis Boott. *Anaesthesia* 1977; **32**: 197–208.
(3) McCall HB. *Some old families*. Birmingham: Watson and Ball, 1890: 105–8.
(4) Miles A. *The Edinburgh school of surgery before Lister*. Edinburgh: Black, 1918: 174–211.
(5) Ellis RH. Early ether anaesthesia: the news of anaesthesia spreads to the United Kingdom. In: Atkinson RS, Boulton TB, eds. *The history of anaesthesia*. London: Royal Society of Medicine, 1989: 69–76.
(6) Boott F. Surgical operations performed during insensibility. *Lancet* 1847; **1**: 5–8.
(7) Annotation. Painless operations in surgery. *North British Review* 1847; **7**: 1609–20.
(8) Syme J. On the use of ether in the performance of surgical operations. *Monthly J Med Sci* 1847; **14**: 73–6.
(9) Simpson WG, ed. *The works of Sir JY Simpson, Bart*. Vol 2. Edinburgh: Adam and Charles Black, 1871: 33.
(10) *Post Office Edinburgh and Leith directory 1847–1848* Edinburgh: Ballantine and Hughes, 1848: **42**; 256.
(11) Hovell BC, Wilson J. The history of anaesthesia in Edinburgh. *J Royal Coll Surg Edin* 1969; **14**: 107–16.
(12) Editorial. Painless operations. *Medical Times* 1846–1847; **15**: 289–92.
(13) Annotation. Operations without pain. *Lancet* 1847; **1**: 77–80.
(14) Simpson Y. *Notes on the inhalation of sulphuric ether in the practice of widwifery*. Edinburgh: Sutherland and Knox, 1847.
(15) Simpson JY. Discovery of a new anaesthetic agent more efficient than sulphuric ether. *London Med Gazette* 1847; **5**: 934–7.

(16) Glover RM. On the physiological and medicinal properties of bromine and its compounds: also on the analogies between the physiological and medicinal properties of these bodies, and those of chlorine and iodine, compounds — Part 5. *Edin Med Surg J* 1842; **58**: 335–64.

(17) *The provincial medical directory.* London: Churchill, 1847; 114.

(18) Furnell MC. The use of anaesthetics. *Lancet* 1871; **1**: 433.

(19) Dilling WJ. David Waldie LRCS (Edin), the prophet of the anaesthetic properties of chloroform. *Liverpool Medico-Chirurgical J* 1934; **10**: 82–98.

(20) Redwood R, ed. *Gray's supplement to the pharmacopoeia.* London: Longman et al., 1847: 633.

(21) Simpson WG. *The works of JY Simpson, Bart.* Vol 2. Edinburgh: Adam and Black, 1871: 158.

(22) Simpson WG. *The works of JY Simpson, Bart.* Vol 2. Edinburgh: Adam and Black, 1871: 177.

(23) Snow J. Remarks on the fatal case of inhalation of chloroform. *London Med Gazette* 1848; **6**: 277–8.

(24) Snow J. On the inhalation of chloroform and ether, with a description of an apparatus. *Lancet* 1848; **1**: 177–80.

(25) Annotation. Death from chloroform in India. *Medical Times* 1848; **18**: 195.

(26) Meggison TN. On the cause of death in the case of Hannah Greener. *London Med Gazette* 1848; **6**: 341–2.

(27) Miles A. *The Edinburgh school of surgery before Lister.* London: Black 1918: 173.

(28) Syme J. Lectures on clinical surgery delivered during the winter session of 1854–55. *Lancet* 1855; **1**: 55–57.

(29) Snow J. Chloroform in London and Edinburgh. *Lancet* 1855; **1**: 108–109.

(30) Snow J. *The manuscript volumes of casebooks (1848–1858). Vol 1.* London: Royal College of Physicians, 448–9.

(31) Snow J. *The manuscript volumes of casebooks (1848–1858). Vol 2.* London: Royal College of Physicians, 159–60.

(32) Bettany GT. Locock Sir Charles (1799–1875). In: Lee S, ed. *Dictionary of national biography.* London: Smith and Elder, 1893: **34**: 55–56.

(33) Bettany GT. Fergusson Sir William (1808–1877). In: Stephens L, ed. *Dictionary of national biography.* London. Smith and Elder 1889; **18**: 365–6.

(34) Farmer L. *Master surgeon. A biography of Joseph Lister.* New York: Harper, 1962: 25.

(35) Lister J. Anaesthetics. In: Holmes T, ed. *A system of surgery, theoretical and practical, in treatises by various authors.* London: Parker and Brown, 1862: 91–107.

(36) Lister J. Anaesthetics. In: Holmes T, Hulke JW, eds. *A system of surgery, theoretical and practical, in treatises by various authors. Vol. 3.* London: Longman Green, 1883: 598–624.

(37) Clover J. Chloroform accidents. *Br Med J* 1871; **2**: 33–34.

(38) Masson AHB, Wilson J, Hovell BC. Edward Lawrie of the Hyderabad Chloroform Commission. *Br J Anaesth* 1969; **41**: 1002–11.

(39) Annotation. The Hyderabad Medical School. *Indian Medical Gazette* 1888; **23**: 21–22.

(40) Syme J. The managers of the Royal Infirmary and Mr Lawrie. *Lancet* 1869; **1**: 888.

(41) Lawrie E. Chloroform. *Indian Medical Gazette* 1879; **14**: 61–63.

(42) Lawrie E. *Chloroform. A manual for students and practitioners.* London: Churchill, 1901.

(43) Annotation. Hyderabad Medical School: Chloroform inhalation. *Lancet* 1889; **1**: 394.

(44) Hehir P. Abstract of the Hyderabad Chloroform Commission's Report. *Indian Medical Gazette* 1889; **24**: 321–6.

(45) Annotation. The Hyderabad Commission on Chloroform. *Lancet* 1889; **1**: 438.

(46) Annotation. The Lancet and the Hyderabad Chloroform Commission. *Lancet* 1889; **2**: 606.

(47) Thornton JL. Sir Thomas Lauder Brunton, 1844–1916. *St Bartholomew's Hosp J* 1967; **71**: 289–93.

(48) Brunton TL. *A textbook of pharmacology, therapeutics and materia medica.* London: MacMillan, 1887: 207, 801–2.

(49) Annotation. The Lancet and the Hyderabad Chloroform Commission. *Lancet* 1889; **2**: 1183.

(50) *Report of the Second Hyderabad Chloroform Commission.* Bombay: Times of India Steam Press, 1890.
(51) Lawrie E. The causation of death during the administration of chloroform. *Br Med J* 1902; **1**: 1058.
(52) Lawrie E. The problem of chloroform. *Br Med J* 1914; **1**: 995.
(53) Gillies J. Analysis of replies to a questionnary on the use of chloroform at the present time. *Anaesthesia* 1948; **3**: 45–52.
(54) Payne JP, Conway C. Cardiovascular respiratory and metabolic changes during chloroform anaesthesia. *Br J Anaesth* 1963; **35**: 588–96.
(55) Raventos J. The action of Fluothane — a new volatile anaesthetic. *Br J Pharmacol* 1956; **11**: 394–410.
(56) Embley EH. The causation of death during the administration of chloroform. *Br Med J* 1902; **2**: 817–21.
(57) Levy AG, Lewis T. Heart irregularities resulting from the inhalation of low percentages of chloroform vapour and their relationship to ventricular fibrillation. *Heart* 1911; **3**: 99.
(58) Thomas KB. Chloroform: commissions and omissions. *Br J Anaesth* 1974; **67**: 723–31.

Anaesthesia in Edinburgh 1850–1900

J Wilson

Original presentation Edinburgh 1989

THE EDINBURGH METHOD

In the 1850s, James Young Simpson virtually left the anaesthetic scene in Edinburgh, except for a few experiments with less attractive agents such as carbon tetrachloride. Chloroform was established as *the* anaesthetic. Its surgical exponents were totally satisfied with what they had. This was a non-scientific method of administering in variable dosage the most potent agent in the field, with the cheapest, simplest and most portable apparatus—which they also considered the most hygienic.

Thomas Skinner, a surgeon of Liverpool, an admirer and former student of the redoubtable Professor James Syme, wrote in 1873: 'If there be an evil more crying, more disgusting, than another in the practice of inducing anaesthesia, it is the use of inhalers. . . . There is not one inhaler, my own excepted, where every patient is not made to breathe through the same mouthpiece, tube and chamber. . . . Sweet seventeen is made to follow a bearded devotee of Bacchus, saturated with the smoke of cigars and exhalation of cognac; the mouthpiece in time becomes loaded with grease and filthy enough to upset anyone's digestion. . . . Speak of refinement! We turn up our noses if we have not a clean table napkin every day, if our knife, fork, spoon and plate be not clean or changed after every dish or course at dinner; . . . . but when we come to inhalation. . . . after 25 years' experience . . . we remain the merest barbarians, everyone breathing after his neighbour. These remarks do not apply to such inhalers as those which are extemporised out of a bedroom towel, linen, flannel, sponge and the like, all of which are readily renewable or easily washed clean' [1].

The original Edinburgh method of chloroforming was variously described by surgeons and obstetricians such as Syme, Lister, Moir and Simpson [2]. It was essentially a piece of cloth, in a single layer or folded, laid across the patient's face as a reservoir and vaporizer for the volatile liquid, with a section raised by the fingers or pins to keep the liquid out of the patient's eyes. This simplest of designs persisted into the 20th century, while the Schimmelbusch-type mask which bears a generic resemblance, was still in British obstetric practice until the 1970s. Apart from the obvious merits of portability, ease of replacement and cheapness, it was claimed to be safe, as the agent could be titrated on to it, or delivered as a large single dose to quickly overwhelm the most resilient patient. Lister claimed the method limited the available chloroform to 4.5%, and John Snow believed that 5% was the concentration above which primary cardiac failure might precede cardiac arrest. In fact my co-author Dr Barry Howell of Hull showed that 10% could be

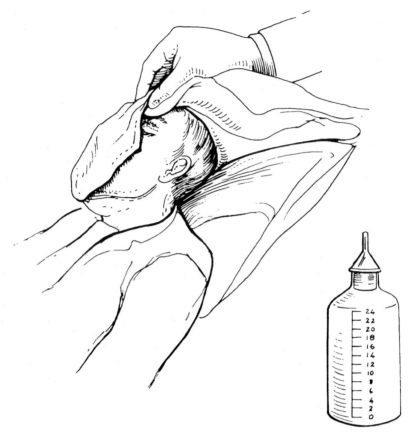

Figure 1   *The Edinburgh Method*

inhaled by this method — a frightening figure for a drug which we now know can cause marked cardiac and respiratory depression at one-tenth of that concentration. In addition, the technique left much to be desired in regard to fresh air supply and freedom of respiration.

EARLY TEACHING

The control of anaesthesia in Edinburgh was jealously retained in the hands of the surgeons and obstetricians. Edward Lawrie, a protégé of James Syme, who was to find fame of a kind in convening the Hyderabad Commissions, put it thus: 'Is it that a surgeon is no longer responsible for the safety of the patient but that the responsibility is to be shared by the man who gives chloroform or ether? In certain eventualities is the anaesthetist to dictate to the surgeon so that the surgeon becomes a mere operator, a subordinate instead of a chief, who under all circumstances retains his supreme command and the entire responsibility in his own hands? This constitutes in my opinion, the tendency to the degradation of surgery against which all surgeons should guard with all their might' [3].

One advantage of the Edinburgh method, and its jealously guarded control, was the ease of teaching. Over the 50 years from 1850 to 1900 its theoretical teaching remained in the hands of two professors of Clinical and Systematic Surgery, who between them gave all of the four lectures per year on the subject, one lasting all of 10 minutes! The practical side of teaching consisted of being one of up to 400 people allowed access to the operating theatre to watch a house surgeon, a dresser, a clerk or even a porter give an anaesthetic at the behest of the surgeon, or being the one selected, probably for reasons of expediency, to be the administrator.

Preparation of the patient for surgery in those days is worth considering. Indifferently, he might be starved for a few hours, or perhaps given some Dutch courage if the forthcoming trial was thought to be too much for him. Some patients, to further protect them from the sight of the throng in the theatre, might have their anaesthetic induced in bed in the ward. They would then be lifted onto a litter (sometimes referred to as a basket) and transported to theatre with the anaesthetic still being given. James Stewart, a Canadian anaesthetist, recalled this in a paper given to colleagues in 1914 [4]. 'The patient was carried in the basket as was our custom, by four students. The way led through a long dim corridor echoing with the sound of many feet. The student who was giving the chloroform could not hear the patient's breathing nor see his face very clearly; indeed I was told that the towel on which the chloroform was poured lay on the man's face all the way; when he was lifted on to the table, he was dead'. Stewart implied in this paper that the Edinburgh method actually afforded greater safety for the patient, and that mortality would have been higher with different agents and more elaborate techniques. Other agents required closer and more precise monitoring and more comprehensive teaching than the syllabus allowed. This is probably the case, and it was the use of other techniques and agents which led to the anaesthetic specialization so feared by earlier surgeons.

MORTALITY, MORBIDITY AND FINANCES

Deaths did occur, but were surprisingly few until the expansion in operating in the 1870s allowed by antisepsis. There will always be arguments over the cause of these early deaths — primary cardiac failure due to over or under administration, secondary failure following respiratory insufficiency, asphyxia from a poorly maintained airway or inhaled stomach contents — the descriptions bear testimony to all of these possibilities, and some make dramatic reading. 'The patient's face grows leaden and pale, sometimes with livid congestion . . .'. The vapour might be given till the breathing became stertorous and the countenance cyanosed. Some would yield easily, others struggled and resisted until overdose and asphyxia caused them to succumb. In these cases death must have been a close companion as tossing and twitching due to hypoxia replaced struggling. One writer as late as the 1880s suggested there were possibly more similarities between hanging and anaesthesia than appearance alone!

The skill and speed of the surgeons must have played a large part in the low mortality rate, but a greater factor probably was the nature of the operations. Of the 1040 performed in 1847, the last year of operating in the old Infirmary, a huge proportion were minor by any criteria, and only a few were not on peripheral sites. Larger procedures included amputations, joint excisions and drainage, removal of malignant and non-malignant tumours, and trauma due to railway and mining accidents. Joseph Bell said 'The lightning-like speed of Liston and other great operators in the pre-chloroform days still lingered as a tradition. . . . Confidence in anaesthetics and still more the devoted worship of the antiseptic fetish have tended to make an operation a very long business. By the time the spray engine was got together in 1892 and the injured limb laved and scraped and shaved and bandaged and every little vessel was tied and lotions at various temperatures were lavished on it . . . by the time drainage tubes were adjusted, double rows of sutures of various materials accurately inserted the surgeon was well into his second hour, and the patient chilled, over anaesthetised and exhausted was put to bed to die the next day without ever having a decent pulse. . . . It is quite possible with smart assistants to amputate both thighs and have the patient back in bed in considerably under half an hour!' [5]. Many great changes were occurring in surgery with refinements in technique, such as radical mastectomy instead of simple excision. Improved medical treatment also decreased the need for some operations, for example lithotomies and surgery for aneurysm.

Other influences on anaesthesia and surgery were improvements in hospital design and in nursing care. The Royal Infirmary, Edinburgh, of 1853 housed 205 surgical beds. Its two operating theatres were only used between noon and 1 pm for elective cases, unless they were part of a clinical lecture. If the surgical team were not present by 10 minutes past noon they lost their slot to the next surgeon in line. With the move to Lauriston Place the number of surgical beds rose to 279, with at least four theatres. The number of surgeons remained at 13, which was the figure agreed with the College of Physicians in the 18th century. But greater utilization of the larger number of theatres allowed an expansion of almost four times in the operative throughput. This increase was aided by better facilities for patient care. In 1854, the average stay was longer but considerably cheaper (42 days at about 53 shillings), compared with 1891 (25 days at 87 shillings). Surgical dressings were blamed for much of this increase in cost, rising from £286 to £2821 per annum. The cost of chloroform never appears in these balances, it being a tiny fraction of the expenses. Not only was the Edinburgh method a simple, portable, easily taught and 'hygienic' means of anaesthetizing, it was also very cheap.

NURSING SERVICES

The Crimean War of 1853–56 lost Edinburgh several of its budding surgeons who volunteered for war service but then died of cholera. On the credit side, the war brought Florence Nightingale to the fore, and gave her the power to change the face of nursing forever. Through her influence, Edinburgh achieved improvements in its hospital buildings, and began its great tradition of nursing. The anaesthetist of today, who relies so much on nurses in the wards and theatre, might ponder the situation in Edinburgh in the first six decades of the 19th century. Joseph Bell, who was house surgeon to Professor Syme in 1854, again gives the picture: 'For the 72 patients I as house surgeon had to look after, distributed in six wards and six little rooms, the nursing staff consisted of nine women, aided in an emergency by the possible services of a drunken old porter who looked after the waiting room. The nine women were: two staff nurses each with about 36 beds to look after, and seven so-called night nurses who also had to do the scrubbing and cleaning of the wards and passages. The two nurses, Mrs Lambert and Mrs Porter, were wonderful women. . . . of immense experience and great kindliness. . . . no two finer specimens of the old school nurse. . . . But the other seven, poor old useless drudges, half charwomen, half fieldworker, rarely keeping their places for any length of time, absolutely ignorant, almost invariably drunk, sometimes deaf . . . had to take care of our operation cases when the staff nurses went off duty. Poor creatures, they had a hard life! Their day's work began at 11 pm, when in a mournful procession, each with a blanket round her shoulder, they walked to the wards from a dormitory, so-called, in the East end of the grounds. There, they were supposed to keep up the fire and nurse the patients until 5 am when they had to set about cleaning the wards, scouring the tins and preparing for the patients' breakfast. During "the visit" they used to prowl about and help at the meals of dinner and tea, and it was not till 5 pm that they were allowed to trudge back to the dormitory. What wonder that at night they snored by the fire . . . and when an accident came in, their blear eyes and stupid heads were of little use except to rouse up one or two tired house surgeons to help the one on duty. Serious operations were doubled in risk by want of ordinary care. Haemorrhages were unnoticed, amputation cases allowed to rise from bed; indeed a zealous house surgeon had his heart ready broken by their unwisdom and neglect . . . The matron was a housekeeper . . . and knew no more of real nursing than the poorest of the scrubbers. Dressers volunteered to look after patients following big operations, on four-hourly watches, and these patients were watched, fed and looked after for the first few days.'

Changes in nursing were attempted in the 1860s but these were mainly trying to train the untrainable. It was not till the 1870s that real improvements occurred in nurse organization, with development of a career structure and the selection of vocationally oriented girls. In 1872 a Lady Superintendent was appointed, with four acting superintendents (two for day and two for night duty). Also appointed were 11 staff (head) nurses, 12 assistant nurses, 16 night nurses and 20 probationers. By 1881 their day was organized as follows: Rise at 6 am, breakfast 6.30, ward at 7 am. Luncheon and tea in their own rooms on the ward. Dine in the nurses' home at 3 pm, supper and prayers 8.45, bed by 10.30. Two hours were allocated 'off duty' each alternate day and friends were only to be seen in these afternoons. A one day and one half-day holiday were allowed each month. Night nurses rose at 7 pm and attended the ward from 8.30 pm to 9.00 am. They got one day's holiday per month. All nurses had 2 weeks holiday a year. These posts were certainly not sinecures, but representative of vast improvements in patient care. It is hardly surprising that the cost of nursing rose from £1100 in 1854 to £4000 in 1892. Considering the increase of the workforce, what is surprising is that the rise was not more — a reflection perhaps on the vocational attitude of the new generation of nurses, and their socio-economic background.

MAINTAINING THE STATUS QUO

While these advances were being made in medicine, surgery and nursing, it is salutary to note what changes occurred in anaesthesia. In the rest of the world during the period 1850–1900 considerable progress was made while Edinburgh clung to the status quo. Outside Scotland (and Edinburgh in particular) vaporizers, some very sophisticated, were introduced for volatile agents. Nitrous oxide was reintroduced in America and Europe, together with oxygen. Klikovitch in St Petersburg even pioneered pre-mixed nitrous oxide and oxygen in obstetrics, and showed graphs of uterine activity demonstrating that nitrous oxide had no deleterious effect on contractions [6]. Chloroform was still in use in Scotland 30 years after its introduction, and without any worthwhile scientific publications. At the Royal Infirmary, the Edinburgh method was still in vogue at the end of the century.

ACKNOWLEDGEMENT

I thank Dr M Barfoot, Archivist for the Lothian Health Board for his kind assistance.

REFERENCES

(1) Skinner T. Anaesthetics and inhalations. *Br Med J* 1873; **1**: 353–4.
(2) Howell BC, Wilson J. The history of anaesthetics in Edinburgh Part 2. *J Roy Coll Surg Edin* 1969; **14**: 165–79.
(3) Lawrie E. The teaching of anaesthetics. *Lancet* 1901; **1**: 64.
(4) Stewart J. Chloroform anaesthesia. *Canadian Medical Association J* 1914; **4**: 1053–65.
(5) Bell J. The surgical side of the Royal Infirmary of Edinburgh 1854–1892. *Edinburgh Hospital Reports* 1893; **1**: 18–34.
(6) Richards W, Parbrook G, Wilson J. Stanley Klikovitch (1853–1910). *Anaesthesia* 1976; **31**: 933–40.

Anaesthesia in Edinburgh 1900–1950

AHB Masson

Original presentation Edinburgh 1989

The transformation of the anaesthetic scene which was started in the 1890s by Silk, Buxton and Hewitt, and spread slowly to the rest of the country. In general, the dentists were much more progressive than their surgical colleagues. The two Scottish founder members of the Society of Anaesthetists, founded by Silk in 1893, were from the Dental Hospitals of Glasgow and Edinburgh. By 1900, when there were no anaesthetists in any of the Edinburgh surgical hospitals, the Edinburgh Dental Hospitals had several to supervise the administration of anaethetics by students. It was not until 1901 that Dr TD Luke, who had sessions in the Dental Hospital, and Dr McAllum were appointed to the Deaconess Hospital and the Royal Hospital for Sick Children respectively.

NEW APPOINTMENTS

The surgeons in the Royal Infirmary viewed these two appointments with interest. At the end of October 1901 it was reported that 'a suggestion had been made that the Managers should appoint an Anaesthetist to the Infirmary, a proposal which met with the approval of the Surgical Staff, but the Medical Managers Committee desired to meet and discuss the matter with the Surgical Staff before making any recommendation to the Board on the subject'. The suggestion had come from one of the gynaecologists, whose letter detailed the advantages of having a 'special and qualified anaesthetist' rather than a senior student to give anaesthetics.

This letter was discussed by the powerful Surgical Staff Committee which consisted of the senior surgeons, headed by Professor Annandale, Lister's successor in the Chair of Clinical Surgery. They met in Annandale's home and a majority, including Annandale, supported the proposal. Three, however, did not. Their reasons were predictable. One doubted if greater safety would accrue since most fatalities occurred in trivial or minor cases. 'It shifted responsibility and when fatalities occurred, it would be found that there was a dual control, no one being personally responsible. It would reflect on members of the staff as having neglected their duty in giving suitable instruction to those whom they have permitted to anaesthetise the patients under their care. It would cause a serious loss of confidence in the relations between the staff and their patients.' But the nub of the matter was clearly spelt out: 'Above all it would lay those surgeons who could not or did not desire the services of the special anaesthetist open to blame and question. And once this disturbing element was introduced, there would be an end to the suitable education of the medical student and the anaesthetist's services would be almost obligatory in every case'.

As a result of this meeting, the managers noted in November that it had been agreed 'practically unanimously' that an instructor on the administration of anaesthetics should be appointed to teach students and to give practical demonstrations on minor, although not major cases. This instructor would be empowered to grant a certificate to all students who attended his demonstrations and then passed a satisfactory examination. They also recommended that all future candidates for the appointment of resident physician or surgeon must hold a certificate of proficiency in the administration of anaesthetics. The managers approved these recommendations and remitted them to the Managers Committee to prepare and submit a set of rules to govern the appointment. However, at the next meeting of the board, it was reported that 'The Medical Managers had had a further meeting with the members of the Surgical Staff, when these gentlemen indicated that they did not desire the appointment of an Anaesthetist who would be at liberty to demonstrate anaesthetics, but merely a teacher on the subject'. Since 'matters of teaching are not dealt with by the Board', the whole subject was dropped.

At the same meeting, a letter from Annandale was submitted requesting Dr Luke to be permitted to act as tutor of anaesthetics in his department. The professor of surgery observed: 'Dr Luke is a thoroughly skilled and experienced anaesthetist and will not in any way interfere with the patients or their treatment (but) simply give tutorial instruction to my class. His remuneration will be arranged by myself.' Another of the senior surgeons had Dr McAllum appointed to his unit. As a result of the Board's decision however, these two anaesthetists had no official status in the hospital and they were not allowed to give, or even demonstrate how to give, anaesthetics. They were graded as clinical tutors, the equivalent perhaps of a senior registrar, the same as the surgical trainees and because of this, they had to apply annually for reappointment. Moreover, although they were unpaid, the maximum term of office was five years.

Luke's five-year term expired at the end of 1906. He had in the meantime been appointed as a university lecturer but he complained to the Board that it was not possible for him to carry out his duties without access to the wards. The managers were adamant. Despite the fact that Luke was manifestly not a trainee and was not even paid an honorarium by the Board, they reluctantly agreed to reappoint him for only one year and that was 'for the convenience of Professor Annandale'.

Luke was intelligent, hard working, an excellent anaesthetist, and a good teacher. He wrote two successful textbooks — *A Pocket Guide to Anaesthetics* and *Anaesthesia in Dental Surgery*. He was also popular; when his appointment was terminated, no fewer than 30 of his surgical colleagues wrote to the Board asking that he and McAllum be appointed as instructors in practical anaesthesia with the same privileges as physicians and surgeons on the staff. This was categorically refused, so when his protector, Annandale, died in 1907, Luke gave up anaesthesia and left Edinburgh. That ended the second attempt to get an anaesthetist appointed to the Infirmary.

A DEATH — AND 'SUPERVISORS OF ANAESTHESIA'

Four years later, there was a third attempt. This time the motivation was different. The Crown Office, with justification, was very critical about the circumstances surrounding the death under anaesthesia of an 8 month old infant who had been admitted for a circumcision. The anaesthetic had been given by the house surgeon.

Crown Counsel directed that the matter, and their opinion, be brought to the notice of the managers.

The managers sent the letter to the Surgical Staff Committee who considered the matter, and informed the Board they believed that, 'in the interests of the Institution' the assistance of officially recognized anaesthetists should be obtained. Since the request this time was prompted by the report from Crown Counsel, it could not be dismissed quite so easily. The Managers recognized that it raised a very important and far-reaching question. If the suggestions of the Staff were carried out, the Minute noted: 'it would in all probability involve the Institution in expense in the shape of salaries'.

It was a year before they reached a decision. They recognized that 'in the surgical wards, it is not always possible to ensure that a qualified medical man is available to devote his whole attention to, and to directly supervise the administration of, anaesthetics' but that 'it is desirable in the interests of the patients that this precaution should always be adopted'; and they decreed that such assistance should be afforded to each surgical charge as well as the out patient department. The managers had the answer. They recommended 'that the seven Surgical Clinical Tutors who at present have no official status on the staff of the Infirmary should be appointed to supervise the administration of anaesthetics at an annual honorarium of £15 each' — the Surgical Clinical Tutors! New regulations were promulgated, which further stated: 'In cases of emergency and when the Supervisors of Anaesthetics are not available, the Resident Physicians and Surgeons shall be held responsible.'

Luke's colleague Dr McAllum died in 1914, just after he had been elected President of the newly formed Scottish Society of Anaesthetists, the oldest national society in the world. For another 20 years there were no further attempts to have an anaesthetist officially appointed to the Infirmary. In practice, there was a very gradual change in that three were working as 'Supervisors of Anaesthesia' by 1920 and five by 1925 and the Board did not now limit the term of their appointments. But when in 1920, Dr J Stuart Ross, a university demonstrator, resigned to take up another appointment, the Board minutes note that 'by the regulations, the Clinical Tutor is the person to occupy the post of Instructor, and the appointment of Dr Ross was made by special arrangement'.

Where anaesthetists were appointed, they had been specifically requested by a senior surgeon and they worked only for him. They were all dentists or general practitioners because anaesthesia in Edinburgh did not generate a sufficient income to allow them to survive on that alone. They did not do any of the emergency work and that was what prompted the next attempt to get a proper appointment. Once again, the move seems to have been triggered by the Crown Office.

UNSUPERVISED ANAESTHESIA

In 1931, the surgical staff asked the managers to appoint two resident anaesthetists 'who would be available at any hour of the day or night' and suggested that two nurses might be trained for this special work. The medical managers rejected the idea of nurses and asked the Board to authorize the appointment of one anaesthetist for night work. A short time after this request was received, the Board received a letter from the Crown Agent which read: 'I am directed by the Lord Advocate to draw the attention of Hospital Authorities and members of the medical profession to the danger of allowing unqualified medical students to administer anaesthetics in cases in which the administration of the anaesthetic is not under the immediate personal supervision of a qualified medical practitioner. It appears from a case which has recently been under his Lordship's consideration that the supervision so exercised may on occasion be merely nominal and that the qualified person may not be present in the room where the patient is being anaesthetised. . . . His Lordship recommends that in no case should an unqualified person be permitted to administer an anaesthetic except in the presence of a qualified medical practitioner and under his immediate personal supervision.'

Where this death occurred I do not know, but it could have been in the Royal Infirmary. Over the years many deaths were recorded under anaesthesia — 'died while being chloroformed in preparation for an operation for whitlow', 'died during an operation for varicose veins', 'died before operation', 'died of heart failure preparatory to an operation being performed' and many similar cases. These were all considered by the Medical Management Committee before being reported to the Procurator Fiscal and in none was any blame attached to the person giving the anaesthetic. The minutes solemnly declared in each and every case that the anaesthetic was carefully administered and everything possible was done for the patient.

A memorandum produced and circulated by the medical superintendent about that time is typical. It is self-congratulatory rather than critical and purports to show that the deaths per thousand anaesthetics had not increased over the years. In no case did the Board discuss or comment on the circumstances of any specific death. The figures are interesting. In the 8 years from 1921 to 1929, there were 74 769 operations with 80 deaths, almost exactly one death/1000 operations. The memo then stated: 'Of the 80 deaths four had been cases of acute emergency and if this number were deducted, the average proportion of fatalities fell to 0.74/1000'. However, not all the deaths were included. Thirteen were excluded because they did not have a general anaesthetic and six because the total number of administrations was unknown!

ANAESTHETISTS FOR EMERGENCY WORK

The Board agreed on one appointment to cover emergencies, and advertised for an anaesthetist to work every night for an honorarium of £200 per year. Dr Sheena Watters bravely applied. Although she was the first person appointed to the Royal Infirmary as an anaesthetist, her status was far removed from that of the physicians and surgeons. Problems soon arose when she had the temerity to go on holiday and a locum had to be sought. It was manifestly impossible for one person to do this night work all year round. Within a year, the work had been split into sessions and divided among three people. The honorarium was increased to £350 per year, shared by the three; that is, a person working two nights a week, every week for a year was paid just over £100!

It should not be thought that the Royal Infirmary was unusual in its anaesthetic mortality or in its attitude to anaesthetists. For example, in 1935 at the Western General Hospital in Edinburgh, 901 operations were recorded, 550 of which were classified as major. But the first anaesthetic appointment to that hospital was not made until 1939 when Dr Frank Holmes, then recently qualified, was appointed as resident anaesthetist at a salary of £150 per annum. For holidays, he had to find and to pay for his locum.

One of the three anaesthetists appointed in 1933 to do the night work at the Infirmary was Dr John Gillies, who had left general practice in Yorkshire to take up anaesthesia in Edinburgh. A year later, Dr Torrance Thomson, the distinguished anaesthetist who had introduced Dr Langton Hewer to nitrous oxide/oxygen anaesthesia in France in 1917, retired from his post as Supervisor of Anaesthesia in the Professorial Unit, and John Gillies was appointed in his place.

JOHN GILLIES

The effect of Gillies' arrival was immediate. Prior to his arrival records were kept rather erratically and techniques were limited to ethyl chloride/ether or chloroform/ether. From the day he started, the anaesthetic book was kept in meticulous detail with his name opposite at least one major case, and that of a student, clearly under good supervision, doing the rest. The techniques were more varied — spinals (done by him, not the surgeon), intravenous agents and the first endotracheal anaesthetics, as opposed to the endotracheal insufflation which had been used on rare occasions.

Even more significant was his impact on his colleagues. In 1938, the Honorary Staff Committee of the Royal Infirmary set up a subcommittee consisting of two surgeons and three anaesthetists — Dr Gillies, Dr David Middleton, a dental surgeon, and Dr Benny Wevill. They recommended that the anaesthetist to each surgical charge should be recognized as a lecturer by the University. They also recommended that there should be an anaesthetist for each surgical charge and that they should be represented on the honorary staff. These proposals were accepted and recognition was achieved at last.

The subcommittee further advocated the appointment of two fulltime junior anaesthetists for emergency work; Dr Wheeler and Dr Leslie Morrison were appointed in 1940, forming under John Gillies' tutelage the original Department of Anaesthetics in the Royal Edinburgh Infirmary. It was also the first department of anaesthetics in Scotland and one of the first in Britain. Not everyone wanted their services. Some of the more elderly obstetricians were particularly resistant to an anaesthetic service and the outpatient department was still a troublesome area. In 1940, a proposal was made to appoint a fourth house surgeon to outpatients to administer anaesthetics but this was over-ruled. Instead, a third resident anaesthetist, Alastair McKinley, was appointed. Like the other two, he was first put on probation for a month without pay. Thereafter, 'provided his work was satisfactory', he was paid £150 per year.

POSTWAR DEPARTMENT

In 1944 the Medical Management Committee, for so long the centre of opposition, considered proposals for the creation of a post of senior anaesthetist who would organize an anaesthetic service, act as Chairman of the anaesthetist staff and organize investigations for anaesthesia. The principle was agreed but as some of the potential candidates were away on service, consideration was deferred until after the war. On 6 July 1946, John Gillies was invited by a delegation from the Infirmary and the University to be Director of Anaesthesia to the Royal Infirmary and also Lecturer (later Simpson Reader) in Anaesthesia to the University. The department which John Gillies started was one of considerable academic excellence. Its membership in the early post-war years included no fewer than seven future professors of anaesthesia, and the work of Gillies and Harold Griffiths on induced hypotension by total spinal sympathetic blockade was a major advance. With Minnitt, Gillies rewrote a *Textbook of Anaesthesia* which was the sixth edition of the book first published by Ross.

John Gillies made his mark both nationally and internationally. In 1943 he was elected to the Council of the Association of Anaesthetists and became its president in 1947. Probably at no other time in its history has that office assumed such importance because that was the year before the start of the National Health Service, when the terms and conditions of the various hospital specialists were under discussion.

The importance of John Gillies to Edinburgh and to the specialty in general was enormous. He shared, as he put it himself, in the rapid and striking progression of anaesthetic practice from a dubious restricted art to a broadbased comprehensive discipline. He fought for and obtained enhancement of the status of anaesthetists in a city traditionally hostile to anaesthetists; and he did it by obtaining the respect of those with whom he worked, by his gentle charm, integrity, good humour and a profound conviction of the importance of 'the integration of training in basic sciences, clinical medicine and surgery with the theory and practice of anaesthetic administration and its important ancillary, patient care.' Anaesthesia had come a long way since 1900.

ACKNOWLEDGEMENT

My thanks to the Lothian Health Board for access to the Minute Books of the Board of Management of the Royal Infirmary of Edinburgh.

Highlights of anaesthesia in Dundee

SW McGowan

Original presentation Edinburgh 1989

In many respects anaesthesia in Dundee developed along conventional lines. Ether was first used in 1847, but soon was entirely superseded by chloroform. Spinals were in vogue in the early 1900s. All anaesthetics were given by non-specialists until 1 January 1914 when the first anaesthetist, Dr Arthur Mills, took up his post. My research in local archives, however, produced records of three features of some interest — two not totally unexpected, the third possibly unique to Dundee.

BEFORE ETHER — NITROUS OXIDE AND ACUPUNCTURE

In 1836, nitrous oxide was used in an entertaining lecture and demonstration. According to Barbara Duncum, such entertainments were popular at that time in England and America [1]. The lecturer at Dundee was Dr Fyfe and the venue was the Watt Institution. This was one of the many Mechanics' Institutes which sprang up in the 1820s in the wake of the industrial revolution. Their purpose was to educate the working classes in basic arithmetic and science. Dundee was an industrial town with flax mills and there was a need for skilled workers. Dr Fyfe's lecture was so popular it was repeated twice. He invited seven gentlemen to come forward and inhale nitrous oxide from a silken bag. Each one reacted differently to the laughing gas, much to the amusement of the spectators. If only the audience had included a dentist with the vision of Horace Wells, inhalation anaesthesia might have been discovered in Dundee.

My second surprise was to learn that acupuncture was used between 1840 and 1843 by a Dundee surgeon, Dr John Crichton, who claimed remarkable success. He treated not only painful conditions such as sciatica, but also swollen joints (hydrops articuli) and hydroceles of the spermatic cord. In the *Annual Report of the Dundee Royal Infirmary 1842–3*, he wrote, 'Hydrocele, in former times requiring a painful operation, with long continued confinement and more latterly the injection of stimulating liquors — has, in all the cases that have presented themselves this last year, been cured by acupuncture alone'.

A POSSIBLE 'FIRST' IN REGIONAL BLOCK

From 1900 onwards, probably as a result of deaths under chloroform, and the adverse reports by various commissions and committees, ether began to be used again, along with mixtures of alcohol, ether and chloroform. Ethyl chloride and

ANÆSTHETIC TABLE.

MEDICAL AND SURGICAL DEPARTMENTS.

General Anæsthetics,

Chloroform, ...	1,085	times.
„ and Alcohol, ...	524	„
„ and Ether, ...	23	„
Ether, ...	10	„
A.C.E. Mixture, ...	23	„
Ethyl Chloride, ...	52	„
Hyoscine, Morphine, and Chloroform,	104	„
Hyoscine, Morphine, and Ether, ...	25	„
Morphine, Atropine, and Chloroform,	34	„
Morphine, Atropine, and Ether, ...	98	„
Atropine and Ether, ...	3	„

Local Anæsthetics.

(a) Cutaneous.

Ethyl Chloride, ...	1	„

(b) Subcutaneous.

Eucaine, ...	4	„
Cocaine, ...	151	„
Novocaine, ...	20	„

(c) Injection into Vein.

Novocaine, ...	1	„
Tropacocaine, ...	1	,

(d) Spinal Injection.

Novocaine, ...	16	„
Stovaine, ...	10	„
Hyoscine and Morphine, ...	8	„
„ „ and Atropine,	1	„

MATERNITY DEPARTMENT.

Chloroform, ...	54	„
	2,246	„

Figure 1   *Dundee Royal Infirmary, anaesthetics for the year 1909–10*

nitrous oxide also came into the picture. The first mention of local anaesthesia appeared in the *Dundee Royal Infirmary Annual Report* for 1908–09, when two Bier's blocks ('injection into vein') were recorded, and 22 spinals using stovaine. The possibly unique development is documented in the *Annual Report* for the following year. Of the 35 spinals listed, novocaine was the agent in 16, another ten used stovaine, but it appears that in eight cases the agents given were hyoscine and morphine, while one patient received hyoscine, morphine and atropine. The apparent injection spinally of hyoscine and morphine continued in the next 4 years, making a total of 57 cases. Although intrathecal morphine is now a standard method of pain relief, the literature on opiates used this way is relatively recent. Contemporary volumes of *The Lancet, British Medical Journal, Edinburgh Medical Journal* and *Proceedings of the Royal Society of Medicine* carry no mention of spinal morphine at the time of these Reports.

We do have to consider the possibility that the injection of hyoscine and morphine was made subcutaneously in patients having a standard spinal anaesthetic. Schneiderlin in 1900 had introduced the use of morphine and hyoscine before surgery [2] and it was a popular combination before both general and spinal anaesthesia. Among its greatest proponents were Professor Kronig in Freiberg, Torrance Thomson in Edinburgh and RC Buist, an obstetrician in Dundee [3].

It is however my considered opinion that the Anaesthetic Tables in these annual reports give a true and accurate record. They were compiled in a most meticulous manner and in great detail. The section on general anaesthetics separates those cases in which chloroform was given alone from those in which it was given after hyoscine and morphine. The hyoscine and morphine is recorded under 'spinal injection' not once, but in 5 successive years. The sub-heading of the anaesthetic table includes medical as well as surgical departments, which may indicate that these agents were given for pain relief, rather than for operations. Although there was no scientific basis for using opiates intrathecally at that time, many drugs and techniques were employed empirically. Meltzer in New York [4] was injecting magnesium sulphate intrathecally to produce spinal analgesia. There is a good case to be made that Dundee was the first centre to use morphine by spinal injection.

ACKNOWLEDGEMENTS

I am grateful for help from Mr Macdonald Black, a dentist of Dundee, from my colleague Dr AL Forrest, and from Mrs Joan Auld, archivist at the University of Dundee.

REFERENCES

(1) Duncum B. *The development of inhalational anaesthesia*. London: Oxford University Press, 1947: 76.
(2) Leedham-Green C. On the scopolamine-morphine narcosis. *Br Med J* 1909; **ii**: 962.
(3) Buist RC. The use of hyoscine-morphine anaesthesia in natural labour. *Br Med J* 1908; **ii**: 808–809.
(4) Meltzer SJ. Spinal anaesthesia with sulphate of magnesium. *Lancet* 1906; **i**: 127, 1057.

Aberdeen, archives and anaesthesia

ID Levack

Original presentation Edinburgh 1989

Founded in 1495, Aberdeen University is the most northerly and one of the oldest universities in Britain. It has an important connection with the beginning of the Scottish chloroform tradition, through a medical graduate and a professor of medicine and chemistry. Later, several luminaries associated with Aberdeen popularized ether against the Scottish enthusiasm for chloroform. In more recent times, the contributions of Michael Tunstall to obstetric and paediatric anaesthesia justify the inclusion of his name along with the earlier pioneers.

THE DISCOVERY OF CHLOROFORM ANAESTHESIA

James Matthews Duncan, after graduation at Marischal College, Aberdeen in 1846, moved to Edinburgh as assistant to James Young Simpson in his midwifery practice. Under Simpson's direction he became involved in the quest for an agent superior to ether for obstetric analgesia [1]. His part in this is recorded in a limited edition biography written by his sister [2] and was recently reviewed in an essay on the discovery of chloroform [3]. In October 1847, Duncan collected a batch of volatile liquids from William Gregory, the Professor of Chemistry at Edinburgh.

Gregory was a contemporary and friend of Justus von Liebig who had been one of the first to synthesize chloroform in 1831. He had spent many weeks in Liebig's laboratory at Giessen, collaborating in studies on organic chemistry, before his first professorial appointment in Aberdeen. From 1839 to 1844 Gregory was Mediciner (Professor of Medicine and Chemistry) at King's College in Aberdeen. From there he moved to the Chair of Chemistry at Edinburgh University.

It was not therefore surprising that the liquids received from Gregory for assessment of their anaesthetic potential included chloroform. Matthews Duncan tested it on himself in his room at Simpson's residence in Queen Street where he lodged. He inhaled the vapour, which made him stuporose, if not unconscious. Convinced that chloroform's properties were ideal, he brought it to the attention of Simpson at the table after supper in the company of George Keith. The famous party followed, although some time before this Simpson had been informed of the possibilities of chloroform by his friend David Waldie [3].

After the discovery, and the glory bestowed on Simpson, whose reputation and position undoubtedly influenced its widespread acceptance, Matthews Duncan was deeply hurt by the lack of recognition given to him by his chief. Initially he continued as Simpson's assistant, and later built up the largest obstetric practice in Edinburgh. When Simpson died in 1870, and the Town Council appointed his nephew as successor to the Chair of Midwifery, it was predictable that Duncan would leave Edinburgh. He eventually did in 1877, to become obstetric physician to St Bartholomew's Hospital. In the same year, Joseph Lister went to King's College Hospital from the Chair of Surgery at the Royal Infirmary of Edinburgh.

GREGORY AND MORPHINE

Subsequently, William Gregory played an important role in devising the means for large scale production and purification of chloroform [4]. This contribution was probably of less value than his early discovery of an inexpensive method of manufacturing salts of morphia [5]. The importance of these developments was inadequately recognized during his lifetime. With chloroform, the personalities of all other workers in the field were obscured by that of Simpson, while Gregory's work on morphine required other developments before achieving full significance. He had produced the muriate (hydrochloride) of morphia in 1831, only 3 years after graduating in medicine [6]. The acetate had been available since 1823, but it was rarely pure, with narcotine the main contaminant. Gregory devised a process to isolate and purify the salt at no greater cost than the equivalent dose of laudanum. However, when taken orally, there was no clear advantage of the pure morphia salt. It was not until 1855, when Alexander Wood of Edinburgh introduced hypodermic injection to medical practice, that the future of morphine salts was secured. The demand would elevate 'Gregory's process' to a commercial scale, but he died within 3 years, and appraisals of his work at the time undervalued the achievements of a remarkable Scotsman.

William Gregory was the sixteenth of the 'academic Gregorys' to hold a Scottish professorship. He was a fifth generation descendant of the Reverend John Gregorie of Drumoak, which is a small parish a few miles to the west of Aberdeen. The family has a renowned hereditary genius [7]. He is buried in a family vault near the entrance of the Canongate Churchyard at the lower end of Edinburgh's Royal Mile.

APPOINTMENT OF A CHLOROFORMIST

William Pirrie, the first Professor of Surgery in Aberdeen, used chloroform during the excision of a breast tumour, 10 days after Simpson read a paper on his experience with chloroform to the Edinburgh Medico-Chirurgical Society in November 1847. Surgical arrogance and rejection greeted a proposal by the Aberdeen Hospital Committee to appoint a staff chloroformist in 1856. It was not until a death under chloroform at the hands of Pirrie in 1871 [8], that a regular chloroformist was appointed. Some insight to this period is available in the biography of Sir Alexander Ogston [9], who was Pirrie's successor, and best remembered as the discoverer of *Staphylococcus pyogenes aureus*. Ogston's short account *How anaesthetics came to Aberdeen* notes that as a student in 1860 he was aware of debate among the surgeons whether chloroform 'the only anaesthetic thought of practically in Scotland' ought to be used in operations — usually it was not. When he graduated 5 years later it was widely used, and one of his duties as a newly appointed hospital doctor was to act as a chloroformist.

Alexander Dyce Davidson became the first designated chloroformist in Aberdeen. He held the post from 1871 to 1875, later being elevated to Professor of Materia Medica. Davidson's successor was Patrick Blaikie Smith, who brought to Aberdeen a completely new approach to anaesthesia.

ABERDEEN VERSUS THE SCOTTISH CHLOROFORM DOCTRINE

Blaikie Smith was a devotee of ether, who described in *The Lancet* a new ether inhaler, accompanied by views on chloroform which were contrary to the established Edinburgh doctrine [10]. Soon after this article was published, John A MacWilliam arrived in Aberdeen as Professor of Physiology. He made an important series of observations, including the first description of ventricular fibrillation [11], and its association with chloroform anaesthesia in various animals [12]. MacWilliam's work was counter to popular medical opinion in Scotland, and to the findings of the Hyderabad Commissions. Much of this background, and an assessment of MacWilliam's contribution is set out in Barbara Duncum's history of inhalational anaesthesia [13]. MacWilliam has also been credited with providing the original concept and experiments on cardiac pacing [14,15].

In practical anaesthesia, the devotion to ether of the Aberdeen school stemmed from Blaikie Smith. A significant advance in the use of open drop ether was made during World War I by Alexander Ogston, a general practitioner anaesthetist who developed his eponymous wire frame mask to achieve a higher inspired concentration, and a more efficient (and economical) use of ether [16]. He was not related to his surgical namesake, who was erroneously credited with this device in the Charles King Collection [17], and in the museum of the Royal College of Surgeons of Edinburgh.

THE MODERN ERA — MICHAEL TUNSTALL

In 1963, Michael Tunstall came to Aberdeen from a senior registrar position in Portsmouth, on the Oxford training rotation under the guidance of RJ Hamer Hodges, who was a founding father of modern obstetric anaesthesia. In the face of considerable commercial hesitancy, Tunstall persuaded The British Oxygen Company to manufacture pre-mixed oxygen and nitrous oxide which came on the market as Entonox [18]. He also made the necessary recommendations [19] on dealing with gas separation due to cold — a requirement of particular significance in the climate of northern Scotland. Among his many other contributions were the Aberdeen 'failed intubation drill' [20] in obstetrics, and the 'isolated forearm technique' [21] to deal with the problem of awareness during Caesarian section. In paediatrics, the Tunstall connector is still widely used to anchor nasal tracheal tubes [22].

Michael Tunstall retired in 1992, but has remained active in research [23]. His efforts, and those of the earlier pioneers were suitably rewarded when in 1993, the University established its first Chair of Anaesthesia.

REFERENCES

(1) Christison R. Anaesthesia and chloroform. In: *The life of Sir Robert Christison, Bart.* Edinburgh: William Blackwood & Sons, 1886; 2: 350–3.
(2) James Matthews Duncan MD FRS — an obituary. Limited edition. Copy held by the Aberdeen Medico-Chirurgical Society.
(3) Simpson D. Simpson and 'the discovery of chloroform.' *Scot Med J* 1990; 35: 151–5.
(4) Gregory W. Notes on the purification and properties of chloroform. *Proc Royal Soc Edin* 1844–50; 2: 316–24.
(5) Colman Green G. William Gregory 1803–58. *Nature* 1946; 157: 456–9.

(6) Gregory W. On a process for preparing economically the muriate of morphia. *Edin Med Surg J* 1831; **35**: 331–8.

(7) Lawrence PD. The Gregory family: a biographical and bibliographical study. PhD Thesis, Aberdeen University, 1971.

(8) Pirrie W. Death of a patient while under the influence of chloroform. *Br Med J* 1871; **2**: 124–5.

(9) Ogston WH. How anaesthetics came to Aberdeen. In: *Alexander Ogston KCVO*. Aberdeen University Press, 1943: 92.

(10) Blaikie Smith P. A new inhaler for the administration of ether. *Lancet* 1884; **2**: 19.

(11) MacWilliam JA. Fibrillar contraction of the heart. *J Physiol* 1887; **8**: 296–310.

(12) MacWilliam JA. Report on an experimental investigation of the action of chloroform and ether. *Br Med J* 1890; **2**: 890–2.

(13) Duncum BM. Hyderabad Commission and its consequences. In: *The development of inhalational anaesthesia*. Oxford: Oxford University Press, 1947: 442–5.

(14) Bloomfield A, Boon NA. A century of cardiac pacing. *Br Med J* 1989; **298**: 343–4.

(15) MacWilliam JA. Electrical stimulation of the heart in man. *Br Med J* 1889; **1**: 348–50.

(16) Ogston A. Notes on the administration of ether by the perhalation method. *Br J Anaesth* 1924; **2**: 76–82.

(17) Thomas KB. *The development of anaesthetic apparatus*. Oxford: Blackwell, 1975: 256–7.

(18) Tunstall ME. Obstetric analgesia: The use of a fixed nitrous oxide and oxygen mixture from one cylinder. *Lancet* 1961; **2**: 964.

(19) Tunstall ME. Effect of cooling on premixed gas mixtures for obstetric analgesia. *Br Med J* 1963; **2**: 915–7.

(20) Tunstall ME. Failed intubation drill. *Anaesthesia* 1976; **31**: 850.

(21) Tunstall ME. Detecting wakefulness during general anaesthesia for caesarian section. *Br Med J* 1977; **1**: 1321.

(22) Tunstall ME, Cater JI, Thomson JS and Mitchell RG. Ventilating the lungs of newborn infants for prolonged periods. *Arch Dis Child* 1968; **43**: 486–97.

(23) Tunstall ME, Ross JAS. Isoflurane, nitrous oxide and oxygen analgesic mixtures. *Anaesthesia* 1993; **48**: 919.

APPARATUS, AGENTS AND TECHNIQUES

The development of the syringe

TB Boulton

Original presentation St Bartholomew's Hospital, London 1987

All modern medical disciplines employ the syringe for one or more of its principal uses, aspiration, irrigation or administration of medication. Medical syringes today are of two types, those with compressed bulbs, which are mainly used for neurosurgical, wound and urological irrigation, and the familiar piston and barrel instruments, universally used in conjunction with the hollow needle for intravenous and parenteral medication. Animal bladders tied to metal pipes or feather shafts have certainly been used for the administration of enemas and for gynaecological and urological irrigation since the heyday of Greek medicine at the time of Hippocrates in the 5th century BC [1].

THE PNEUMATIC PRINCIPLE

The pneumatic principle of a piston running in a cylinder is said to have originated in the barber shops in the Greek colonial city of Alexandria, on the coast of Egypt, about 280 BC. Vetruvius, the Roman author and architect tells us that Ktesibios, the inventive son of the barber, used the device with a weight running in a tube to enable a mirror to be adjusted to any desired height. Ktesibios noted that the compression of the air both slowed the descent of the weights and caused a hissing sound as it escaped from the joints between the segments [1].

Ktesibios went on to use the pneumatic principle of the piston and tube in several devices, 'including a water pump for extinguishing fires'. This was the first known use of valves — so important to the specialty of anaesthesia today. He also built a water flute, or organ, and from this came the word 'hydraulics' to join 'pneumatics'. We do not know whether Ktesibios invented the first piston and barrel syringe, but one is described by Heron, also of Alexandria, about a century later. He cited this as an example of the application of pneumatics to surgery for the aspiration of pus from wounds; hence the Greek 'pyulkes' (the pus puller) later latinized to pyulcus [1].

There is little reference to the piston and barrel syringes during the Dark Ages. The early medical functions of the syringe, such as the administration of enemas, were usually carried out by the more easily constructed bladder and tube devices. By Tudor times, syringes re-emerged as much prized instruments of the surgical armamentarium [2,3].

Essays on the history of anaesthesia, edited by A Marshall Barr, Thomas B Boulton and David J Wilkinson. 1996: International Congress and Symposium Series No. 213, published by Royal Society of Medicine Press Limited.

THE SIXTEENTH AND SEVENTEENTH CENTURIES AD

Two small metal syringes were found in the surgeon's chest of Henry VIII's recently salvaged man-of-war, the *Mary Rose*, which sank in 1545. One is brass, and the other is pewter with a brass nozzle. Surgeon Vice Admiral Sir James Knott believes that the presence of such instruments at that time probably indicate that the surgeon of the *Mary Rose* was a Master Surgeon of the recently formed Barber Surgeons Company. He would have been temporarily recruited for the campaign on which the ship was about to set out. The works of Ambroise Paré suggests that besides the aspiration of pus, the syringes would be used for the irrigation of wounds, fistulae and of the urinary tract, and also in the treatment of bladder stones and of gonorrhoea which by that time had reached Europe from the New World [3].

Syringes had become standard ship surgeons' equipment by Stuart times. Woodall, in his famous book, urges cautious use of the syringe for irrigation with mercury sublimate for the treatment of gonorrhoea and the need for great cleanliness in the use of the instrument [4]. Sir Christoper Wren and Sir Robert Boyle used a syringe made of a dog's bladder and a goose quill to inject both wine and opium into the veins of dogs in 1656 [5,6]. They were not the first to experiment in this way, the Austrian, Lausitz, predated them. Major, Professor of Medicine at Kiel, was probably the first to make a deliberate intravenous administration of opium to man in 1662, followed by another German, Johann Sigmund Elsholtz, in 1665 [5]. They were ahead of their time.

The world had to wait until 1872, 30 years after inhalation anaesthesia had been introduced, for Pierre-Cyprien Oré of Bordeaux, to inject chloral intravenously, for the treatment of tetanus and for the induction of anaesthesia [7]. By this time the familiar piston and barrel syringe was already well established for intramuscular and subcutaneous injection [8].

EARLY BLOOD TRANSFUSION

James Blundell, Professor of Physiology and of Obstetrics at the Southwark United Hospitals of St Thomas' and Guy's, used a glass-barrelled syringe with a metal piston and an intravenous cannula to withdraw blood from a donor and inject it into a recipient in his pioneer blood transfusions of 1818. He later incorporated a barrel and piston syringe and valves into his 'blood impellor' which he described in 1824 [9].

SUBCUTANEOUS MEDICATION

The danger of absorption of centrally acting poisons from snake bites and remote soft tissue wounds had been known from time immemorial. Did not Achilles die from the central effects of a poison arrow in his vulnerable heel? Interest in administration through the skin developed at the beginning of the 19th century, in parallel with the chemical preparation of various alkaloids, including morphia. Vesicants, such as cantharides, which denuded the epidermis, were first used and then barbs and lancets. Sir Robert Christison recommended a phial of cyanide fixed to a harpoon to kill whales; history does not relate whether this was actually done. Lafargue of Paris reported in 1838 on the effects of inoculating morphia subcutaneously using a vaccination lance dipped in powdered morphine paste mixed with a little water [6,8,10].

The first use of the syringe for subcutaneous medication was probably by two New York physicians, Taylor and Washington. They were reported to have made an incision and used a syringe and blunt lacrimal duct cannula to administer subcutaneous morphine in 1839 [6]. In 1845, Dr Rynd of Dublin used an eye dropper and an elaborate spring-loaded trochar and cannula to introduce morphia mixed with creosote subcutaneously. He placed this in the vicinity of the branches of the trigeminal nerve in an effort to treat neuralgia. Rynd's retrospective description of this use of his trochar and cannula led to him being erroneously credited with the invention of the piston syringe and hollow needle for hypodermic medications [6,8,11].

MR FERGUSON AND DR ALEXANDER WOOD IN 1853

Metal syringes are listed intermittently in early 19th century catalogues and later on, glass and metal instruments were offered for various purposes including syringing the lacrimal duct. However, we are concerned with a certain glass syringe which the Edinburgh physician, Dr Alexander Wood, described as 'one of the elegant little syringes constructed by Mr Ferguson of Giltspur Street, London'. This was designed for injecting acid solutions of perchloride of iron through a hollow needle to sclerose naevae. It was Dr Wood who was inspired to use this syringe, with its hollow needle, to inject morphia subcutaneously in 1853, making parenteral medication a practical and universally applicable technique [10].

No catalogue picture of Mr Ferguson's elegant little syringe survives, however a broken syringe said to have been used by Wood is preserved at the Royal College of Surgeons of Edinburgh. This, from Wood's description, could well be the original. The syringe is not graduated, it has a glass barrel and a glass piston which is wrapped around with cottonwool to give it a better fit. It has a metal cone with a male screw for mounting a hollow needle which has not survived [6,8].

Wood's original purpose in injecting morphine through the skin into the tissues was to place the drug in the vicinity of the nerves responsible for chronic neuralgia — he was aiming at local anaesthesia. He published his successful results of nine cases in 1855 in the *Edinburgh Medical and Surgical Journal* [10]. His paper was well received locally and a coterie of enthusiastic practitioners of the new technique of subcutaneous injection was rapidly established in Edinburgh. This group included James Young Simpson who, besides introducing chloroform as an inhalation anaesthetic, had also experimented with the topical application of chloroform in an attempt to produce local anaesthesia. Several eminent visitors, notably Bertrand from Germany and Fordyce-Barker from the USA, were also initiated into the technique [6].

It was Wood's second paper in the *British Medical Journal* in 1858, which triggered world-wide acceptance of subcutaneous medication [12]. Wood, like Lafargue, Rynd and others, was interested initially in the local effects of the injected drugs. He was aiming at local anaesthesia of peripheral nerves. He was, however, well aware of the remote effects due to the absorption of morphia from the cellular tissues into the blood stream, and his papers reveal a detailed knowledge of work done by Magendi, Brodie, Christison and others on this subject. Wood seemed at first to have regarded such central actions as tiresome side effects. He records, for example, that he was, as he put it, 'a little annoyed' to find that his first patient, an old woman suffering from cervical brachial neuralgia, was still sleeping 12 hours after the subcutaneous injection of what he calculated to have been 25 mg morphine [10,12]!

After the publication of Wood's second paper in 1858 [12], Charles Hunter, house surgeon at St George's Hospital, London, was rapidly in print [13]. He wrote at first in support of Wood's local injections but then, 2 weeks later, correctly stressed the overriding importance of the central action of the injection of morphine [14]. Hunter coined the word 'hypodermic' in contrast to Wood's 'subcutaneous' and claimed priority for a different technique [15]. Wood, at least partially, accepted Hunter's hypothesis of the primary importance of central action, but pointed out that he had already considered the possibility in his article [10,16]. A most unseemly and wordy public argument over priority ensued between Wood and Hunter, with Ryan and others, including Claude Bernard himself, claiming priority [6,8,14,16]. It is of interest that Wood never corrected the printer's error in his second paper in 1858, in which the date of his first subcutaneous injection is given as 1843 instead of 1853 [12]. Whether this was an oversight, or intentional, we do not know, but such a date would have given him undisputed priority over everybody else. The controversy of local over central action persisted for many years. As late as 1895 the eminent pharmacologist, Karl Binz, advised injection as close as possible to the site of the pain [6].

Many texts attribute the invention of the syringe and hollow needle and the introduction of subcutaneous medication to Charles Gabriel Pravaz of Lyon, and there is a statue of him with an inscription to that effect in that city. This is untrue and, to do him justice, Pravaz never made any such claim [6,8]. He was interested in the possibility of coagulation of blood in arterial aneurysms by the injection of perchloride mercury. He conducted experiments in sheep using a silver syringe screwed to a cannula, which was first introduced into an artery with the aid of a trocar [17]. The confusion may have arisen because Behier, another Frenchman, reported the use of the same equipment for subcutaneous medication with acknowledgements to Pravaz in 1859, the year after the publication of Wood's second paper [18]. The syringe used by Pravaz and Behier had a screw mechanism for advancing the plunger [6], which was cumbersome but useful in estimating dosage when the barrel was made of opaque metal. It is of less practical value when the plunger is visible through glass. Hunter used a similar mechanism in the syringe which he devised, perhaps in an effort to emphasize that his technique was different from Wood's.

Wood continued to use the simple sliding piston and he and the instrument makers made many improvements including adding graduations and reducing the size of the needle. These syringes were widely advertised as the subcutaneous technique increased in popularity [6,8,12].

LUER AND RECORD FITTINGS

The push fitting for the needle was introduced by Luer of Paris in 1869, and a similar but smaller Record fitting by a Berlin instrument maker in 1906 [6].

Older anaesthetists will remember the confusion which the existence of these two sizes caused right up to the 1960s when disposables with the standard Luer mounts were introduced. Adaptors were much prized and often lost. There were few more frustrating experiences than, when having successfully obtained cerebrospinal fluid, finding that the syringe did not fit the needle and that no adaptor was available.

LOCAL ANAESTHESIA

Koller introduced reversible pharmacological anaesthesia by the topical application of cocaine to the eye in 1884, but its rapid exploitation by injection by Halsted and others in the same year depended on the syringe and hollow needle, and, incidentally brought with it the scourge of syringe-drug abuse [19]. It is an interesting coincidence that Alexander Wood died in 1884, the same year as a drug capable of producing local analgesia was introduced, the effect he was originally attempting to obtain [8].

INTRAVENOUS ANAESTHESIA

The German Johann Sigismund Elsholtz injected a solution of opium intravenously to produce unconsciousness in man in 1665, and Pierre-Cyprien Oré of Lyons, France used a piston and barrel syringe to induce anaesthesia by injecting chloral hydrate intravenously in 1872.

Intravenous anaesthesia was slow to develop, however, chiefly because no very suitable agents were discovered until the barbiturates became available in the 1920s [20].

ANTISEPSIS AND ASEPSIS

It is difficult to appreciate that subcutaneous medication predated Lister's antiseptic technique by a decade. References to local iatrogenic abscesses are surprisingly rare, and there does not seem to have been much hazard as long as a reasonable social cleanliness was employed [6].

A major revolution in the history of the syringe has occurred in the author's professional lifetime; when he was a student and a house surgeon in the 1940s, morphia injections were prepared by dissolving a tablet in a heated spoon while solutions of procaine were made by dropping tablets into boiling water [21]. Syringes were decontaminated with alcohol and those for spinal anaesthesia were sterilized by boiling. The battles, first for the establishment of sterile syringe services, and then for the introduction of disposable syringes, are early examples of the unfortunate struggles which professionals have had with administrators and politicians since the establishment of the National Health Service.

MECHANICAL SYRINGES

Finally, mechanically operated syringes were introduced. The 1947 *Pye's Surgical Handicraft* illustrates one which was designed for the continuous injection of penicillin [21] and they are now, of course, familiar pieces of equipment in the intensive care unit, in the operating theatre and for pain control.

CONCLUSION

This paper has covered 23 centuries and mentioned a number of characters in the history of the development of the syringe and its uses. Nobody knows exactly who invented the piston and barrel syringe, nor who joined it to the hollow needle, but anaesthetists should surely pay tribute to Dr Alexander Wood of Edinburgh for his new use for Mr Ferguson's 'elegant little syringe' which was produced in the street adjacent to St Bartholomew's Hospital, and which led to parenteral medication, intravenous general anaesthesia and to local anaesthesia [10].

REFERENCES

(1) Majno G. *The healing hand. Man and wound in the ancient world.* Cambridge, Massachusetts: Harvard University Press, 1975.
(2) Rule M. *The Mary Rose. The excavation and raising of Henry VIII's flagship.* Leicester: Winward, 1983.
(3) Knott J. Surgeons of the Mary Rose. The practice of surgery in Tudor England. *The Mariner's Mirror* 1983; **69**: 3.
(4) Woodall J. *The surgions mate or treatise discovering the due contents of the surgion's chest.* London, 1617.
(5) Davidson MHA. *The evolution of anaesthesia.* Altringham: Sherratt, 1965.
(6) Howard-Jones M. A critical study of the origins and early development of hypodermic medication. *J History Med* 1947; **2**: 201.
(7) Oré PC. Des injections intraveneuses de chloral. *Bulletin de la Société de Chirugie de Bordeaux* 1872; **1**: 400.
(8) Boulton TB. Classical File. Alexander Wood, MD (1817–1884) and the use of the syringe and hollow needle for practical medication. *Survey Anesth* 1984; **28**: 346.
(9) Boulton TB. Classical File. James Blundell MD, FRCP, and the introduction of human blood to man. *Survey Anesth* 1986; **30**: 100.
(10) Wood A. New method of treating neuralgia by direct application of opiates to the painful points. *Edin Med Surg J* 1855; **82**: 265.
(11) Rynd F. Description of an instrument for the subcutaneous introduction of fluids in affections of the nerves. *Dublin Q J Med* 1861; **32**: 13.
(12) Wood A. Treatment of neuralgic pain by narcotic injections. *Br Med J* 1858: 721.
(13) Hunter C. On narcotic injections in neuralgia. *Medical Times Gazette* 1858; **2**: 457.
(14) Hunter C. Correspondence. *Medical Times Gazette* 1858; **2**: 457.
(15) Hunter C. Practical remarks on the hypodermical treatment of disease. *Lancet* 1863; **2**: 444.
(16) Wood A. Correspondence. *Medical Times Gazette* 1865; **1**: 639.
(17) Pravaz CG. Sur un nouveau moyen d'opeer la coagulation du sang dans les artères applicable à la guerison des aneurismes. *Compte rendu de l'Académie des sciences. Paris* 1853; **36**: 88.
(18) Behier LJ. Method endermique. Injections médicamenteuses souscutanées. *Bulletin général de thérapeutique médicale, chirurgicale, obstetricale pharmaceutique* 1859; **57**: 49.
(19) Boulton TB. Classical File. *Survey Anesth* 1984; **28**: 150.
(20) Dundee JW, Wyant GW. *Intravenous anaesthesia.* Edinburgh: Churchill Livingstone, 1974.
(21) Bailey H. *Pye's surgical handicraft.* 15th ed. Bristol: Wright, 1947.

The Alcock chloroform vaporizer—
The prototype discovered

D Zuck

Original presentation Croydon 1989

In 1988 I described the Alcock vaporizer [1], a production model of which was found in the Museum of the Academy of Medicine in Toronto. NH Alcock (1871–1913) was a lecturer in physiology at St Mary's Hospital Medical School, Paddington and had worked with AD Waller on animal experiments investigating death and morbidity associated with chloroform anaesthesia. His fully-developed 'new apparatus for chloroform anaesthesia' was described in 1908—a calibrated plenum vaporizer with a facility for temperature compensation [2]. A prototype of this device has now been discovered.

In the early 1980s the authorities at St Mary's Hospital deposited a collection of items that had been associated with Professor AD Waller in the store of the Science Museum, South Kensington. Among these were an example of his chloroform balance, some of the devices based on toy clockwork trains that he had used to transport film while recording the electrical activity of the heart, a Dubois anaesthetizing machine, presumably the one he described using during his research, and an apparatus made out of sheet copper to which no one was able to attach an identity or a purpose.

Dr Alan Sykes, a retired lecturer in physiology and an active historian, inspected the collection of Walleriana while researching the life of AD Waller. I had previously supplied Dr Sykes with photographs of the Alcock vaporizer found in Toronto, and he told me that he had seen something in the collection which bore a resemblance to the apparatus in my photographs, but was rather different. I visited the store, which is in the old Post Office Savings Bank Headquarters at Olympia, and was able to confirm that the apparatus was indeed a prototype of the Alcock vaporizer. It conforms to the original description published by Alcock: '. . . a circular copper vessel 5" in diameter and $4\frac{1}{2}$" deep which contains 150 cc chloroform. One and a quarter inches from the bottom is fixed a shelf, closed except for two oblong holes. Immediately above and touching this shelf is a movable circular plate pierced by two triangular holes. This can be rotated by a hollow central rod, so as to vary the size of the openings into the space below. Air supplied either from a small foot bellows or an electric blower, enters the chamber by a tube opposite one aperture, and leaves by another . . .' The prototype differs from the production model in being calibrated not in percentages of chloroform, but arbitrarily from one to ten, and in not having a water jacket together with a thermometer in the central rod, to

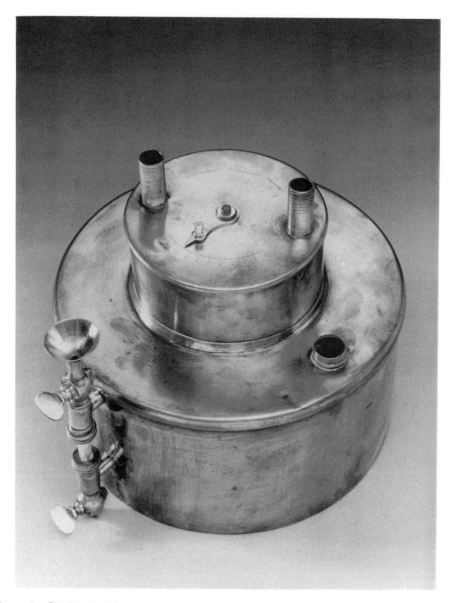

Figure 1 *Caption opposite*

allow for temperature compensation. Otherwise it corresponds exactly to the description, and even has the name of the manufacturer, CF Palmer, stamped on the top. The photographs show the structure of the vaporizing chamber and controls.

ACKNOWLEDGEMENTS

I am indebted to Dr Alan Sykes, to Mr Tim Boon of the Science Museum, and to the Science Museum Photographic Department.

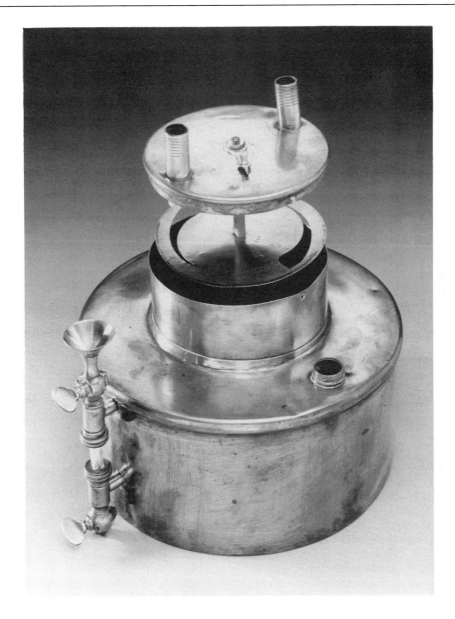

Figures 1 and 2   *Prototype Alcock vaporizer in the Science Museum store*

REFERENCES

(1) Zuck D. The Alcock chloroform vaporizer. *Anaesthesia* 1988; **43**: 972–80.
(2) Alcock NH. A new apparatus for chloroform anaesthesia. *Br Med J* 1908; **ii**: 372–3.

The etherometer, or 'how to use the Phillips ether vaporizer'

C Foster

Original presentation London 1987

Bryn Thomas has an illustration of the Phillips Automatic Ether Vaporizer circa 1925 in his book (Fig. 1). Hugh Richard Phillips, MD Edinburgh (1874–1932) was chloroformist to the Italian Hospital in London from 1902, and on the staff of the hospital until 1931. He also worked at Great Ormond Street Hospital for Sick Children for 10 years [1].

His ether vaporizing bottle of brown glass marked 'Wellcome Chem Works' has a neck fitted with an elaborate metal collar into which screws a cap and dip tube. An inlet tube with a ball valve permits pressure from a hand bulb or oxygen cylinder to pass into the bottle via a tiny passage. Ether liquid is thus forced up the dip tube, the upper end of which is occluded by a metal pin fixed to an upper collar. If this is rotated on its screw thread, space is made for the liquid to pass through two small holes in the pin, up a curved hollow tube under a glass dome. On being released from this tube the ether presumably vaporizes and passes again through minute passages onwards to the patient. A description of this piece ends: 'The "automatic element" was no doubt given since it would be possible by rotating the upper collar, automatically to control within small limits the amount of ether liquid to be vaporised. However, it has proved impossible to make the apparatus perform in this way. Liquid ether appears at the outlet tube!'

On glancing through old books, looking for pictures of apparatus, I discovered a picture in Blomfield's book [2] on anaesthesia with text which says 'The etherometer is a useful contrivance for supplying ether by drops in an automatic manner. When pressure within the bottle has been worked up by the handpump, the anaesthetist has merely to regulate the rate of flow of the drops by turning the screw top of the bottle.' Thus, this apparatus was designed to deliver liquid ether to the mask to be vaporized.

The measurement of the flow rate of ether was useful, rather than just having a bottle and dropping it on. It also freed one hand, an innovation which Magill used in his second endotracheal apparatus of 1927, and, again, in 1932. Bryn Thomas's book notes that 'This piece is something of an oddity because it appears to have been an attempt to copy the vaporisers of Magill — see No. 43, P. 194 in which the glass dome method was also used'. In fact, this is not true — Magill's 1921 endotracheal apparatus does not have the glass dome. This was added by him to improve the apparatus so that the rate of drops of the ether 'can be easily seen from any angle' [3].

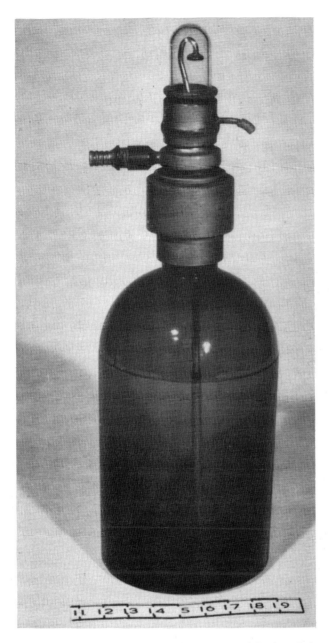

Figure 1 *Phillips etherometer. Reproduced by kind permission of the Association of Anaesthetists of Great Britain and Ireland*

REFERENCES

(1) Thomas KB. The development of anaesthetic apparatus. Oxford: Blackwell Scientific Publications, 1975: 197–8.
(2) Blomfield J. *Anaesthetics in practice and theory. A textbook for practitioners and students.* London: William Heinmann, 1922.
(3) Magill IW. Improved anaesthetic apparatus. *Lancet* 1927; **ii**: 396.

The anaesthetist's table

KA Stewart

Original presentation Leicester 1988

Anaesthetic rooms are a relatively recent development. There were few before the introduction of the National Health Service in 1948 (the use of small anterooms for induction is recorded in two hospitals in the 19th century [1,2]). They only became a standard feature of theatre suites in the UK during the 1960s. Indeed they are not yet universal. Throughout the world many suites are built without anaesthetic rooms — to save money, to save space, to avoid reduplicating equipment, and more recently to avoid moving the anaesthetized patient and compromising the continuity of monitoring by multiple electronic devices. A trend is developing towards an earlier simplicity — but without the same simplicity of equipment.

Prior to the introduction of anaesthetic rooms, patients were transferred conscious from a trolley in the theatre and anaesthetized on the operating table. The anaesthetist's table was a standard piece of equipment. It was made of tubular enamelled metal and was some three feet high and about 18 inches square with a galleried top. There were usually two removable plate-glass shelves and occasionally a drawer beneath the bottom shelf. The whole table was mounted on castors.

WHAT DID THE TABLE HOLD?

Surprisingly, anaesthetic books of the time give little indication of how the anaesthetist's table was furnished. For example, in the 1911 edition of Boyle's *Practical Anaesthetics* [3] the table was not mentioned. However, as always, our surgical colleagues were glad to instruct. Alexander Miles, an Edinburgh surgeon, published a book on surgical ward work and nursing which also issued advice on all aspects of theatre procedures and techniques [4]. In the 1899 edition of 280 pages he devoted a complete chapter to the anaesthetist's table. Admittedly the chapter was only two pages long, but it does provide interesting details of contemporary furnishings, and a list of items which should appear and be readily available: two bottles of chloroform and two bottles of ether (presumably a backup for each in case a bottle ran out or was dropped), alcohol for mixing with ether, a dropper bottle, a folded towel, a Schimmelbusch-type mask, an ether inhaler — either a Clover or a Junkers — a small bottle of Vaseline to protect the face from the effects of volatile liquids, tongue forceps, clean towel, small basin, a hypodermic syringe charged with ether, several more syringes, a bottle of eucalyptus oil for sterilizing the syringes, two glasses — presumably for measuring — a strong solution of ammonia (presumably equivalent to smelling salts), capsules of amyl nitrate, and very strong cocaine solutions for local anaesthesia by injection.

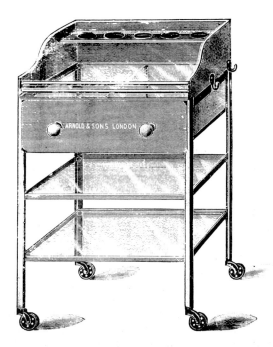

Figure 1   *Anaesthetist's table, from Arnold & Sons 1904 catalogue*

Anaesthetists brought up in the pre disposable syringe era will appreciate the author's comment on hypodermic syringes — 'There should always be several of these on the table; it is quite exceptional to find a hospital syringe fit for use' — a poignant reminder of the difficulties in matching barrels and plungers, and the constant mix-ups that occurred between Record and Luer fittings. Miles described two uses for the syringe: one, to inject morphine and atropine before the operation, which was supposed to make the rapid administration of chloroform safer by diminishing the sickness, and secondly to inject ether subcutaneously, should the patient feel pain, or the heart's action become feeble. The sterilization of the syringes is also worthy of notice. Eucalyptus oil diluted with olive oil in a ratio of 1:6 was said to be a fairly reliable antiseptic and less irritating than carbolic.

FORTY YEARS ON

Some 40 years later another surgeon, Harold Burrows, in the 1939 edition of his book on surgical instruments and appliances [5], again described the anaesthetist's table and astonishingly little had changed. The table itself was exactly as before, except it now had a drawer at the top, and the addition of an earth chain. The list of items recommended to be placed on the table looks extremely familiar — Junkers' inhaler, a 'nasotracheal inhaler', ethyl chloride, a bottle of anaesthetic ether, bottles of chloroform, a measuring glass, a mask for administering alcohol, chloroform, ether (ACE) mixture, chloroform drop bottles as before, another dropper for ether, gauze and lint of special size, tongue forceps, throat swabs, hypodermic syringe tested beforehand, tablets of morphine, atropine, strychnine

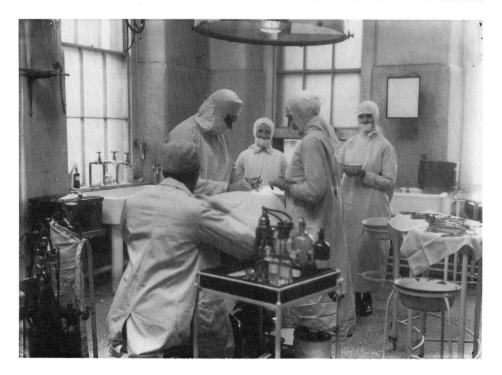

Figure 2 *Operating theatre, Royal Berkshire Hospital, about 1928, courtesy Photography Department, Royal Berkshire Hospital*

and ergotine, ampoules of pituitrin, capsules of amyl nitrate and coramine, clean towel, receiver, Vaseline, stomach tube. . . . Of the 20 items recommended, 14 were on the 1899 list. We certainly cannot claim a rapid advance in the agents and equipment for the anaesthetist. The injection of ether subcutaneously is no longer mentioned. New arrivals include ethyl chloride, Coramine as an all-purpose analeptic, and a stomach tube. The outstanding omissions to the later list appear to be apparatus for suction and for airway control. The importance of suction did not occur to most anaesthetists until the enquiry some 12 years later by the Association of Anaesthetists into deaths under anaesthesia, which showed regurgitation and vomiting to be the most common contributory cause [6]. Airways, however, and Magill's laryngoscope and endotracheal tubes were well in use by 1939 and had been in all the surgical instrument catalogues for years. The 'nasotracheal inhaler' was probably for pharyngeal insufflation. The author was somewhat out of date, but corrected the omissions in his 1941 edition which includes 'a set of airways' and 'Magill's tube and introducer'.

The next forty years saw the gradual demise of the anaesthetic table. By 1979, 80 years after Miles' early description, the anaesthetist's table had disappeared, to be replaced by superior 'furnished accommodation'. With the improved status of the anaesthetist, the lowly table which served the profession for so long has been forgotten. The anaesthetist of today, surrounded by complex machines and state-of-the-art equipment, might say, with varying degrees of enthusiasm: 'My table thou hast furnished, . . . and my cup overflows'.

REFERENCES

(1) Anon (quoting correspondence from CS Tomes). The administration of ether in America. *Br Med J* 1873; **1**: 297.
(2) Reports of medical and surgical practice in the hospitals and asylums of Great Britain. Chloroform and ether as anaesthetics. *Br Med J* 1876; **1**: 12–13.
(3) Boyle HEG. *Practical anaesthetics*, 2nd ed. London: Hodder & Stoughton, 1911.
(4) Miles A. *Surgical ward work and nursing*, 2nd ed. London: The Scientific Press, 1899.
(5) Burrows H. *Surgical instruments and appliances used in operations*, 10th ed. London: Faber & Faber, 1939.
(6) Association of Anaesthetists committee report. Deaths associated with anaesthesia. Report on 400 cases. *Anaesthesia* 1952; **7**: 200–5.

Developments in thermoplastic tracheal tubes

CA Russell

Original presentation Leicester 1988

Intubation has a recorded history back to Egyptian times. In 1543 Vesalius passed a reed or cane into the trachea of a pregnant pig. In 1871 Trendelenberg [1] was well ahead of his time using a tracheostomy tube with an inflatable cuff made from thin sheets of natural rubber. The air line even incorporated a rubber balloon to indicate cuff inflation.

A milestone was Macewen's device of 1880, introducing a 3/8" brass tube via the mouth [2]. Outstanding among German workers was Franz Kuhn, who in 1902 devised an endotracheal tube of metal strap coiled to form an airtight flexible cylinder which fitted the glottis. His tube allowed the passage of a small aspirating catheter — the first recorded use of the technique.

In 1910 the work of Elsberg and colleagues marked the beginning of anaesthesia by endotracheal insufflation. Rowbotham and Magill [3] in 1917 used narrow gum elastic tubes, one to insufflate with ether/air, the other to carry away the expired gases. By 1928 Magill was using a single, wide bore, uncuffed red rubber tube [4]. Insufflation died promptly, and Magill's technique is still in use today. The inflatable cuff descibed by Dorrance in 1910 was reintroduced by Guedel and Waters, who slid the cuff onto the tube prior to use [5].

WAR-TIME DEVELOPMENTS — PORTEX LTD

Dr Sydney Leader, a dental surgeon at the Dental Hospital, London, set up a company based in his flat in Great Portland Street in 1940. He called the company Portland Plastics Ltd, renamed Portex Ltd in 1967.

This Austrian-born entrepreneur with degrees in both medicine and dentistry, was marketing artificial eyes and teeth. He was desperately searching for materials to replace ceramics and glass which were in short supply because of the war. Plastic materials were known before World War II, but the war was the catalyst for development of the modern-day plastics industry. Polyvinyl chloride (PVC), polyethylene and acrylic were produced as substitutes for natural materials like rubber, gutta percha and shellacs which were all difficult to obtain. Dr Leader was in the right place at the right time to experiment with these new materials for dentures, artificial eyes and flexible dental tubing.

In the summer of 1943, Leader visited Major Thornton, a Royal Army Medical Corps anaesthetist at Basingstoke General Hospital which had a wartime plastic and maxillo-facial surgical unit. Their discussions resulted in the use of PVC as a substitute for rubber in making tracheal tubes. The first clinical trial was published in 1944 [6], followed by Major RA Gordon's paper in 1945 [7], reporting the results of his use of the new tubes with the Royal Canadian Medical Corps, also at Basingstoke.

The tubing was supplied in various sizes, the 7 mm–9 mm being popular as satisfactory for the average adult male. It was presented in coils of 10″ diameter, which interestingly corresponds almost exactly to our current 140 mm Magill radius of curvature — today's international standard. It is worthy of comment that the British Standard for Magill tracheal tubes was only published in 1986, almost 60 years after their invention.

At first, Portland Plastics through M&IE Ltd simply supplied lengths of tubing, and the anaesthetist had to prepare a tube by cutting off the desired length, fashioning a bevel with scissors, smoothing the tip with a hot spatula and polishing with a chloroform-soaked cloth. Gordon noted,'The rubber Magill tube is not ideal; it kinks in the nasopharynx and movement of the head and neck will obstruct it. It also deteriorates rapidly on sterilization. The PVC tube, however, remains patent when acutely flexed; this is more marked at body temperatures since the tubing becomes softer and more malleable as the temperature rises.' Thornton had also observed that the thermoplastic PVC tubes, after withdrawal from the patient, remained moulded to the form it had taken in the respiratory tract. This has been one of the major advances of the PVC tube, which softens and moulds to the patient's anatomy, without exerting undue pressure on the larynx.

Developments of the tube have shown many other advantages. PVC cuffs expand uniformly, without the herniation of latex rubber; medical grade PVC is non-toxic, now passing stringent implantation tests, while natural rubber tubes release toxic and irritant substances, leading to reactions of varying severity. On-site formulation and processing had major advantages, and Portex today still manufactures its own PVC compounds. PVC is the largest tonnage plastic material in the world, so costs are low. It can be moulded and extruded to very high accuracy and tolerances, unlike rubber which swells to several times the cross-sectional area of the die. Natural rubber tubes could never be produced at low enough prices for them to be considered for single use. PVC tubes are disposable, and the hazards of cross-infection together with costs of recycling provide strong arguments for their use.

LONG-TERM INTUBATION

The qualities of PVC made long-term intubation feasible for the first time, and the work of Wally Guess [8] was important in this area. From the early 60s to the present day, development has concentrated on one of the most important components of tracheal tube design — the inflatable cuff. The first integral PVC cuff was introduced by Portex in 1964. It was essentially a copy of the rubber cuff. It was quite thick and when inflated resembled a rubber boot! By about 1973 its diameter had been increased and thickness reduced to obtain a more elastomeric cuff.

The basic design remains to this day as the 'standard' Portex cuff in the range of 'Blue-Line' endotracheal tube products. In the late 60s, however, anaesthetists were becoming concerned with injury to the trachea following prolonged intubation, and particularly over damage to the delicate ciliated epithelium lining the trachea. Lomholt introduced the concept of a high-volume, low-pressure cuff in 1967 [9]. Geffin and Pontopiddon in 1969 [10] pre-stretched the standard cuff in boiling water to give a larger diameter floppy cuff which was successful in reducing tracheal injury. The development of the high-volume, low-pressure cuff had begun. Products such as alternately inflated double cuffed tracheotomy tubes were no longer required. The Portex 'Softseal' square-shaped cuff became available in 1973.

TRACHEAL INJURY

In the 1970s, explanations were sought as to why tracheal damage was not eliminated by these bigger cuffs. The pressures inside the cuff applied to the tracheal wall were the key. Crawley and Cross [11] found that in high-pressure cuffs the pressure remained constant during the ventilation cycle, whereas with the high-volume, low-pressure cuffs there was cycling of the pressure with the distal end of the cuff being compressed by the ventilator pressure. Therefore it was not necessary to apply peak airway pressure into the cuff to maintain a seal, and the minimum pressure seal during the cycle would prevent aspiration. This understanding led us to the view that the front part of the square shaped cuff simply added to the bulk — a distinct disadvantage on intubation. A seal in the trachea depends upon the pressure at the seal point, not the length of the seal. Industrial lip seals/'O' rings are clear examples of the principle. Hence a large cuff in contact with the trachea does no more sealing than one of minimum length and is bound to cause damage in proportion to the area of contact. These arguments resulted in the pear-shaped 'Profile' cuff introduced in 1976. Originally this was assembled on to the tube the opposite way, but it was turned around so that the slope of the cuff would ease intubation. In 1977, Nordin [12] demonstrated in rabbits that an intra-cuff pressure above 40 cm water restricted blood flow in mucosal capillaries, leading to necrosis and stenosis [12]. More recent work [13,14] has reduced this critical level which must not be exceeded, to 30 cm water.

The final study which helped to explain the different mechanisms of sealing between high and low pressure cuffs, was Mackenzie's work in the 80s on dimensions of the human trachea [15–17]. Low-volume, high-pressure cuffs inflate as a highly stretched spheroid. They seal by distorting the trachea to the same circular shape. The modern cuffs have sufficient circumference to totally fill the lumen without distending the trachea. The cuff seals when its pressure is sufficient to prevent gas forcing its way past the contact area. Because the cuff is not stretched, the pressure within the cuff is identical to pressure exerted on the tracheal wall. Also, more importantly, the pressure can be measured and monitored. These data allow cuff diameters to be optimized. Excessively large diameter cuffs cause creases and folds on sealing, which act as pathways for fluid aspiration, and require extra pressure to compress the folds and achieve a seal. Mehta showed that the intra-cuff pressure should exceed the hydrostatic pressure that can be generated by a column of liquid collecting above the cuff [13].

TUBES OF THE FUTURE

It is interesting to consider why anaesthetists should require such a large number of sizes of tracheal tubes [18]. It is clear that in an adult, the cuff diameter, and hence circumference, is the most important dimension. The ideal tube size is the compromise between being large enough for adequate ventilation, and small enough to prevent laryngeal damage by pressure on the tissues. It has been suggested that only two tubes are required for use in adults, a 7.5 mm for females and 8.5 mm for males. With optimally dimensioned 'Profile' cuffs, these should be suitable for 99% of the population. Perhaps in a few years time, the anaesthetist will simply ask for a male or female tube, possibly coloured blue for male, pink for female!

REFERENCES

(1) Trendelenberg F. Beitrage zuden Operationen on der Luftwegen. *Arch Klinische Chirurgie* 1871; **12**: 112.
(2) Macewen W. Clinical observations on the introduction of tracheal tubes by the mouth instead of performing tracheostomy. *Br Med J* 1880; **2**: 122–144, 163–165.
(3) Rowbotham ES, Magill IW. Anaesthetics in the plastic surgery of the face and jaws. *Proc Royal Soc Med* 1921; **14**: 17–27.
(4) Magill IW. Endotracheal anaesthesia. *Proc Royal Soc Med* 1928; **22**: 83–88.
(5) Guedel AE, Waters RM. A new intratracheal catheter. *Current Researches in Anesthesia and Analgesia* 1928; **7**: 238.
(6) Thornton HL. Vinyl 'Portex' tubing. *Br Med J* 1944; **2**: 14.
(7) Gordon RA, Ainslie EH. Experience with vinyl-plastic endotracheal tubes. *Anesthesiology* 1945; **6**: 359–61.
(8) Guess W. Safety evaluation of medical plastics. *Clin Toxicol* 1978; **12**: 77–95.
(9) Lomholt N. A new tracheostomy tube cuff with controlled pressure on the tracheal mucous membrane. *Acta Anaesth Scand* 1967; **11**: 311.
(10) Geffin B, Pontopiddan MD. Reduction of tracheal damage by the pre-stretching of inflatable cuffs. *Anesthesiology* 1969; **31**: 462.
(11) Crawley BE, Cross DE. Tracheal cuffs — a review and dynamic pressure study. *Br J Anaesth* 1975; **30**: 4.
(12) Nordin U, Lindholm CE, Wolgas TM. Blood flow in the rabbit tracheal mucosa under normal conditions and under the influence of tracheal intubation. *Acta Anaesth Scand* 1977; **21**: 81.
(13) Mehta S. Safe lateral wall pressure to prevent aspiration. *Ann Royal Coll Surg Eng* 1984; **66**: 426–7.
(14) Seegobin RD, Van Hussett GL. Endotracheal cuff pressure and tracheal mucosal flow; endoscopic study of effects of four large volume cuffs. *Br Med J* 1984; **288**: 965–8.
(15) Mackenzie CF, Shin B, Whitley N, Helrich M. Human tracheal circumference as an indicator of correct cuff size. *Anesthesiology* 1980; **53**: ASA Abstract S414.
(16) Mackenzie CF. The relationship of human tracheal size to body habitus. *Anesthesiology* 1979; **51**: ASA Abstract S378.
(17) Mackenzie CF, Hallisey J, Clark D, Steinberg S, Helrich M. Adult tracheal and laryngeal dimensions as an indication for correct tracheal tube use. *Anesthesiology* 1982; **57**: 500.
(18) Chandler M, Crawley BE. Rationalization of the selection of tracheal tubes. *Br J Anaesth* 1986; **58**: 111–16.

The history of extracorporeal circulation

KG Lee

Original presentation Southend 1988

Prior to the 1950s, cardiac surgery was limited to closed procedures and operations outside the heart, including ingenious attempts at revascularizing the ischaemic myocardium. This limitation was due to the inability to maintain a blood supply to the body on opening the heart. Open heart surgery using moderate hypothermia and temporary inflow occlusion was first performed successfully in 1952, but this only gave a modest increase in the time allowed for the surgery, and complex intracardiac surgery remained impossible. The advent of cardiopulmonary bypass, first used successfully in 1953, revolutionized the scope of cardiac surgery. Extracorporeal circulation is now used in many other fields, including neurosurgery, oncology and intensive therapy, but its origins go back much further than the early 1950s.

EARLY PHYSIOLOGISTS

The concept of artificial circulation and life support is as old as that of anaesthesia. European physiologists of the late 18th and early 19th centuries realized that the vital properties of organs could be temporarily restored after apparent death by allowing fresh blood to pass through them. The French physiologist Nysten injected gaseous oxygen into hearts quickly removed from guillotined criminals after execution in 1803, demonstrating some evidence of restoration of irritability in the myocardium. In 1811, he published the results of experiments in which he injected oxygen into the great veins of unanaesthetized dogs in an atmosphere of nitrogen; he was able to prolong their survival from 4 to 12 minutes [1]. Le Gallois experimented with perfusion and ventilation of decapitated rabbits using syringes, and in his book published in 1812 he was the first to mention the idea of artificial circulation [2]. He contended that life may be preserved in any part of an organism by external perfusion, despite it being separated from the rest of the body. Kay, in 1828, showed that the irritability of dying muscle could be temporarily restored by artificial perfusion while in 1849, Loebell was the first to attempt artificial perfusion of isolated kidneys.

The work of Brown-Sequard in the mid-19th century advanced the knowledge of artificial circulation considerably. He demonstrated the necessity of oxygenating the perfusing blood, by whipping it in air. By the same process of whipping and filtering the blood, he was able to render it incoagulable by defibrination, and show the desirability of anticoagulation in perfusion work. He successfully perfused various organs, producing some evidence of return of reflex activity after apparent death. These included mammalian heads, and even the limbs of freshly guillotined criminals at the stage of rigor mortis (for the latter he used his own artificial blood) [3]. The production of artificial perfusion apparatus for laboratory use began, as indeed did the legend of Frankenstein. (Mary Shelley wrote the novel in 1818).

In 1868, Ludwig and Schmidt described an apparatus for constant pressure infusion of arterialized blood into an isolated organ from a reservoir. Von Schroder reported improvements in oxygenation in 1882, including the bubbling of air through a bottle of venous blood; the first attempt at bubble oxygenation. In 1885, Von Frey and Gruber described the first apparatus to allow constant aeration of the blood without interruption of flow to the perfused organ; they used a thin film of blood exposed to gas on the inside of a slanted, rotating metal cylinder. This was the first apparatus to resemble the modern pump oxygenator in principle [4].

These early experiments suffered from many shortcomings. A large volume of blood was needed to prime the apparatus; this usually came from a large animal; a readily available and plentiful source. Blood from a horse or sheep might therefore be used to perfuse a dog or cat, and the experiment would then be severely affected by transfusion reaction. The trauma to the blood from mechanical handling, whipping and aeration was severe, it would have been devoid of clotting factors, and would have contained cell debris, free haemoglobin, denatured proteins and vasoactive compounds. Gaseous and particulate emboli would have been plentiful. At best these machines could only oxygenate a few hundred millilitres of blood per minute to some 90% saturation, making them suitable only for bench perfusion of isolated organs.

EARLY 20TH CENTURY ADVANCES

Around the turn of the century, attempts were made to improve on this apparatus. In 1895, Jacobj was the first to use an excised, ventilated animal lung as an oxygenator, and he showed good oxygenation with reduced damage to the blood. An apparatus designed by Brodie in 1903 required no additional blood for perfusion [5].

An alternative approach to laboratory perfusion work also used at the time was to make a heart-lung preparation of an animal with which to perfuse the excised organ. The organ would be placed in circuit between the aorta and vena cava of the preparation. This method was used by Frank and Starling, and was cheaper and more readily available than artificial apparatus. However it was subject to variability in performance. This led to greater understanding of cardiovascular physiology.

1920s TO 1950s

During this period, particularly after World War II, science and technology advanced steadily. New materials became available. Stainless steel was found to be more physicochemically inert than the copper and brass of the 19th century physiologists. Transparent plastics began to replace red rubber as a blood carrier. High quality glass was manufactured for the first time. Silicones were developed and found many uses in blood handling because of their inertness and unwettability. Their effect on the surface tension of liquids also made them ideal antifoaming substances, effectively dispersing gas bubbles in blood.

Heparin was discovered quite incidentally in 1916 by Jay McLean, then a student at Johns Hopkins Medical School, Baltimore. He was given a research project to study the properties of thromboplastic material extracted from animal brain tissue — coagulant phospholipid compounds known as cephalins. He went on to explore extracts of other tissues for similar substances, and unexpectedly found an extract of dog liver which had the opposite effect — preventing coagulation. He mentioned this finding in his results, but it was put to one side [6]. McLean gave it the name 'heparin' from its liver origin, and it was subsequently investigated by others in the USA. It was also found to be present in other organs, including the lungs. During the ensuing years it was purified, its bioassay was standardized and it was marketed for clinical use in 1935. Heparin gave, for the first time, predictable, self-limiting anticoagulation without damaging the blood, and the later development of protamine made it fully controllable.

Greater understanding of haematology, blood incompatibility, clotting mechanisms, physiology and pharmacology was acquired throughout this period. Parallel advances were also being made in the fields of surgery, anaesthesia and supportive care. Cardiac surgery was progressing rapidly, the operations of closure of the patent ductus arteriosus, correction of coarctation and the Blalock–Taussig shunt all being described between 1939 and 1945. The factor still preventing open heart surgery was the lack of a circulatory support apparatus for use in man.

THE ARTIFICIAL LUNG

Progress in the development of oxygenators before 1950 consisted mainly of improvements on the original 19th century ideas, incorporating 20th century technology. The excised animal lung still provided the standard for comparison. Since the physics of gas transfer across a liquid surface were not fully understood until the early 1960s, development of artifical oxygenators had to be empirical, done on a trial and error basis. Because of the difficulty in defoaming blood before the introduction of silicones in 1950, the most promising area for the researchers was in filming the blood, to increase the surface for gas exchange. Larger and more complex rotating cylinders were devised, but they were limited by the tendency to damage and foam blood. Rippling the blood over a stationary screen increased its surface area by causing turbulent flow, without foaming the blood, but a steady thickness or flow of blood was needed for useful oxygenation. Materials tried for the screen included silk, nylon, glass bulbs and stainless steel mesh. The use of rotating discs for spreading the blood originated with Hooker in 1915, but the first to devise a machine suitable for use in large animals was Bjork in Sweden in 1948. This principle was later used very successfully in humans, but has since been superseded. Other methods included the use of rotating spirals, screens and cones, and many other combinations and permutations of the above principles [7].

The use of silicones in the debubbling chamber made the bubble oxygenator safe, and it became universally accepted from 1955 onwards. Modern development of the semipermeable membrane oxygenator is in turn threatening the position of the bubble oxygenator.

THE ARTIFICIAL PUMP

Surprisingly, development of successful pumps lagged behind that of oxygenators. Early workers had first used constant flow perfusion from a reservoir, which had a limited duration. For longer perfusions, they used syringes and systems of non-return valves, and the syringes were later driven mechanically. The potential value of pulsatile flow was first recognized by Ludwig and Schmidt in 1868. This was achieved by Jacobj in 1890, by intermittent compression of a balloon placed in the circuit, on a 'bag-in-bottle' principle. Dale and Schuster designed a more modern version of this pump in 1928, which was repeatedly adapted and widely used until the 1950s [8]. Ingenious ideas included the adaptation of an Austin 7 engine to drive a four-cylinder blood pump of this type in 1933 [9]! The emphasis on pulsatile flow persisted until the 1950s, and probably discouraged the development of other types of pump; it then subsided only to be resurrected again in more recent years.

Other principles explored included the centrifugal pump and the Archimedean screw, but few of these ideas achieved any widespread application. Devices which used external compression of a flexible tube were of some value. The Sigmamotor pump utilized a row of metal fingers to sequentially compress a tube, driving blood along it; it was first used in 1949, and was very successful. The pump generally used now is the familiar roller pump. Its origin is difficult to pinpoint, since the basic design is old. Roller pumps were first used for handling blood in the 1920s, but De Bakey's description of a manually operated roller pump for rapid transfusion in 1934 is perhaps the most well known [10]. There have been many adaptations since the 1920s, but the roller pump was not incorporated into extracorporeal circulation apparatus until 1953. All the early bypass attempts in man (including the first success) used Dale and Schuster pumps.

Centrifugal pumps were never widely used, because of their tendency to damage the blood, but the recently introduced vortex pump is based on the same principle, of spinning a stream of blood into an orifice, creating pressure and flow. These new pumps are said to be less traumatic to blood than modern roller pumps.

EXTRACORPOREAL CIRCULATION IN MAN

The first worker to perfect a pump oxygenator which could be used to perfuse whole intact animals and feasibly humans, was the Russian, Brukhonenko. He described the 'Autojector', which used an excised animal lung for gas exchange in 1929, however this was not well known in the West. The credit for the idea of using artificial circulation as an adjunct to cardiothoracic surgery is given to John H Gibbon Jnr, a Philadelphia surgeon. Even so, it was not the prospect of open heart surgery that initiated his research.

In the early 1930s, Gibbon was dismayed at the appalling mortality of pulmonary embolectomy (Trendelenberg's operation) — an operation best described in those days as a 'premorbid autopsy', since it was never contemplated until the patient was near death and there had been only nine survivors out of the 142 operations reported. He worked in the laboratory on a means of artificially maintaining the circulation during temporary occlusion of the pulmonary artery in cats. He adapted the available apparatus, including a rotating cylinder film oxygenator and his own adaptation of the Dale and Schuster pump, and performed an autopsy on the cats after each experiment. He published his initial results in 1937 [11]. He later allowed the cats to survive, and began to see encouraging results. Meanwhile, heparin and dicoumarol became clinically available and were used to treat pulmonary embolism effectively, but Gibbon saw the potential for his technique in cardiac surgery. His work was interrupted by World War II, but he and others carried on the quest for human cardiopulmonary bypass after the war. Gibbon obtained engineering help from the International Business Machines Company (IBM), but was unable to make a rotating cylinder oxygenator large enough for human use. By changing to a vertical stainless steel screen oxygenator, he obtained immediate success in trials on larger animals between 1949 and 1952. Gibbon was not, however, the first to attempt bypass surgery in man.

Dennis and his co-workers had been working on a pump oxygenator in Minnesota, using a rotating screen disc oxygenator. They performed open heart surgery on a 6-year-old girl on April 5 1951. Unfortunately, on opening the heart she was found to have a common atrium—a much more serious problem than had been anticipated, and, although the bypass performed well, the surgery failed, and the patient died [12]. There were at least two other failures, including one by Gibbon, before the first successful bypass operation was performed, also by Gibbon in Philadelphia, on May 6 1953. The operation was the closure of an atrial septal defect on an 18-year-old girl, bypass time was 26 minutes, and the patient went on to live a normal life [13].

John H Gibbon was later nominated for a Nobel prize, but it was considered that his ideas were not sufficiently original to justify the award. Interestingly, successful pulmonary embolectomy using bypass was not reported until 1962!

OTHER APPROACHES

Cardiac surgery with bypass after 1953 still carried a very high mortality rate, and was not uniformly accepted. Gibbon was unable to reproduce his remarkable success in patients with more complex congenital ventricular defects. He became disillusioned and stopped using his bypass apparatus. Hypothermia with venous occlusion gave enough time to complete atrial septal defect repair and valvotomy, and was being increasingly used. Many researchers looked at other approaches to the problem of open heart surgery. Perfusion from a reservoir was limited in duration by the size of the reservoir, without refilling. Intravenous injection of gaseous oxygen or hydrogen peroxide (endogenous oxygenation) caused pulmonary gas embolism. Single pumps substituting for the right or left heart only were tried. The use of two separate pumps substituting for the two ventricles and the patient's own lungs for gas exchange (autogenous lung oxygenation) proved complex, but achieved some success. This was the basis of Drew's profound hypothermia technique [14]. The use of an animal lung for gas exchange (autologous lung oxygenation) continued, but this was limited in duration by the formation of interstitial oedema in the animal lung leading to oxygenation failure.

Andreasen and Watson, working in England, demonstrated in 1952 that life could be temporarily supported by a blood flow as low as 10% of the resting cardiac output, if directed primarily to the brain and kidneys. They obtained low flows in dogs by occluding the vena cava and allowing only azygos venous drainage into the heart [15]. Before that workers in extracorporeal circulation had concentrated on equalling the resting cardiac output. The azygos flow concept triggered new thinking and groups in England and the USA began to work with controlled cross circulation. This consisted of one animal providing a circulation for a second by vascular connections, with a flow control to prevent the donor from exsanguinating into the recipient. This principle was applied to humans by Lillehei in Minnesota in 1954, with remarkable success, leading to a number of cardiac surgery 'firsts', including the correction of Fallot's tetralogy and atrio-ventricular canal. He operated on children with congenital heart disease, using an anaesthetized, compatible parent as the circulatory donor [16]. The reason for the spectacular success of the technique probably lay in the donor's ability to correct any physiological derangement in the circulation during the procedure. This was not realized at the time, since understanding of the effects of acid/base and other physiological abnormalities was poor or non-existent. The technique was controversial, because of the risk to the normal donor. One critic described it as the first operation in history with the potential for 200% mortality. Cross-circulation fell into disrepute after the death of a donor. A safe, simple, disposable bubble oxygenator was introduced by De Wall in 1955.

REFINEMENTS

Total cardiopulmonary bypass gradually became accepted as the safest and most useful aid to open heart surgery. The refinements which followed ensured that bypass would supersede the other techniques. These included the perfection of the bubble oxygenator, the use of moderate hypothermia with bypass, the introduction of elective cardiac arrest ('cardioplegia') by Melrose at the Hammersmith Hospital in 1955, advances in sterilization and technology of plastics, and the development of a small, compact membrane oxygenator. Pulsatile flow is now readily available, thanks to the microprocessor, but its value and necessity are still being questioned.

CONCLUSION

Extracorporeal circulation is an old idea, but a new science in man. It developed by trial and error in a haphazard way, by many individuals working independently, trying to achieve rapid progress without a full understanding of the underlying physical and physiological principles involved. As a result, emphasis has been on the mechanical approach to artifical circulation, within the bounds of the available technology of the day, rather than on the physiological response to it.

Cardiopulmonary bypass is now used routinely to replace cardiopulmonary function for increasing periods of time, but the physiological insult caused by it has not changed in nature — merely in severity. Cardiopulmonary bypass still remains a crude physiological exercise, which cannot easily be continued for more than a matter of hours without detriment to the patient.

The principles of extracorporeal circulation are now finding new applications in medicine, and the technology of bypass is constantly progressing. Many of the older approaches are also being reappraised, such as partial left or right heart bypass for cardiac support, and autogenous lung oxygenation. There are many advances yet to come in the field of artificial circulation.

REFERENCES

(1) Nysten PH. *Recherches de physiologie et de chemie pathologique*. Paris: JA Brasson, 1811.
(2) Le Gallois JJC. *Expériences sur le principe de la vie*. Paris: D'Hautel, 1812.
(3) Brown-Sequard E. Recherches expérimentales sur les propriétés physiologiques et les usages du sang rouge et du sang noir et leures principaux elements gazeux, l'oxygene et l'acide carbonique. *J Physiol De l'Homme (Paris)* 1858; 1: 95–122, 353–67, 729–35.

(4) Von Frey M, Gruber M. Untersuchungen uber den stoffwechsel isolierter organe. Ein respiration-apparat für isolierte organe. *Arch F Anat W Physiol (Phys Abthy)* 1885; **9**: 519–32.

(5) Hewitt RL, Creech O. History of the pump oxygenator. *Arch Surg* 1966; **93**: 680–96.

(6) McLean I. The discovery of heparin. *Circulation* 1959; **19**: 75–134.

(7) Galletti PM, Brecher GA. *Heart-lung bypass. Principles and techniques of extracorporeal circulation.* New York: Grune and Stratton, 1962: 47–120.

(8) Dale HH, Schuster EHJ. A double perfusion pump. *J Physiol* 1928; **64**: 356–64.

(9) Daly I de B. A seven horse power Austin engine adapted as a blood pump. *J Physiol* 1933; **77**: 36–37P.

(10) De Bakey ME. A single continuous flow blood transfusion instrument. *New Orleans Med Surg J* 1934; **87**: 386–9.

(11) Gibbon JH Jnr. Artificial maintainance of circulation during experimental occlusion of the pulmonary artery. *Arch Surg* 1937; **34**: 1105–31.

(12) Dennis C, Spreng DS, Nelson GE, *et al.* Development of a pump oxygenator to replace the heart and lungs; an apparatus applicable to human patients, and application to one case. *Ann Surg* 1951; **134**: 709–21.

(13) Gibbon JH Jnr. The development of the heart-lung apparatus. *Rev Surg* 1970; **27**: 230–44.

(14) Drew CE, Cliffe P, Scurr CF, *et al.* Experimental approach to visual intracardiac surgery using an extracorporeal circulation. *Br Med J* 1957; **2**: 1323–9.

(15) Andreasen AT, Watson F. Experimental cardiovascular surgery. *Br J Surg* 1952; **39**: 548–51.

(16) Lillehei CW. A personalised history of extracorporeal circulation. In: Sketty KR, Parulkar GB, eds. *Proceedings of the World Conference on Open Heart Surgery*, Bombay 1985. New York: McGraw Hill, 1985.

Memories of early days of open heart surgery in the UK and India

Ruth E Mansfield

Original presentation Southend-on-Sea 1988

These memories are mainly from the Brompton Hospital in the UK where I was privileged to work with such pioneers as Brock, Tubbs and Cleland, and later, after 1969, from my time in India. Tribute must also be paid to my teachers in anaesthesia, the late Sir Ivan Magill for his endotracheal tube and many techniques, and to the late Michael Nosworthy [1] for controlled ventilation of the lungs. Both of these men helped to make thoracic, and later heart surgery safe.

In the 1950s moderate hypothermia of 28–30 °C was used, which gave up to 10 minutes cardiac arrest in open heart procedures, enough for a closure of an atrial septal defect (ASD) or pulmonary valvotomy. This was achieved by surface cooling or veno-venous cooling. For surface cooling, the patient was anaesthetized sufficiently to prevent shivering, usually with a sleep dose of 2.5% thiopentone given slowly, a relaxant and nitrous oxide mixture. Nasopharyngeal, oesophageal and rectal temperature probes and ECG leads were put in place. A large bath of water and ice was brought alongside the patient who, complete with IV drips and connected to the anaesthetic apparatus, was then immersed. To balance a Water's cannister on the side of the bath and hand ventilate, while vigorously massaging the patients' limbs to get even cooling, was quite a feat. Because of the after-drop in temperature of approximately 4 °C and with the risk of ventricular fibrillation, the patient was removed from the bath at a nasopharyngeal temperature of 32 °C, dried and placed on a warming/cooling blanket already on the operating table. At 28 °C the open heart surgery was begun, while warming was started by the warming blanket. However, if after the chest was closed the temperature was still under 36 °C, then the patient was placed in a warm bath.

It was little wonder that Brock favoured veno-venous cooling. He stated that 'Immersion was aesthetically and surgically unattractive.' Using the technique developed at Guy's by Ross in 1954–1956 [2], the chest was opened under normothermia and diagnosis confirmed. A cannula was inserted into the superior vena cava and another into the inferior vena cava. Hypothermia was achieved by hand-pumping the blood from the superior vena cava through a cooling coil and returning it at a temperature of 31 °C to the inferior vena cava. The advantages of this method over surface cooling were that cooling and rewarming were quicker, the temperature achieved was more controllable with an after-drop of only 2 °C, and if during the cooling resuscitation became necessary, it could be immediate as the chest was already open.

PROFOUND HYPOTHERMIA

Profound hypothermia of 15–12 °C gave up to 60 minutes operating time without brain damage. Tubbs used the Drew technique, developed at Westminster

Hospital by Drew, Keen and Benazon in 1959 [3] which used two pumps to take over the two ventricles during cooling. Blood from the right atrium was collected in a right reservoir and then pumped into the pulmonary artery through a cannula inserted through the infundibulum of the right ventricle. This blood passed through the lungs, which were ventilated with 30% N_2O in oxygen, to reach the left atrium. A left atrial drainage tube then carried this oxygenated blood to the left reservoir. It was then pumped from the left reservoir by the left pump into the heat exchanger. The cooled blood was returned to the patient via the femoral artery and clamps were applied when the heart stopped beating, usually at about 15 °C. After surgery the blood temperature could be raised by using the heat exchanger as a blood warmer. The heart was defibrillated at 30–32 °C and heparin was reversed once the patient was off-bypass.

Drugs and techniques for anaesthesia were similar for most cardiac surgical procedures at the time. During cooling at 28 °C, nitrous oxide could be turned off and 100% oxygen given for ventilation. Since carbon dioxide production falls in parallel with the reduced metabolic rate of hypothermia, 5% CO_2 was added to the mixture during the cooling process and 7% CO_2 when 15 °C was reached in order to keep a normal PCO_2, however during rewarming CO_2 was not added. At a temperature of 15–12 °C ventilation of the lungs was unnecessary. They were kept inflated with oxygen during the surgery on a quiet non-beating dry heart. On rewarming, above 30–32 °C it became necessary to administer anaesthetic drugs again. It was important to monitor nasopharyngeal, oesophageal and rectal temperatures, as the latter lagged behind.

The two major advantages of this technique were that fewer 'pump lungs' occurred when using the patient's lungs as the oxygenator, and coronary perfusion was not needed for operations on the aortic valve. The disadvantages of profound hypothermia were the need to cannulate both systemic and pulmonary circulations, the long perfusion times for cooling and rewarming, and the time limit of 60 minutes for aortic clamping.

THE DISC OXYGENATOR

The Melrose disc oxygenator was used at the Brompton Hospital in 1960 after its development at the Hammersmith Hospital [4]. Venous blood from the right heart was exposed to a gas mixture of 97% oxygen and 2.5% carbon dioxide in the disc oxygenator and returned via the femoral artery. The rotating steel discs of the oxygenator were difficult to clean and, of course, had to be sterilized between each use. It was usual to notify the blood bank of any expected cases as often ten units of fresh blood were required. The oxygenator was primed with blood depending on the body surface area. Bleeding during closure, and postoperatively, was a frequent complication. Calculation of loss was by swab weighing and measurement of drainage. With the Melrose technique, cardiac arrest was achieved with potassium at a normal temperature. The administration of anaesthetic intravenous drugs was necessary during the period of cardiac arrest since blood circulation through the patient was maintained by the pump throughout surgery. The lungs were kept in a state of inflation with oxygen, but not ventilated during the cardiac procedure. It was a pioneering method, sufficiently successful for Cleland's team of Melrose, Beard the anaesthetist and the theatre sister to be invited to Russia to demonstrate.

THE BUBBLE OXYGENATOR

Bubble oxygenators, such as the Rigg bag, Temprol and others with a heat exchanger incorporated in the circuit were developed. Entry of air into the circuit was minimal, while oxygen was bubbled through blood and Hartmann's solution in the bag. With haemodilution, it was found unnecessary to prime with so much blood. Indeed, it was possible to use clear prime depending on the patient's haematocrit, provided fresh acid-citrate-dextrose blood was available for possible haemorrhage. Blood loss was calculated from the central venous pressure, and blood could be infused into the patient from the oxygenator as necessary. Postoperatively, the patient was transferred to the intensive care unit (ICU), hand ventilated, tube in place, and put on a ventilator at least overnight and until the condition was stabilized and breathing adequate. A tracheotomy, with its possible complications was hopefully avoided.

MEMORIES OF INDIA

When I arrived in India, in 1969, open heart surgery had already been performed at the Christian Medical College and Hospital, Vellore, 90 miles inland from Madras. It was a teaching hospital of 1,100 beds with seven operating theatres, but no anaesthetic rooms. Dr Gwenda Lewis had organized the Anaesthesia Department with staff, trainees and technicians, but sadly caught poliomyelitis resuscitating a child. In spite of this she carried on from her wheelchair until she handed over to one of her trainees, Dr George Varkey, just before my arrival.

The drugs available were basic, such as novacaine, xylocaine, morphia, thiopentone, ether, halothane, suxamethonium, and d-tubocurarine. Supplies of nitrous oxide and oxygen were better than in many parts of India as the Indian Oxygen Company had a plant in Madras and there was a delivery of large and small cylinders to the gas bank at the Christian Medical College engineering department. This was rebuilt before the 14 new theatres and seven anaesthetic rooms in 1973, to supply piped oxygen, nitrous oxide and oxygen to recovery rooms and the cardiac ICU. In the latter there was also compressed air to run the ventilators.

Ventilation was by hand until we got a Blease Pulmoflator. Monitoring at first was with a blood pressure cuff, arterial and venous lines and a Sambourne ECG machine. Electrolytes with potassium samples were sent to the biochemical laboratory by messenger. Drip sets were home-made with rubber tubing and glass, and steel needles sharpended in the Central Sterile Supply Department. Disposable needles, cannulae and drip sets were sorely missed until some disposable supplies came through. There was a blood bank and donors were paid 10 rupees for a pint of blood, although relatives were told 'No donation, no operation'.

At first a Melrose disc oxygenator was used (with the usual blood loss). This was sterilized and run by the cardiac technicians with advice from consultants. Later disposable bubble oxygenators became available. Rheumatic infection was the commonest problem, with stenosis and incompetence even occurring in those under 10 years of age. Many mitral valvotomies were done by Stanley John [5], by the Brock method and valve replacements reserved for incompetence and aortic disease. There were also many congenital cases — ASD, ventricular septal defect

(VSD) and tetralogy of Fallot, some with a haemoglobin of up to 24 gm/dl that had to be haemodiluted preoperatively.

After a visit by Mr Christoper Lincoln we started using cardioplegia, the solution being prepared in the pharmacy, and did a study on the effects on cases with and without cardioplegia with the facilities available.

INTERESTING INCIDENTS

When the new theatres were built at the Christian Medical College, we had trolleys with separate, movable tops and base sections, so that the patient could be transferred from the ward base directly on to the theatre base over a barrier. This was to minimize infection as there had been cases of tetanus in the old theatres. During an electricity cut, we had to bring a patient back due to bleeding. While hand ventilating in the ward, one of the surgical assistants lifted the top section of the trolley off the base, there was a difficult moment until it was secured and the lights came on in time to use the lift.

One evening when visiting the cardiac ICU we found two patients on ventilators in distress and realized that the compressed air had failed, so had to connect them to pure oxygen. Being unable to contact the engineering department by telephone, I decided to go the quarter mile to that department to solve the problem. Luckily I met one of the anaesthetic technicians en route and we found that one of the engineering staff had, unrealizingly, turned off the supply. In spite of a reprimand from the chief engineer this happened twice again, until a fine of 10 rupees was threatened.

In 1980 one of Stanley John's postgraduate trainees, James Thomas, asked if I would be available while he restarted the cardio-thoracic unit at Miraj Medical Centre, another teaching hospital founded in 1888. It was more of a challenge than Vellore as the pump oxygenator was 16 years old and had to be rewired and its output checked before use. We decided at first we would start with the short procedures and relatively small patients. Our first patient was a teenage girl with an ASD. All was well until we went on bypass and the cardiac sucker did not function, instead of the blood being returned to the machine it was wasted. The porter standing by to bring fresh blood seemed to have gone to lunch! We had to use Hartmann's solution in the meantime. Fortunately, James Thomas closed the ASD in record time and all was well until we took her to the ICU only to find they had a case of septicaemia which had been admitted into the same room. No wonder there was trouble with her wound!

We learned by our mistakes. It was obvious that the cardiac unit should have its own ICU if infection was to be avoided. In the meantime the coronary care ward was used until the cardiac ICU was ready. As the pharmacy only opened at 8 am and we started operating at 7.30 am we had to have all possible drugs, drip sets, cannulae, syringes purchased by the patient the night before and brought to the theatre with him.

On visiting the Miraj Medical Centre in 1985, we were glad to see how far and how well the unit had progressed.

REFERENCES

(1) Nosworthy MD. Anaesthesia in chest surgery, with special reference to controlled respiration and cyclopropane. *Proc Royal Soc Med* 1941; **34**: 479–506.

(2) Brock RC, Ross DN. The clinical application of hypothermic techniques. Arteriovenous cooling. *Guy's Hospital Reports* 1955; **104**: 99.

(3) Drew CE, Keen S, Benazon DB. Profound hypothermia. *Lancet* 1959; **1**: 745–7.

(4) Melrose DG. A mechanical heart-lung for use in man. *Br Med J* 1953; **2**: 57–62.

(5) John S, Bashi VV, Jiairaj PS, *et al.* Closed mitral valvotomy, early results and long term follow up of 3724 consecutive patients. *Circulation* 1983; **68**: 891–6.

COMPLICATIONS AND SAFETY

John Snow — an early intensivist

RS Atkinson

Original presentation Southend 1988

John Snow lived in an era long before the invention of intensive care units and by no stretch of the imagination can he be referred to as an intensivist. Why then this title? The aim is to draw attention to how John Snow thought about medical treatment, and how he was ahead of his time in applying some of the principles of anaesthesia as then understood, to the care of the ordinary medical patient. Some of his patients had near fatal conditions and there was nothing to lose, so why not try some anaesthetic principles and some chloroform? He didn't have to worry about medico-legal considerations in those days!

It is important to consider other things about Snow besides his anaesthetic career, most important amongst these being Snow himself. We are indebted to Benjamin Ward Richardson for much of the biographical details we have [1]. Richardson was his friend and biographer and tells us that Snow was born in York on 15 March 1813 and studied in Newcastle. It is well known that he treated cholera at Killingworth Colliery. After some time at Burnup Field in Newcastle and Pateley Bridge in Yorkshire, he came to London. He took a circuitous route through Liverpool, trudging on foot through Wales, visited an uncle in Bath, and finally arrived in London in 1837. We know something about him as a person. He is said to have been of middle height and of slender build, of sedate expression and he had a reserved manner with strangers. In short, he was introverted and devoted himself to scientific experimentation and rational clinical work.

In London, he took the various examinations then available and joined the Westminster Medical Society (WMS), where he was an active participant at meetings. In 1841 — at a time some 5 years before the introduction of anaesthesia — he was also interested in the principles of resuscitation. He gave a paper to the WMS entitled 'Asphyxia — on the resuscitation of newborn children' and his aim was to describe a double air pump invented by a Mr Read of Regent's Circus.

He spoke at many WMS meetings and wrote papers on various subjects — for example, paracentesis of the thorax — some of which were published in the *Medical Gazette*. When anaesthesia arrived in London at the end of 1846, Snow was quick to take an interest. He had a lively mind and was adaptable to new ideas.

Essays on the history of anaesthesia, edited by A Marshall Barr, Thomas B Boulton and David J Wilkinson. 1996: International Congress and Symposium Series No. 213, published by Royal Society of Medicine Press Limited.

SNOW AND ANAESTHESIA

Richardson suggested that Snow enjoyed the rational nature of anaesthetic administration and its humane aspects and appreciated its basis in physiological knowledge. Snow started to design an improved ether inhaler and experimented with anaesthetics on animals and on himself.

He attended outpatients of St George's Hospital where he used anaesthesia for tooth extraction. Eventually Richardson tells us the ether practice in London came almost exclusively to Snow, though, of course, ether soon gave way to chloroform. Snow kept a diary of his clinical practice, from 17 July 1848 until 5 June 1858, covering the last ten years before his untimely death. These diaries occupy three exercise books, which on Snow's death, came into the possession of Richardson and his family. Richardson's daughter-in-law, Mrs Audrey Richardson, presented them to the Royal College of Physicians of London where they now reside in the library [2].

RESUSCITATION

It is interesting to read some of the extracts from the diaries, and particularly those which are quite unconnected with surgical operations. Snow attempted resuscitation of newborn babies and in one of his entries he described his only case of cardiac arrest during anaesthesia, and what he did to try to resuscitate the patient. It is stimulating to discover that he also had several cases of what we might describe today as 'near misses'.

He did a lot of obstetrics and it is quite clear that practice was rather crude in the mid 19th century. It is well known that both the maternal death rate and perinatal death rate were high. It is fascinating to read some of the descriptions of obstetric practice, of how chloroform was administered and how, in the absence of proper antenatal care the babies were often delivered in perilous states. Snow described several attempts to revive stillborn or hardly breathing newborn babies. It seems that as a last resort he passed a gum elastic catheter into the larynx and attempted to inflate the lungs by blowing down it.

In another patient, Snow described how he passed a female catheter into the glottis but was unsatisfied with his attempts to resuscitate the patient and took it out again. He remarked that his fellow practitioners achieved much better results by blowing directly into the baby's mouth.

Snow's one anaesthetic death was during administration of amylene, a drug about which little is known today but one which he used in a number of patients to produce anaesthesia. He gave a fairly honest description and he noted that his attention was distracted from the anaesthetic for a few seconds while he was watching the surgery. When he looked back he found the valve of the face piece had moved so as to occlude the aperture, presumably giving the patient a higher than usual concentration of amylene. He discontinued the anaesthetic at once and felt for the pulse which was not present in the left wrist and only a slight flutter in the right. Although the patient was breathing well, the respirations gradually became slower and deeper. Snow drew the surgeon's attention to this and they threw cold water on the patient's face which did not work very well. The patient was now becoming livid and gasping, and they began to perform artificial respiration according to the method of Marshall Hall. They pressed on the chest, the face being turned to one side and Snow noted that air could be heard going in and out of the lungs freely. In other words, he checked that the technique was actually working. He also noted that care was taken that the tongue did not fall back and he was very particular to notice the timings — 4.46 inhalation commenced, 4.48 unconscious, 4.49 surgery commenced, 4.54 called Mr Fergusson's attention to the fact that all was not well, 5.00 deep inspirations were still occurring and they apparently felt some kind of pulse. They continued for one and a half hours before they gave up.

At post mortem they did not find much to account for the death. Although, it is interesting to note that the patient is said to have drunk a pint of bottled ale a quarter of an hour before the operation! The significance of this is unknown. However the patient was only 33, and presumably healthy.

What about his 'near misses'? It is interesting to read that it was quite common for a state of syncope or fainting to occur. For instance, during the extraction of four molar teeth which required immense force in removal, Snow said, '. . . I felt the face was rather cold during the extraction of the second and subsequent teeth and at the end of the operation there was a little cold sweat on the forehead. He appeared faint and a minute or two afterwards the pulse could hardly be felt. He was laid on a sofa and recovered from the faintness very slowly. It was upwards of ten minutes before he became conscious, after which he felt very drowsy and it was more than half an hour before he felt able to go'. The relatively detailed records that were kept are very interesting when considered in the context of the times when they were made.

TETANUS

What about other medical diseases? If as a general practitioner, as Snow was, you came across a patient who was dying , was about to die, was likely to die, or there was no other known therapy, why not try an inhalation of chloroform? For example, on 7 March 1858, Snow administered chloroform at St Mark's Hospital to a man aged 52 with tetanus. 'He was operated on by Mr Salmon on Monday last for prolapsed ani and haemorrhoids by ligature, and the tetanus commenced on Friday evening. The patient was conscious and able to speak. He said he was not in pain but complained of twitchings. Spontaneous contractions came on almost every minute causing him to start and his muscles remained contracted between these. The abdomen was hard, he was able to show the tip of his tongue between his teeth. He had not been able to swallow anything since yesterday. His pulse was 148 full and strong and his breathing 30 in a minute'. Snow commenced his chloroform 'I had only just placed the face piece on with the valve wide open (presumably to allow plenty of air to get in) when his breathing became embarrassed and I removed it. The chest became fixed and his breathing stopped, his lips became very blue and he became unconscious, the pulse becoming very slow and somewhat feeble. Mr Salmon said he thought the man was dying. The nurse, however, told us that he had had a similar attack before in the course of the morning. In a minute or two the muscles of the chest became relaxed and he made gasping inspirations at intervals and in about a minute his breathing was natural and his lips a proper colour again and his pulse as quick as before'. Snow continued 'I now re-applied the chloroform'. They removed a bit of sloughing tissue while the patient was asleep. '. . . the patient slept for about 20 minutes after the operation, then he had a little spasm on his anus being touched, and the chloroform was repeated and he slept the same time as before. I endeavoured after he awoke to get him to take some egg and brandy but he spluttered it out after attempting to swallow and had a bad attack of spasm.' Of course, the patient subsequently died in St Bartholomew's Hospital—even in those days patients were transferred.

In another case on 11 November 1853 'Administered chloroform at 10 Mansfield Street, to a son of Mr Morris, aged 10, who was affected with lockjaw. The jaws could only be opened sufficiently to get the tip of a spoon betweeen his teeth. Chloroform was administered so as to make him unconscious. He still couldn't open his jaw . . . the chloroform was repeated a second time and then a third time, no relaxation of jaw was effected although I carried the effect of chloroform to insensibility and as far as seems safe in such a subject'.

CONVULSIONS, MANIA, TYPHOID, CHOLERA

Snow administered chloroform to treat convulsions in a child aged 2 years 11 months who was presumably in status epilepticus. The chloroform only had a temporary effect and the child later died.

Viscount Hinton, aged 34, suffered from acute mania—'He could not be persuaded to breathe the chloroform so he was seized by three keepers and held while I administered it, first on a towel and afterwards with the inhaler. When he found he was gassed and the chloroform was beginning to take effect, he became somewhat tractable and desired that it might not be given too strong'.

He used chloroform to treat typhoid; patients with typhoid have some abdominal pain and the anaesthetic was given to ease the pain. After taking chloroform the delirium never became quite as violent as before.

He even used it to treat a patient with cholera. '. . . She had severe cramps and almost constant vomiting. The pulse was small, feeble and frequent. The patient inhaled from a small inhaler to the extent of being made just unconscious and when she woke up in a few minutes the inhalation was repeated to the same extent. Soon after I left she fell into a natural sleep which lasted two and a half hours and she continued afterwards to improve'.

These are just a few extracts from Snow's diaries and are quite fascinating. They show that Snow was not afraid to try unconventional methods in those patients who had very little hope of recovering otherwise. He wasn't afraid to try the effect of chloroform and see what it would do. He was willing to utilize his medical and anaesthetic skills on patients who were otherwise certain to die in an attempt to provide a lessening of their symptoms and hopefully a long term cure. He was truly an early intensivist.

REFERENCES

(1) Richardson BW, Snow J. A representative of medical science and art of the Victorian era. *The Asclepiad (London)* 1887; **4**: 274–300. Reprinted in *Snow on Cholera*. New York: Hafner Publishing Company, 1965.
(2) Atkinson RS. The *'lost'* diaries of John Snow. *Progress in Anaesthesiology*. Amsterdam: Excerpta Medica Foundation, 1970: 197–9.

The adult respiratory distress syndrome: an old disease

JF Searle

Original presentation Edinburgh 1989

Ashbaugh, Bigelow, Petty and Levine published a paper in *The Lancet* in 1967 entitled 'Respiratory distress in adults' [1]. They showed that the lungs respond in a similar way to a wide variety of insults. This paper was the first of an ever increasing flood of papers on the adult respiratory distress syndrome, which has continued unstemmed ever since.

Ashbaugh *et al.* described 12/272 patients receiving respiratory support who did not respond to the then usual methods of treatment. These patients all had pulmonary oedema. Had their left atrial pressures been measured it is likely that they would have been normal or low. Postmortem examination of the lungs in seven patients showed hyperaemia, dilated engorged capillaries and areas of alveolar collapse. Interstitial and intra-alveolar haemorrhage and oedema were common. Hyaline membranes were present in six patients. Two patients who died after a protracted course had diffuse fibrosis of the lungs.

This clincial picture was certainly known to Osler. He described congestion of the lungs in his textbook *The Principles and Practice of Medicine* first published in 1892 [2]. He recognized that it occurred not only in heart disease, but also when very hot or irritating substances were inhaled as well as following drunkenness, exposure and cold. He had also seen it in debilitating illnesses, brain injury and morphine poisoning. He observed that in all forms there was transudation of serum from engorged capillaries chiefly into the air cells but also into the alveolar walls.

However, the credit for recognizing the response of the lung to disease and injury both within and without the respiratory system belongs to Virgil H Moon, pathologist at Jefferson Medical College and the Army Institute of Pathology, Washington DC. He described what he called the pathology of secondary shock in a classic paper in the *American Journal of Pathology* in 1948. The term 'secondary shock' was used at that time to describe shock arising from causes other than major bleeding [3].

Moon examined the records and pathology slides of 129 men whom he regarded as a representative sample of the thousands of deaths which had occurred in US Army personnel during active service and training. There were 30 cases of trauma from car accidents and wounds from gunfire or shells, ten patients had been burnt, 20 cases of poisoning including such substances as mapharsen, phosphorus, mercury and arsenic, one death occurred after a bout of protracted drinking, ten fulminating infections, 15 deaths from asphyxia — five unfortunately when their oxygen supply failed at 23 000 feet, 12 men collapsed in the heat during marching or drill. There were a few patients with intestinal obstruction or pancreatitis and a further miscellaneous group.

The common finding in the lungs (as in many other organs) was of hyperaemia and oedema. There were capillary haemorrhages and leucocyte infiltration.

These findings were no surprise to Moon, 16 years earlier in 1932 he had published the results of experiments on dogs [4]. The hind legs of dogs were extensively bruised under ether anaesthesia, and the appearance of the lungs was the same as in the American service men who had died in action or training. The early pathology of the lung following serious illness or accident was known long before 1967, and nearly 40 years before what was wrongly described in the 1960s and 70s as 'respirator lung'.

How much was known about the pathogenesis of such changes? The carnage of World War I generated a huge amount of research into the effects of trauma and, its most dreaded complication, infection. Many explanations were offered for the circulatory failure following trauma where there was not obvious bleeding, but gradually the evidence pointed to the capillary circulation.

By 1923, in the Oliver-Sharpey Lecture to the Royal College of Physicians of London [5], Sir Henry Dale, referring to bacterial toxins, could say, 'when poisons like these are formed in such quantities as to be distributed in effective amounts through the circulation so that all or a large proportion of the capillaries lose their tonus, there arises the peril of circulatory collapse due to peripheral stagnation of the blood'. He went on to observe that loss of tonus was followed by an increase in the permeability of the capillary adding 'unfortunately, methods of dealing effectively with dilated and permeable capillaries are not easy to find'.

The importance of leaky capillaries in so-called secondary shock was thus well recognized by the late 1920s. Lt Col W B Cannon summarized it succinctly in 1927 in the reports of the Medical Department of the United States Army in the World War: 'the theory of secondary shock which has the strongest support both in clinical observation and laboratory experiments is that of a toxic factor arising from damaged and dying tissues and operating to cause increased permeability of the capillary walls' [6].

Early researchers had some pieces of the jigsaw of the pathogenesis of the adult respiratory distress syndrome. More has been discovered since then, but the puzzle is not yet completed.

REFERENCES

(1) Ashbaugh DG, Bigelow DB, Petty TL, Levine BE. Respiratory distress in adults. *Lancet* 1967; 1: 319–23.
(2) Osler W. *The principles and practice of medicine*. 1892. Edinburgh: Young and Pentland, 1892.
(3) Moon VH. The pathology of secondary shock. *Am J Path* 1948; 24: 235–73.
(4) Moon VH, Kennedy PJ. Pathology of shock. *Arch Path* 1932; 14: 360–71.
(5) Dale HH. The activity of the capillary blood vessels. *Br Med J* 1923; 1: 1006–10.
(6) Cannon WB. *Wound shock*. Washington DC: The Medical Department of the United States Army in the World War, 1927; 11: 186.

Solutions to medical problems may be found in writings from the past

J Rupreht

Original presentation Croydon 1989

It is not uncommon in medicine for ailments to be treated on the basis of symptoms, rather than treating their cause. This is all that can be done if a disease is not understood. It is, however, worthwhile considering the possibility that a previously effective aetiological treatment may have been forgotten. Because in the past a condition was not understood in present day terms, useful knowledge from that period may remain unnoticed and unused. I would like to explore this hypothesis in two instances, of interest both in anaesthesia and resuscitation. In each case, an excellent solution to the problem had been described, only to be forgotten, and rediscovered at a much later date.

CENTRAL ANTICHOLINERGIC EFFECTS AND TREATMENT WITH PHYSOSTIGMINE

Following Fraser's description in 1863 of the 'ordeal' poison from Calabar beans [1], Dr Kleinwächter from Prague used the bean extract in atropine poisoning, and reported his findings in the amazingly short time of 22 days [2]. He explicitly mentioned that reversal of atropine toxicity was no coincidence but a clear pharmacological action, and recommended that this specific treatment should replace the then current and inefficient symptomatic treatment. However, for some reason, Kleinwächter's findings were forgotten, and the treatment of poisoning by atropine and other centrally acting anticholinergics remained symptomatic for decades to come. As late as 1970, the 4th edition of *The Pharmacological Basis of Therapeutics* advocated only symptomatic treatment [3]. By 1975, this book had updated its recommendations to include the use of physostigmine salicylate, which is the chief component of Calabar bean extract.

We all know that anticholinergic poisoning has been quite common, with patients suffering post-operatively from the central nervous system effects of premedicants. Yet no anaesthetist or surgeon investigated a solution to the problem. This is curious, since cholinergic central nervous transmission was fully established early this century, with physostigmine playing the major role as an investigatory tool. Fortunately, in psychiatry, atropine-induced coma was treated with physostigmine [4], and it was the psychiatrists who in 1970 stressed that central anticholinergic effects of drugs should be recognized, and could be treated with physostigmine [5]. From then, the concept was widely published, and began to enter the standard anaesthetic literature [6,7]. In 1982 the 9th edition of *Synopsis of Anaesthesia* included information on the central anticholinergic syndrome (CAS),

117

and the use of physostigmine in anaesthesia and intensive care. Knowledge of CAS and its management had become widespread by 1989, when the 5th edition of *General Anaesthesia* provided a full chapter on 'CAS in the post-operative period'.

In 1988, *Anaesthesia* published an historical paper [8] describing the early knowledge of physostigmine treatment, with a translation of Kleinwächter's paper from the German. The title is 'Observations on the effect of Calabar bean extract as an antidote to atropine poisoning'.

CLOSED CHEST CARDIAC COMPRESSION

It is commonly believed that closed chest cardiac compression in resuscitation from apparent death is a recent innovation. Nothing could be further from the truth. Early in the era of surgery under chloroform, such a technique was known and applied, with success.

In 1892, Dr Maass, a surgeon in training at the Göttingen Clinic, described two cases of chloroform death. He referred to the book published in 1889 by his teacher, Prof Koenig [9]. He noted that Koenig advocated closed-chest heart compressions for chloroform deaths, at a rate of gasping respirations. Maass in his paper [10] 'The method of resuscitation in cardiac death after chloroform', reported that in his two cases, the slow rate of compression advised by Koenig was unsuccessful, and the patients were considered to be lost. In a side room, Maass, 'somewhat agitated', continued cardiac compressions but at a higher rate, at least 80–100 per minute. Both resuscitations were fully successful, and Maass recommended the application of this high rate of closed chest compressions. The article is of further interest in its description of the 'blue' and 'white' appearances of the patients in whom chloroform 'syncope' occurred.

It is difficult to understand why this report of successful closed chest resuscitation was not acted upon. For years to come the accepted technique was open chest heart massage, even in cases far away from the surgical environment. Modern guidelines for cardiac resuscitation began with the paper by Kouwenhoven *et al.* in 1960 [11]. Their recommendation was for about 60 closed-chest compressions per minute. Combined with adequate ventilation provided simultaneously, the success of this approach has been self-evident. Further studies however, have shown a greater improvement in circulation is obtainable by increasing the rate of compression to 80–100 per minute. This was one of the key alterations in the guidelines published by the American Medical Association in 1986 [12].

The circle is closed again. In the past, a correct observation on the value of a treatment was lost, only to be rediscovered and widely applied at a later date. How many people died unneccessarily in the meantime. How many survived resuscitation, but with cerebral damage?

LESSONS TO BE LEARNT

Many discoveries from the past could have been used if only practitioners had been aware of them, or of their significance. Another well-known example in anaesthesia is curare. It was widely known that an animal given curare had survived by artificial ventilation. Every doctor and physiologist knew that Claude Bernard had established its site of action as outside the central nervous system. Yet nobody thought of applying curare during surgery. Was it ignorance of basic pharmacological knowledge? Was it lack of imagination by surgeons and anaesthetists alike? Once again it was psychiatrists who used curare first, before Harold Griffith took it up and revolutionized anaesthesia.

It is worth contemplating why medical men do not apply existing knowledge for the benefit of their patients. Osler was surprised at how little knowledge was needed for one to practise medicine. The author of this paper is surprised how conservative and often ignorant, doctors can still choose to be. One wonders how many other much-needed treatments have long ago been discovered, applied and described, all unknown to the self-assured contemporary medical community. It is suggested that curiosity for medical writings of the past may be of value in resolving some present day medical enigmas. Other circles might be closed, and answers given to correctly formulated questions. The main difficulty lies in keeping an open mind.

REFERENCES

(1) Fraser TR. On the characters, actions and therapeutical uses of the ordeal bean of Calabar (*Physostigma venenosum*, Balfour). *Edin Med J* 1863; **9**: 36–56, 123–32, 235–48.

(2) Kleinwächter I. Beobachtung über die Wirkung des Calabar-Extracts gegen Atropin-Vergiftung. *Berliner Klinische Wochenschrift* 1864; **1**: 369–71.

(3) Goodman LS, Gilman A. *The Pharmacological basis of therapeutics*, 4th ed. London: Macmillan, 1970: 1604–42.

(4) Forrer GR, Miller JJ. Atropine coma; a somatic therapy in psychiatry. *Am J Psych* 1958; **115**: 455–58.

(5) Granacher RP, Baldessarini RJ. Physostigmine. *Arch Gen Psych* 1970; **32**: 375–80.

(6) Atkinson RS, Rushman G, Lee JA, eds. *Synopsis of anaesthesia*, 9th ed. London: John Wright & Son, 1982: 127.

(7) Rupreht J, Dworacek B. The central anticholinergic syndrome in the postoperative period. In: Nunn J, Utting J, Burnell Brown R, eds. *General anaesthesia*, 5th ed. London: Butterworths, 1989: 1141–8.

(8) Nickalls RW, Nickalls EA. The first use of physostigmine in atropine poisoning. *Anaesthesia* 1988; **43**: 776–9.

(9) Koenig F. *Lehrbuch der allgemeinen Chirurgie*. Berlin: Verlag von August Hirschwald, 1889: 59–65.

(10) Maass D. Die Methode der Wiederbelebung bie Herztod nach Chloro-formeinatmung. *Berliner Klinische Wochenschrift* 1892; **12**: 265–8.

(11) Kouwenhoven WB, Jude JR, Knickerbocker GG. Closed-chest cardiac massage. *JAMA* 1960; **173**: 1064–67.

(12) Standards and guidelines for cardiopulmonary resuscitation and emergency cardiac care. *JAMA* 1986; **225**: 2841–3044.

Cotton Process Ether (CPE) and Hewer's Ethanesal Examples of believing is seeing

JB Stetson

Original presentation Edinburgh 1989

Times change; human nature remains the same. Many can remember the photographs and cine footage of Neville Chamberlain stepping from the aeroplane waving a bit of paper and plagiarizing his elder half brother's (Sir Austen Chamberlain) line 'Peace in our times'. He wanted to believe. The persistent refusal to believe chloroform can cause unexpected death is a well known tale. When McKesson taught primary and secondary saturation with nitrous oxide, promising safe abdominal relaxation; his followers wanted to believe. The reverse can also be true; the condemnation of curare in the 1950s is a recent example. People did not want to believe that they could misinterpret observed results.

This review will recount the desire of Cotton in North America and Hewer and Wallis in the United Kingdom to believe that diethyl ether is not an anaesthetic, but is a volatile solvent that carried other gases or chemicals that were the true anaesthetics. Two commercial preparations were concerned, Cotton Process Ether (CPE) in North America manufactured by the American company DuPont, and Ethanesal marketed by Savory and Moore. Zuck published a paper explaining how these products came to be produced and how the theory that pure ethyl ether is not an anaesthetic came to be promulgated [1]. This account gives further consideration to this extraordinary episode and provides additional details particularly concerning the North American aspect of the story.

JH COTTON AND COTTON PROCESS ETHER (CPE)

Biographical information about Cotton is sparse. He was born in 1891, and died 21 November 1952. He received both an AB and MA from the University of Toronto. He qualified in medicine in 1915, practised in Toronto until 1935, then moved to Willowdale, a suburb of Toronto.

Less than two years after qualifying he gave a talk and ether demonstration on 14 June 1917 before the Canadian Association at the Royal Victoria Hospital, Montreal [2]. He asserted that, 'ether, ethyl ether, with which we are so familiar, is not an anaesthetic, and the analgesia which comes from the administration of commercial ether is not due to ether, but rather to the impurities occurring in it'.

He called some of the impurities 'irritants' and categorized them according to the site where he claimed they acted (anterior nasal, nasopharyngeal, etc). He also divided the 'effective' pharmaceuticals or impurities into two groups, firstly 'narcotics' (producing peripheral congestion and drunkenness) and secondly 'analgesics' (producing loss of sensation and peripheral vasomotor spasm). 'Absolute ether' (made by Cotton by a method which was not detailed) was a narcotic but not an analgesic, therefore an analgesic needed to be added to act with it. The analgesic which he added was carbon dioxide. 'Absolute ether' was compared to nitrous oxide, and although McKesson was not mentioned by Cotton one wonders if Cotton had read McKesson's 1915 report on partial rebreathing [3]. However, Cotton noted Henry Hill Hickman's 1823 use of carbon dioxide as an anaesthetic.

Cotton constructed a can that acted as a syphon bottle to carbonate ether. He then 'discovered' that ethylene was a synergist with his 'absolute ether' and added it to his armamentarium. The qualities utilized were not reported. The schedule of the June 14 demonstration was listed in the report: '8.45 am a cat received absolute ether saturated in ethylene. . . . cat relieved of all sensation yet capable of walking. 8.55 am a middle-aged Chinaman received absolute ether with carbon dioxide; Infected upper arm. Eight incisions were made over biceps. Patient free from sensation but not at all unconscious. 9.10 am same cat, absolute ether, cat hyperaesthetic. 9.20 am a middle-aged Englishman received absolute ether-ethylene 15 minute operation. Resection splintered bone from elbow. Patient capable of carrying on conversation and yet was entirely free from sensation'. Cotton concluded that absolute gas-free ethyl ether was not an anaesthetic. He believed that it was a vehicle for analgesic gases such as carbon dioxide and ethylene, and a narcotic stimulant.

The next year Cotton spoke in Indianopolis, Indiana [4]. He noted that alcoholics required 25–75% more ether than non-alcoholics. He considered anaesthesia as analgesia (blocking of sensory impulses from the periphery) plus narcosis (or sleep). George Crile and Lower had published their book entitled *Anoci-Association* in 1914 [5]. Yandell Henderson had published an article on his acapnia-shock theory in the 1915 *Yearbook of Anesthesia and Analgesia* [6]. Cotton may have unconsciously melded these recently published concepts with McKesson's to develop his theories.

Cotton now had CPE (Cotton Process Ether) which the manufacturers stated was composed of absolute d-ethyl ether with ethylene, carbon dioxide and alcohol added, prepared in one ounce glass ampoules. He had also developed a closed system with a vaporizer, but no CO_2 absorption; however the section of Cotton's report labelled 'Analgesia' contains a tantalizing but confusing paragraph. It is captioned: 'Exhibit B — Rebreathing of oxygen' and it reads 'The ether container was filled with caustic potash sticks in order to absorb any accumulation of carbon dioxid[sic]. An excess of oxygen was given, 10 to 20 litres per hour, and the blood pressure readings were closely followed in 20 cases'. War wounds were being treated. Had the cases received ether first? Was this closed system ether anaesthesia (or analgesia) with CO_2 absorption? Other workers had used CO_2 absorption with oxygen and nitrous oxide [7–9], but, if Cotton's patients had also received ether, he was probably the first to have administered ether and oxygen using CO_2 absorption.

ETHER ANALGESIA

Cotton opened an address before the Dental Society of the State of New York (Albany, 13–15 May 1920) with the comment, 'Ether analgesia of complete type was practically unknown a short time ago' [10]. Cotton had either become very proficient at administering ether analgesia or had become an expert at hypnosis without knowing it. The technique of ether analgesia employed by Artusio in the 1950s [11] was different from that used by Cotton. Artusio specified that he took '. . . ether-oxygen anaesthesia to the first plane of the third stage (surgical anaesthesia)'. Patients were intubated at that stage and then lightened to stage 1 (Artusio divided Stage 1 into three planes). Hewer's clinical work with Ethanesal will be detailed in the next section of this essay, but as his development of ether analgesia was similar to that of Artusio, he may be quoted. 'It is sometimes possible to procure perfect analgesia without anaesthesia, and, if a long extra-abdominal operation is being performed, such as an extensive tendon transplantation, the patient can usually be allowed to become exceedingly light, and may even be blinking his eyes, but will remain quite motionless, breathing quietly, and not feeling pain' [12]. Cotton's demonstration of dental analgesia with his nasal mask, CPE and air is reminiscent of the N_2O/oxygen/trichloroethylene analgesia used in the 1950s and 60s with a demand flow apparatus.

A representative of the DuPont Company was present at the dental meeting held in Albany. He reported CPE was '. . . absolute di-ethyl ether, with 2% of ethylene, ½% volume of carbon dioxid[sic], and 1% by weight of alcohol to keep it from frosting on a mask'. In his clinical directions Cotton noted he used oil of rose or another essence to hide the odour of the ether (a system introduced by Gwathmey who liked oil of bitter orange). Cotton had developed an inhaler by attaching a nasal mask to a double tubed 1 oz (28 ml) CPE Bottle. He claimed his system was safe '. . . even for fools', and that his patients never vomited.

In the same year that Cotton spoke to the dentists (1920), Dr Joseph E Lumbard of New York City presented 'Remarks on Cotton Process Ether from personal experience and the reports of Other Observers' at the Eighth Annual Meeting of the American Association of Anesthetists in New Orleans [13]. Lumbard tried to obtain CPE analgesia, '. . . in a few cases, and my experience has been that of others, some [administrations] appeared to be quite successful while others passed into surgical anaesthesia . . .'. He had used CPE 400 times and felt CPE was a stronger ether during induction but he failed to notice any differences during maintenance. Recovery '. . . seemed less disturbed'. 'CPE was less irritating, but there was more of a tendency to cyanosis'. The paper provoked a lively discussion [13].

The last article published about CPE appears to be that of Paul Cassidy DDS, of Cincinnati, Ohio. It was 'Read by proxy during the Joint Meeting of the Canadian Interstate and New York Anesthetists with the Ontario Medical Association, at Niagara Falls, Canada, June 1–3, 1921' [14]. Cassidy provided a chart of the loss of ethylene from the opened cans in which CPE was supplied by DuPont. Cassidy developed an apparatus made of copper that allowed opening of the cans within the closed machine so none of the gases were lost. An electric light bulb '. . . hermetically sealed from the CPE was employed to keep the anaesthetic at . . . a very even temperature'. This was '. . . to produce an even flow of the entire mixture as originally compounded, which is after all, the only excuse for its being utilized'.

A critique of Cassidy's article entitled 'Sixty-seven years ago in anesthesia and analagesia' was published in 1989 [15]. The reviewer wrote: 'The theory was that ethylene (an explosive N_2O if you will) speeds induction of anaesthesia and decreases the amount of ether needed to maintain anaesthesia while the CO_2 assures that the patient keeps breathing'. It is obvious the reviewer was not familiar with Cotton or CPE. In retrospect one wonders if, in a closed system, the ethylene and carbon dioxide would bubble off (especially with the aid of the warm electric light bulb), and at the time of induction present to the patient anaesthetic gas mixtures with high partial pressures of ethylene and carbon dioxide. The resulting hyperpnoea (never noted by Cotton or the few others who recorded their results) would allow a rapid adjustment to a high inspiratory level of ether.

RL MACKENZIE WALLIS, C LANGTON HEWER AND ETHANESAL

RL Mackenzie Wallis (1886–1929) was a chemical pathologist who initially worked in the laboratories at St Bartholomew's Hospital in London from 1911–1914 [16]. At the outbreak of war he left to join the Royal Army Medical Corps and was drafted to India; while in India he began to study purity and decomposition of anaesthetic ethers. Wallis returned to St Bartholomew's after the War and continued his interest in di-ethyl ether and the impurities present in commercial preparations by distilling with 'finely divided potassium permanganate' and identified a mixture of impurities which included alcohol, water, acetone, mercaptans, thioethers, aldehydes, peroxides and acids [1,12].

It was apparently at this point that Wallis was approached by C Langton Hewer (1896–1986) [17] who had recently been demobilized from the RAMC and had subsequently been appointed to the staff of St Bartholomew's at the age of 24. Hewer had an evil smelling specimen of ether which had caused respiratory difficulties in two patients. Wallis identified mercaptans as the impurity and gave Hewer some of his own highly purified ether. Hewer reported that it was not possible to induce anaesthesia with this specimen, and concluded that pure ether was not an anaesthetic but merely a solvent and that the purification had removed a vital ingredient. Wallis then became aware of Cotton's work with CPE and he experimented by adding CO_2 and ethylene to his purified ether. Wallis reported that successful animal trials were conducted (although these were never described in detail) and Hewer used the preparation on 100 patients [1,12]. Further experiments and analysis of residues convinced Wallis that ketones were the essential ingredient in anaesthesia, but that they were so potent that it was necessary to use a volatile solvent (ether).

Wallis and Hewer described their experimental and clinical findings at a meeting at the Royal Society of Medicine on 1 April 1921 and published their papers in *The Lancet* 3 months later [1,12]. Meanwhile Hewer had written a short paper in the *St Bartholomew's Hospital Journal* [18] reporting in detail on 200 cases. He had anaesthetized 500 patients aged between 3 months and 70 years with durations of anaesthesia between 5 and 165 minutes and 48% had no vomiting. This finding is rather interesting, the patients all received atropine before the anaesthetic, morphia was not administered before the anaesthetic '. . . unless very excitable or nervous . . .' however morphia was administered '. . . just before the patient regains consciousness . . .' [1,12].

Hewer's monograph *Anaesthesia in Children* was published in 1923 [19]. The chapter on Ethanesal contained illustrations of his continuous flow dripper and bottle for endotracheal insufflation. He reported 3000 Ethanesal anaesthetics in $2\frac{1}{2}$ years. The same chapter appeared in *Practical Anaesthetics* (3rd Edition 1923), co-authored with H Edmund Boyle, Hewer's senior colleague at St Bartholomew's [20].

Boyle went to North America during the summer of 1921 as the representative of the Anaesthetic Section of the Royal Society of Medicine. He spoke at the meeting held in Niagara Falls, Canada, at which, as noted above, Cassidy's paper on CPE was read by proxy [14]. Boyle's topic was N_2O:oxygen: Ethanesal:chloroform anaesthesia. He spoke of 'The anaesthetist of today' and 'the era of newer anaesthetics' [21]. Boyle noted he induced with 10:1 N_2O:oxygen, then passed the gases over chloroform and Ethanesal (equal parts), and after the patient was stabilized cut back to 4:1 N_2O:oxygen. He considered N_2O:oxygen with rebreathing the basic anaesthetic, the vapours were adjuvants. If diathermy was to be employed for treatment of carcinoma of the tongue, fauces or tonsil, only chloroform was employed. He emphasized that the patient's colour must always be pink. Boyle stated he had been using Ethanesal for 3 months and liked it (prior to the use of Ethanesal he had employed ether in the manner he now used Ethanesal). An updated version of the paper was published in 1923 [22].

Hewer and Boyle continued to be enthusiastic about Ethanesal. Hewer, like Cotton, had the clinical ability to bring the patients into a state of ether analgesia, but the tide of opinions of others was flowing against them. The American Medical Association (AMA) had forced DuPont to reveal the contents of CPE and treated CPE and Ethanesal as quackery (a review of the AMA's actions appears later). In the USA there were no critical and objective studies of CPE, but in Canada, England and Holland critical objective studies of CPE and Ethanesal were performed, pure ethers prepared, and the clinical utility of pure ether demonstrated.

AN INQUIRY BY THE COUNCIL ON PHARMACY AND CHEMISTRY OF THE AMERICAN MEDICAL ASSOCIATION AS TO THE NATURE OF CPE

The February 21, 1920 issue of the *Journal of the American Medical Association* carried the note, 'About January 20, the News Service of the EI Du Pont De Nemours and Co Inc circularized the press of the country with what it was pleased to term a good filler; this particular piece of press agent work dealt with the New Du Pont Ether' [23]. The news release prompted queries to the AMA from members. The Secretary of the Council on Pharmacy and Chemistry asked DuPont Chemical Works for the composition of the new ether, DuPont's response was evasive. The AMA warned physicians, 'it is many times more serious for a physician to employ a secret or semi-secret substance as an anaesthetic'.

Three months after the first notice, information was received from DuPont and the following analysis was published, 'An improved anesthesia ether consisting of highly refined diethyl oxide $(C_2H_5)_2O$), plus approximately two volumes of ethylene, half volume of carbon dioxide, and 1% by weight of ethyl alcohol' [24]. If Ethanesal had been marketed in the United States it would have received the same treatment; it is, perhaps, unfortunate that the British Medical Association did not have an equivalent department to the Council of Pharmacy and Chemistry. The essence of the report of the composition of CPE was reprinted in the AMA publication *The Propaganda for the Reform of Proprietary Medicines* in 1922 [25]. The BMA did not have an equivalent department.

THE RESULTS OF CRITICAL UNBIASED EVALUATIONS OF PURE ETHER AS AN ANAESTHETIC

Wesley Bourne, the first recipient of the Henry Hill Hickman Medal of the Royal Society of Medicine (1935) enlisted the assistance of Raymond L Stehle, of the McGill University Laboratory of Pharmacology in his quest to produce a pure ether [26]. They produced a pure ether by combining sodium ethylate with ethyl iodid [sic]. Bourne, after animal testing, used the ether to anaesthetize five surgical patients and one obstetric patient (Bourne's specialty). He noted 'good analgesia was obtained intermittently for each pain over a period of forty minutes of normal labor'. Bourne could obtain analgesia without the magical CPE or Ethanesal. The pure ether was also a proper anaesthetic. The date of publication (*Journal of the American Medical Association*, 1922) was long before Boyle's final article on Ethanesal in the *British Medical Journal* in 1923 [22].

In 1923 a report entitled: 'The anaesthetic action of pure ether' by Dale, Hadfield and King appeared in *The Lancet* [27]. H King of the British National Institute for Medical Research, prepared an ethyl alcohol-sulphuric acid ether by multiple distillations and washings. The leading pharmacologist (Sir) Henry Dale (1875–1968) carried out animal tests and found the drug satisfactory. CF Hadfield (1875–1965) [28] another senior colleague of Hewer's at St Bartholomew's Hospital used the ether to anaesthetize eight patients with excellent results. King then examined commercial samples of Ethanesal and found they contained 95.5% ether, 4% n-butyl alcohol and 0.5% 'of a mixture of ethyl alcohol and an aldehyde . . .' but no ketones [27]. Wallis and Hewer were invited to comment on this report. Wallis stated, 'We are quite at a loss to explain the above observations of Dale and his co-workers . . .', Hewer added 'I have no doubt of the accuracy of the work of Dale and his colleagues, . . . I have now used Ethanesal in over 4000 cases, and am convinced that, whatever may be its exact chemical composition, it gives, on average, better results than any anaesthetic ether that I have tried'.

Professor W Storm van Leeuwen, Director of the Pharmacotherapeutical Institute of the University of Leyden (Holland), also investigated ethers. He prepared pure ether by crystallization of ether with benzidine, followed by distillation [29]. He added known impurities to his pure ether and tested the drug on cats and mice. When methylethyl ketone, the supposed active ingredient in Ethanesal, was tested, it was found to be toxic! '. . . all the cats died after being narcotized two or three times. In all cases we found multiple haemorrhages of the lungs, liver, kidney, peritoneum'. Commercial Ethanesal was next examined by van Leeuwen. When the containers were opened, carbon dioxide escaped. Analysis revealed no ketones, reaction for ethylene 'slightly positive', considerable amounts of normal butyl alcohol and a small amount of isoamyl alcohol. When he examined CPE, he found ethylene, but 'little or no carbon dioxide' [29].

The *Journal of the American Medical Association* carried a one page summary headlined: 'Claim that pure ether has no anaesthetic properties, without foundation' [30]. CPE and Ethanesal were discussed and the '. . . painstaking investigations' of Dale, Hadfield and King [27] and Stehle and Bourne [26] reviewed. The officials of the AMA considered CPE and Ethanesal quackery.

An extensive discussion followed van Leeuwen's presentation of his data at the Royal Society of Medicine. Hewer tried to turn black to white. Hadfield was forceful in pointing out the numerous differing pronouncements by Wallis concerning ketone type and percentage. Wallis had previously stated methylethyl ketone was expensive; a discussant pointed out: '. . . large quantities were available as a by-product at a very low cost'. Boyle closed the discussion with slides on the 10 000 Ethanesal administrations performed by Boyle and Hewer; almost all had had preliminary nitrous oxide or ethyl chloride and over a quarter were in combination with chloroform [29].

TEXTBOOK EVALUATIONS OF ETHANESAL
AND COTTON PROCESS ETHER

Henry Robinson, the editor of the fifth edition of Hewitt's British textbook *Anaesthetics and Their Administration* (1922) presented a terse evaluation of

Ethanesal, 'I have been unable to discover any advantage possessed by this anaesthetic over ether . . . . . . considerably the more expensive of the two' [31]. Blomfield in *Anaesthetics in Practice and Theory* (1923) stated 'my own observations do not support this contention [that Ethanesal can be used] on patients suffering from respiratory affections . . ., and other observers also have found that Ethanesal is quite potent in causing mucous and salivary secretion' [32].

Gwathmey's encyclopaedic *Anesthesia* Second Revised Edition [33] (United States, 1925) contained information about the Boothby–Cotton gas:oxygen:ether-apparatus developed by Frederic J Cotton and Walter M Boothby (both of Harvard Medical School and Boston City Hospital) but nothing about James Cotton of Toronto, C Langton Hewer, CPE or Ethanesal. *Practical Anaesthesia*, a handbook published in Australia in 1932, noted, '. . . Ethanesal has passed out of vogue' [34].

THE ALLEGED RELATIONSHIP BETWEEN THE USE
OF ETHANESAL AND THE INTRODUCTION OF
ETHYLENE AS AN ANAESTHETIC

Hewer was already well known amongst British anaesthetists at the time of the Ethanesal controversy, despite being comparatively young. He ultimately became one of the most respected figures in British anaesthesia, the founder editor of the journal *Anaesthesia* (editor 1946–1966). He was elected in 1959 to deliver the prestigious Hewitt Lecture at the Royal College of Surgeons in London which he entitled 'Forty years on' [35]. He did not mention Ethanesal but he did state, 'Mackenzie Wallis also showed that ethylene dissolved in di-ethyl ether altered its narcotic effects and this led to a thorough investigation of the gas which was carried out mainly in America by Luckhardt, Carter and others' [35].

The impression which may be created by Hewer's assertion is unfortunately erroneous. AB Luckhardt of the University of Chicago Physiology Department [36] was not influenced by Wallis, Hewer or Cotton. He had learned of ethylene's noxious effect on carnations about 1907 and felt that if the gas could put buds to sleep, it could have a similar effect on animals. His early research was interrupted by World War I. After the War, with his student J Bailey Carter (later Professor of Internal Medicine, Rush Medical College), he investigated and recorded the effects of ethylene on animals, themselves, and other members of the Physiology Department of the University of Chicago. The agent was taken up by Isabella Herb, Chief of Anesthesiology at the Rush Medical College who began to use it clinically [36]. Luckhardt and Carter published their first paper on the 'new gas anaesthetic' in 1923 [37].

William Easson Brown of Toronto also investigated ethylene. Brown qualified at the University of Toronto in 1916. He served in the Royal Canadian Army Medical Corps (RCAMC) during World War I and worked in the Department of Anesthesiology, Toronto General Hospital after the War. He reasoned, 'Owing to the fact that ethylene is said to be one of the active constituents of a certain commercial ether, it was thought that this would be a good gas to experiment with'. He does not specify CPE or Ethanesal, but Cotton did work in Toronto. Brown's first paper on ethylene [38] was published in the same month as Luckhardt's [37].

CONCLUSION

For the centennial of ether anaesthesia, Wesley Bourne's presentation: 'Pure ether and impurities: a review', was the leading article of the November 1946 issue of

Anesthesiology [39]. It was a complete review of the subject, including the investigations of the 1940s demonstrating the safety of using ether from large bulk containers.

Wallis, Hewer and Boyle were undoubtedly slow to admit that they were wrong. Memories are the yarn with which we weave the tapestry of our past life as we wish it to be seen. Hewer's 1959 Hewitt Lecture did not refer to Ethanesal, and in respect of Wallis he mentioned his interest in ethers and that he had '. . . showed that minute quantities of impurities could have toxic effects'. There was no mention of ketones! [35]. There is no mention of Ethanesal in the obituaries of either Wallis [16] or Hewer [17]. Hewer, despite their professional differences over Ethanesal, wrote two appreciative obituaries about Hadfield [17,40]; they do not refer to Ethanesal either! It is, however, of interest to record that they had collaborated in a joint paper concerned with the introduction of trichloroethylene to the United Kingdom in 1941 [41].

REFERENCES

(1) Zuck D. Faith against science. The ethanesal mystery. In: Atkinson RS, Boulton TB, eds. *The history of anaesthesia*. London: Royal Society of Medicine Services and Parthenon Publishing, 1989: 207–13.
(2) Cotton JH. Anaesthesia from commercial ether—administration and what it is due to. *Canadian Med Assoc J* 1917; 7: 769–77.
(3) McKesson EI. Fractional rebreathing in anaesthesia—its physiologic basis, technich and conclusions. *Am J Surg* 1915; **29**: Anesthesia Supplement, 51–7.
(4) Cotton JH. Cotton process ether and ether analgesia. *Am J Surg* 1919; **33**: Anaesthesia Supplement, 34–43.
(5) Crile GW, Lower WE *Anoci-association*. Philadelphia: WB Saunders, 1914.
(6) Henderson Y. Some considerations of respiration in relation to apnea, anoxemia, acapnia and anesthesia. In: McMechan FH, ed. *The American yearbook of anesthesia and analgesia*. New York City: Surgery Publishing Co, 1915: 95–106.
(7) Jackson DE. A new method for the production of general analgesia and anesthesia with a description of the apparatus used. *J Lab Clin Med* 1915; 1: 1–12.
(8) Anonymous. Re: Mr Coleman, hydrate of lime. *Br J Dental Sci* 1868; **11**: 253.
(9) Rendle R. On the use of protoxide of nitrogen gas. *Br Med J* 1869; ii: 412–13.
(10) Cotton J. Cotton process ether for dental operations. Reprinted from the *Dental Cosmos* for January 1921: 3–18.
(11) Artusio JF. Di-ethyl ether analgesia: a detailed description of the first stage of ether analgesia in man. *J Pharmacol Exper Therap* 1954; **111**: 343–8.
(12) Wallis RLM, Hewer CL. A new general anaesthetic. *Lancet* 1971; **1**: 1173–8.
(13) Lumbard JE. Remarks on Cotton Process Ether from personal experience and the reports of other observers. *Am J Surg* 1920; **34**: Anesthesia Supplement, 118–21.
(14) Cassidy P. Experimental and clinical observations on Cotton Process Ether. *Am J Surg* 1922; **36**: Anesthesia Supplement, 73–5.
(15) Anonymous. Sixty-seven years ago in anesthesia and analgesia. *Anesth Analgesia* 1989; **68**: 19.
(16) GERL Mackenzie Wallis. *St Bartholomew's Hosp J* May 1929: 118–19.
(17) Boulton TB. Editorial; C Langton Hewer. *Anaesthesia* 1986; **41**: 469–71.
(18) Hewer CL. A few points about ethanesal. *St. Bartholomew's Hosp J* May 1921: 124.
(19) Hewer CL. *Anaesthesia in children*. New York: Paul B Hoeber, 1923: 36–53.
(20) Boyle HEG, Hewer CL. *Practical anaesthetics*, Third edition. London: H Frowde and Hodder and Stoughton, 1923: 97–103 and 133–9.
(21) Boyle HEG. Gas-oxygen-ethanesal-chloroform combined anesthesia for nose and throat and abdominal surgery. *Am J Surg* 1922; **36**: Anesthesia Supplement, 17–21.
(22) Boyle HEG. Anaesthesia by the gas-oxygen-ethanesal and gas-oxygen-chloroform-ethanesal combinations. *Br Med J* 1923; ii: 806–8.

(23) Queries and Minor Notes. The new Du Pont ether. *JAMA* 1920; **74**: 544.

(24) Queries and Minor Notes. Cotton process ether. *JAMA* 1920; **74**: 1474.

(25) Anonymous. *The propaganda for reform in proprietary medicine.* Volume 2. Chicago: Press of American Medical Association, 1922: 421–2.

(26) Stehle RL, Bourne W. The anesthetic properties of pure ether. *JAMA* 1922; **79**: 375–6.

(27) Dale HH, Hadfield CF, King H. The anaesthetic action of pure ether. *Lancet* 1923; **1**: 424–9.

(28) CLH. Charles Frederick Hadfield. *St Bartholomew's Hosp J* 1965; September: 349.

(29) Van Leeuwen WS. On the narcotic action of purest ether. *Proc Royal Soc Med* 1924; **17**: 17–34.

(30) Anonymous. So-called "improved" ethers. *JAMA* 1923; **81**: 1040.

(31) Robinson H. *Anaesthetics and their administration* (Hewitt). 5th ed. London: H Frowde and Hodder and Stoughton, 1922: 335.

(32) Blomfield J. *Anesthetics in practice and theory.* Chicago: Chicago Medical Book Co, 1923: 32–3, 156–7.

(33) Gwathmey JT. *Anesthesia.* 2nd ed. New York: Macmillan, 1925.

(34) Anaesthetic staff of the Alfred Hospital, Melbourne. *Practical anaesthesia.* Glebe, New South Wales: Australian Medical Publishing Co, 1932: 67.

(35) Hewer CL. Forty years on. *Anaesthesia* 1959; **14**: 311–30.

(36) Stetson JB. Arno Benedict Luckhardt and the introduction of ethylene. In: Atkinson RS and Boulton TB, eds. *The history of anaesthesia.* London: Royal Society of Medicine Services and Parthenon Publishing, 1989: 595–601.

(37) Luckhardt AB, Carter JB. The physiologic effects of ethylene. A new gas anesthetic. *JAMA* 1923; **80**: 765–70.

(38) Brown WE. Preliminary report: experiments with ethylene as a general anaesthetic. *Canadian Med Assoc J* 1923; New Series **13**: 210–11.

(39) Bourne W. Pure ether and impurities: a review. *Anesthesiology* 1946; **7**: 599–605.

(40) CLH. Obituary Charles Frederick Hadfield (1875–1965). *Anaesthesia* 1965; **20**: 514–15.

(41) Hewer CL, Hadfield CF. Trichloroethylene as an inhalation anaesthetic. *Br Med J* 1941; **1**: 924–5.

A case of repeated anaesthesia

OP Dinnick

Original presentation Croydon 1989

This case concerns the patient of an unnamed, presumably American physician, whose activities circa 1860 were recorded by J Marion Sims.

In his book on uterine surgery [1] Sims devotes a section to vaginismus — a term by which he meant 'an excessive hyperaesthesia of the hymen and vulvar outlet, associated with such involuntary spasmodic contraction of the sphincter vaginae as to prevent coition'. It was in the context of this subject that Sims wrote as follows (parts of his lengthy account have been omitted):

'I will here relate a most remarkable case that fell under my observation a few years ago. A lady aged 30 was married at 21. Vigorous attempts at copulation were made fruitlessly for five or six weeks. The husband and wife were both young and, of course, ignorant on the subject and were not surprised that there was difficulty at the beginning; but soon they began to debate the point of asking for medical advice. At last the wife became worn out with the oft-repeated and painful attempts at coition. . . . The family physician was called . . . and advised sexual intercourse while the wife was etherised. This was soon done and the wife knew nothing of it, but when the act was attempted the next day, and the next, it was found to be utterly impossible. After a week's fruitless trial, the physician was sent for again, and again she was etherised and coition effected with the greatest ease. But it was subsequently impossible when she was not etherised.'

Sims then digresses, and after finding no fault with the husband's performance, he continues: 'Suffice it to say that it became the business of the physician to repair regularly to the residence of this couple two or three times a week to etherise the poor wife for the purpose above alluded to. They persevered, hoping that she would become pregnant and that delivery would cure her. This etherisation was continued for a year, when conception occurred. But during the whole period of utero-gestation, etherisation was necessary to coition. After the birth of the child there were a few copulations without ether — but it was exceedingly painful . . . and they were compelled to resort to ether again. At the end of another year of ethereal copulation, there was another conception, which resulted in an abortion at the third month. After this, she was etherised constantly for another year, when at last they saw no hope of a cure and, becoming alarmed at the frequent repetition of anaesthesia, they concluded to give it up altogether. And when they consulted me, there had been no effort at copulation for three or four years.'

This strange story had a happy ending. Sims operated on the wife, after which 'sexual intercourse was performed for the first time without pain.'

The case has several points of particular interest for anaesthetists. The woman conceived twice under 'complete anaesthesia' (Sims' phrase) and the fetus was repeatedly exposed to ether. That she aborted once is not surprising, but that she had a full term child is astonishing. Unfortunately we do not know if the child had any congenital anomalies. It is tempting to think that it did not, as Sims was a meticulous reporter. The mother appears to have had no side-effects suggestive of liver damage, or other toxic complications, although she must have had in just over $3\frac{1}{2}$ years, at least 350 anaesthetics, and possibly over 500.

Snow wrote [2] that 'Many patients have inhaled this agent (chloroform) hundreds of times . . .', but the three examples he gave were not his own patients, and their inhalations several times a day were self-administered for the relief of pain. One patient with 'neuralgia of the uterus' followed this practice for about 15 months when she gave it up as her condition had resolved. How long the other two continued to inhale is not assessable though a woman with 'a painful cancer' did so 'day and night for a very long time'.

However, such administrations are not directly comparable with those received by Sims' patient, where even the lowest estimate of 350 administrations must surely constitute a record for the number of anaesthetics given by one physician to the same patient.

REFERENCES

(1) Sims JM. *Clinical notes on uterine surgery*. London: Robert Hardwicke, 1866: 326–45.
(2) Snow J. *On chloroform and other anaesthetics*. London: John Churchill, 1858: 343–4.

PEOPLE AND PLACES

Memorabilia of Wells and Morton in New England: The relics of injustice

JAW Wildsmith

Original presentations Reading 1986 and London 1994

The 'discovery' of anaesthesia resulted from the work of many men. Joseph Priestley, Thomas Beddoes and Humphry Davy each played a part, but clinical development was due to two dentists, Horace Wells and William Thomas Green Morton. Neither life nor history treated them equally. Morton died an eminent man, in spite of the controversies his work produced, but Wells died young and at his own hand, without receiving the credit that was his due. It was he who recognized the clinical significance of the analgesic action of nitrous oxide and then performed an appropriate experiment on himself before promoting his method freely for the benefit of others. Unfortunately, his public demonstration was not a success, and he later became a victim of his own mental illness and of the greed and ingratitude of others.

Morton helped Wells with his work on nitrous oxide, having been at various times both his student and his partner. Morton deserves credit for persevering with the principle of inhaled anaesthesia, for finding an alternative agent and for perfecting its use sufficiently to allow a successful public demonstration. However, his subsequent resistance to giving any credit to Wells for the discovery of anaesthesia was ingratitude indeed to one who had been both teacher and banker. The motive was, almost certainly, Morton's attempt to patent not only the use of ether, but also the process of anaesthesia by inhalation as a principle.

'SHRINES' IN NEW ENGLAND

New England, comprising the north-eastern states of the USA, was very much the birthplace of general anaesthesia. The Connecticut River forms the spine of New England and much of the lives of both Wells and Morton were lived out on its banks. It is a measure of the youth of anaesthesia that the memorabilia of its pioneers are very often still accessible, and well worth visiting. New England has many attractive areas and a tour of what may be called the 'shrines' of anaesthesia is an entertaining way of seeing them. Many visitors to Boston, Massachusetts

Essays on the history of anaesthesia, edited by A Marshall Barr, Thomas B Boulton and David J Wilkinson. 1996: International Congress and Symposium Series No. 213, published by Royal Society of Medicine Press Limited.

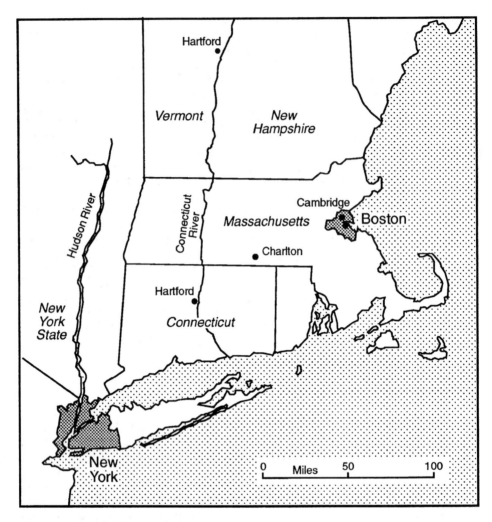

Figure 1   *Sites of the 'shrines' of anaesthesia*

visit the Ether Dome in the original Bullfinch Building at the Massachusetts General Hospital, but few are aware of the many other interesting sites that may be reached easily from Boston [1]. The birthplaces of both Wells and Morton remain standing and are relatively easy to find. Wells was born in a house in School Street, Hartford, Vermont which lies on the west bank of the Connecticut River, 140 miles north-west of Boston, near White River Junction. Alongside the door is a plaque placed by the American Society of Anesthesiologists at the centenary of nitrous oxide. It unambiguously credits Wells with the discovery of anaesthesia.

Downstream 120 miles is Hartford, Connecticut where Wells spent most of his adult life and where his ill-starred work on the inhalation of nitrous oxide took place. Today, Hartford (Connecticut) is a typical American city with its original centre almost lost under a maze of freeways, but you can still find the line of Main

Street where Horace Wells had his office and where stood Union Hall, the site of the fateful public demonstration given by Gardner Quincy Colton on 10 December 1844. As a result of that demonstration Wells discussed with Colton, and an associate called John Riggs, 'pushing' the gas further than ever before. They convened the following morning in Wells's office where he inhaled the gas until he lost consciousness, and Riggs extracted a molar tooth. The site of this office is marked, and Hartford contains many other places of interest. Still standing on Main Street is the First Church of Christ in which Wells met, and later married, his wife, and the church has a stained glass window depicting them. Nearby Bushnel Park has a splendid memorial statue, and just to the south of the city centre is Cedar Hill cemetery where Wells and his family are buried. On the front of the tomb is the epitaph 'There shall be no pain', while at one end is the inscription 'I sleep to dream' and at the other 'I awaken to glory'. The chapel of Trinity College, which is on the road to Cedar Hill cemetery, has a carved pew-end with a profile of Wells.

The other major site is the Menczer Historical Museum of the Hartford Medical and Dental Society at 230 Scarborough Street. It has many treasures, but its heart, literally and metaphorically, is a room dedicated to Horace Wells and his memorabilia. There is his practice day book (which also records his dealings with Morton), the passport Wells used for his trip to the French Academy in Paris to try and obtain recognition for his priority in the field of anaesthesia by inhalation, and also a certificate of recognition from the UK which was produced when nitrous oxide anaesthesia was re-introduced at the end of the 1860s [2].

INJUSTICE TO WELLS

These relics bring into sharp relief how badly Horace Wells was treated in his own time — and since, for subsequent historians have not set the balance right. Consider what Stanley Sykes had to say in his *Essays* [3]: 'We know that he (Wells) was irresolute, wayward and volatile for he kept abandoning his dental practice in order to make a living in strange and unusual ways, such as buying pictures in Paris to sell in the United States, and other queer ventures. . . . 'What really possessed Horace Wells that he had such an unhappy and unsuccessful life and such a tragic death? As I see it, he was a man who was easily depressed and discouraged, too easily led and influenced by others; for after one partial public failure, he completely abandoned his attempts to publicise nitrous oxide anaesthesia which had already been satisfactory in his hands in a number of cases.'

Although some of the facts support these interpretations [4] more recent publications aim to set the record straight [5]. Consider Wells's curriculum vitae. He studied dentistry in Boston for 2 years and then set up practice in Hartford in 1836. Within 2 years he was successful enough to get married and within four he had published his *Essay on Teeth*, as definitive an account of dentistry at the time as there is. In 1842 he devised a child's dental regulator, making him a pioneer of orthodontic practice as well as of anaesthesia. In the same year he started to train others (not only Morton) and in 1843 the City of Hartford awarded him a prize of $100 (then a significant sum of money) for best dentistry. He was also active as an inventor. This is not an 'irresolute, wayward and volatile' individual. The death notice in the *Connecticut Courant* hardly confirms Sykes' view either, even allowing for the traditional kindness of the obituary writer: 'The death of this gentleman has caused a profound and melancholy sensation in this community.

He was an upright and estimable man, and has the esteem of all who knew him. Of undoubted piety, simplicity and generosity of character, enthusiastic in the pursuits of science, and having just been acknowledged as the discoverer of etherisation in surgical operations, he was regarded with the highest respect by all our citizens, and there was no-one who seemed less likely to meet the sad fate that has befallen him.'

However, there was a darker side to Horace Wells. Advertisements in the press of the time reveal periods of suspension of his practice because of 'ill-health', and the sordid nature of his final offence — assaulting a prostitute — implies mental derangement. An obituary notice in the *Newhaven Journal*, further away from home, was perhaps nearer to the mark. 'He was subject to great mental depression amounting almost to disease.' Consider also, some quotes from his suicide notes: 'I cannot proceed — my hand is too unsteady, and my whole frame is convulsed in agony. My brain is on fire.' 'I feel that I am fast becoming a deranged man, or I would desist from this act. I cannot live and keep my reason, and on this account God will forgive the deed. I can say no more.' Surely this poor man was a manic depressive.

MEMORABILIA OF MORTON

With this sobering thought in mind, the tourist can begin the journey back to Boston and to some memorabilia of WTG Morton. Just off the main road from Hartford, Connecticut to Worcester, Massachusettts is Charlton, Massachusetts. On the south side of Route 20 is a memorial to Morton, about 100 yards east of the farm track that leads to the house where he was born. There is a plaque to the right of the doorway. Returning to Boston, all of the buildings associated with the two dentists have been swept away under modern development, but Tremont Row may still be found. It was at number 19 Tremont Row that Morton probably first used ether. A little to the west of there lies the Boston Public Garden, in the north-west corner of which is the Ether Monument. Because of the great controversy between Morton and Jackson the name of the discoverer was originally left blank, resulting in it being known for a while as the 'Either' Memorial! Finally the interested tourist should visit Mount Auburn cemetery in Cambridge, on the north side of the Charles River. This is the burial place of Morton, and of many of the witnesses to his historic demonstration.

REFERENCES

(1) *An historical guide to New England pertaining to the discovery of anaesthesia*. Wood Library-Museum, Park Ridge, Illinois: American Society of Anesthesiologists, Inc, 1972.
(2) Wildsmith JAW, Menczer LF. A British footnote to the life of Horace Wells. *Br J Anaesth* 1987; **59**: 1067–9.
(3) Sykes WS. *Essays on the first hundred years of anaesthesia — volume 2*. Edinburgh: E & S Livingstone, 1961.
(4) Menczer LF, Mittleman M, Wildsmith JAW. Horace Wells. *JADA* 1985; **110**: 773–6.
(5) Wolfe R, Menczer LF. *I awaken to glory: essays celebrating the sesquicentennial of Horace Wells's discovery of anaesthesia*. Canton: Science History Publications, 1994.

Sights and sites in Edinburgh

D Wright

Original presentation Edinburgh 1989

There are many places in Edinburgh of historical interest to anaesthetists. As to definitions—a sight is a spectacle, an object of special interest and a site is the situation, especially of a building. Some places are indeed objects of specific interest in themselves; other places merely mark where something has been in the past. Knowing what was there, however, allows us to retain our historical perspective and may help to preserve other important features of our past.

Figure 1 shows a map on which the sites are shown and the appendix has some helpful hints about access and transport. All the places are within 2 or 3 miles of the centre of Edinburgh and several are much closer.

The list of places starts with two sites within 300 yards of South Bridge; unfortunately the original buildings no longer stand. Joseph Black lived at 58 Nicholson Street and James Syme ran a surgical hospital in Minto House in Chambers Street. Joseph Black, one of the great figures of eighteenth century Scottish science, lived from 1728–1799 and was best known for his discoveries of carbon dioxide in 1754 and the principle of latent heat in 1762.

As one of the characters of Edinburgh medicine he was much admired for his science—and for the general character of his life. He was described by Lord Cockburn as a 'striking and beautiful person, tall, very thin and cadaverously pale: his hair carefully powdered though there was little of it. He wore black speckless clothes, silk stockings, silver braces and either a slim green umbrella or a genteel brown cane. The general frame and air were feeble and slender. No lad could be irreverent towards a man so pale, so gentle, so elegant, so illustrious'.

'He died while sitting at table with his usual fare, a few prunes, some bread and a little milk diluted with water. Having the cup in his hand and feeling the approach of death, he sat it down carefully on his knees, which were joined together and kept it steadily in his hand in the manner of a person perfectly at ease, and in this attitude, and without a writhe on his countenance, he expired placidly, as if an experiment has been wanted, to show his friends the ease with which he could die'.

He lived for a number of years at 58 Nicholas Street and afterwards the house became the Asylum for the Blind in 1807. There has over the years been widespread change in this street and the site, about 100 yards south of the College of Surgeons is now occupied by a Cooperative supermarket. One might remember Black when passing, because of the CO_2 in COOP.

James Syme moved into Minto House in 1829. Syme, who lived from 1799–1870, was Professor of Clinical Surgery from 1833 and is probably best known to students of the history of anaesthesia as the subject of scathing attacks by Stanley Sykes in his *Essays on the First 100 Years of Anaesthesia*. Earlier in 1820, Syme had failed to get on to the staff of the Royal Infirmary when a vacancy arose. Piqued,

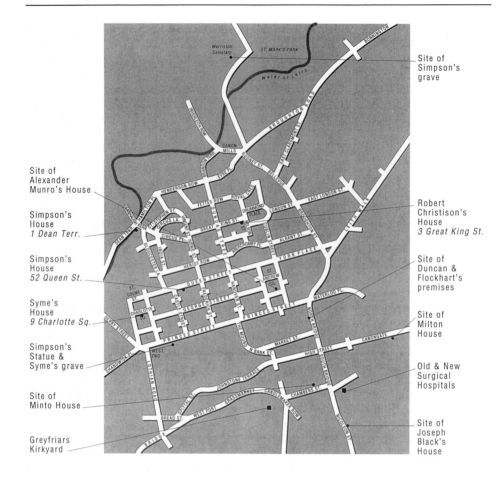

Figure 1 *Map of central Edinburgh showing sites of anaesthetic interest*

he decided to open his own hospital, and, collecting money by subscription, bought and equipped Minto House. It was at this time a three storeyed building of 15 rooms, surrounded by a garden and situated to the north of Argyle Street. This overlooked the Cowgate with an entrance from Horse Wynd. Two house surgeons, John Brown and Alexander Peddie, paid Syme £100 each for the privilege of working with him and the hospital took public patients, particularly those involved in accidents. It rapidly became popular, developing an international reputation, and was a major factor in Syme's advancement to the Chair of Surgery. John Brown became amongst other things, an author of some note and is perhaps best known for his short story 'Rab and his friends', which poignantly describes an operation carried out in Minto House by Syme in those pre-anaesthetic days. In 1833 Syme was successful in his application for the Chair and Minto House closed as a surgical hospital, being a medical charity for some years until in 1852 it became, for 4 years, the Maternity Hospital. Minto House was finally demolished during the construction of the present Chambers Street, which started in 1871.

In parenthesis we may consider where the Maternity Hospital was between 1846 and 1852. Milton House, which like Minto House, no longer exists, stood in the Canongate, to the east of Moray House, near where Milton House School now stands. This is where the first hospital use of chloroform in obstetrics took place. By 1848 the hospital report, presented by James Simpson, was able to state 'Since the use of chloroform became general, in the Maternity Hospital, shortly after the discovery of chloroform, 95 women in all have been delivered in this house under its influence. . . . The women have been invariably found deeply grateful for the relief to their sufferings afforded by the anaesthetic influence of chloroform'.

At either end of Chambers Street can be found sites of considerable antiquity, relatively unchanged, both of which are worth visiting. At the east end of Chambers Street, across the South Bridge, is Infirmary Street. Walking down Infirmary Street there is a view of what started its life as the High School and was converted in 1832 into what became known as the Old Surgical Hospital.

It was in this hospital that the first operation was performed using chloroform as an anaesthetic, with Professor James Miller as the surgeon and Simpson holding the patient, a 4 or 5 year old gaelic speaking child with osteomyelitis of the radius. Also attending were Robert Christison and, by chance, Professor Dumas of Paris (who had first ascertained chloroform's chemical composition in 1835).

The building started life on 24 June 1777, the foundation being laid of what was to be the second High School (the first had been built in 1578). One of the first pupils, in 1779, was the young (Sir) Walter Scott. By 1828 the school decamped to its third site, newly built on Calton Hill, and the disused school house was sold to the managers of the Royal Infirmary for £3500. It was adapted to form a surgical hospital and opened in 1832 with 32 surgical beds, an operating theatre having been built on the back. The New Surgical Hospital was added to the Old, when in 1853, a purpose built extension was opened with a further 128 beds. The Infirmary also purchased or leased other houses in and around the area of Surgeon's Square and it was in this complex of assorted and often unsuitable buildings that Simpson, Syme and Lister worked.

Today the buildings appear almost unchanged from the outside, the same patterns of lichen blackened stones are visible in old photographs which span some 136 years. The Old Surgical Hospital is part of the University's Dental School and the New Surgical Hospital, the Geography Department. The area behind the Old Surgical Hospital was called Surgeon's Square and the old Surgeon's Hall of 1697 still stands there. On the west side of the Square used to stand the dissecting rooms that Robert Knox used and which were supplied with bodies by the infamous Burke and Hare. Next door to this were the rooms of the Royal Medical Society.

These buildings, the Old and New Surgical Hospitals and the old Surgeon's Hall can be viewed from the outside and are well worth a visit, the atmosphere on a quiet weekend is most impressive. No noise but a clamouring of memories.

At the other end of Chambers Street is the Kirk of the Greyfriars, the first church to be built after the Reformation and opened in 1620. The National Covenant was signed in the church in 1638 and many famous Edinburgh inhabitants were buried in the churchyard in succeeding centuries. Two graves of interest to anaesthetists are those of Joseph Black and Alexander Monro. Black's is in a part of the churchyard now kept locked, but Monro's grave, with that of his father, is easily found by taking the path which goes due south from the south-west corner of the Kirk. The grave of father and son is a little way down on the right. Monro secundus (1773–1817) is known from anatomy as the namer of the foramen of Monro, but he is also important for his thoughts on resuscitation.

William Cullen wrote in a letter to Lord Cathcart 'concerning the recovery of patients drowned and seemingly' dead which was published in *Journals of the Board of Police* in 1774. 'Dr Monro informs me, it is very practicable to introduce directly into the glottis and trachea, a crooked tube, such as the catheter used for a male adult. For this he offers the following directions. The surgeon should place himself on the right side of the patient and introducing the forefinger of the left hand at the right corner of the patient's mouth, he should push the point of it behind the epiglottis, and using this as a directory, he may enter the catheter, which he holds in his right hand at the left corner of the patient's mouth till the end of it is passed beyond the point of the forefinger and it is then to be let fall, rather than pushed into the glottis, and through this tube, by a proper syringe attached to it, air may be with certainty be blown into the lungs'.

Greyfriars Kirkyard has an atmosphere of its own. The older seventeenth century graves and their carvings have an eerie sensation with the carvings of skeletons and latin mottoes usually of the 'cras mihi, hodie tibi' type.

Leaving Greyfriars, one can then walk to the New Town. Although parts of the town seem quite unchanged, there is no trace of Alexander Monro's house in St Andrew Square. He lived at 30 and 32 at various times. Number 32 has been replaced by an insurance office and number 30 is now the entrance to the bus station.

Princes Street has several sites of interest. James Syme was born at 56 Princes Street in 1799. The house is now an hotel. The Scottish Society of Anaesthetists was founded in the Balmoral Hotel on February 20 1914. The hotel is now a Littlewoods store, to the west of the foot of the Mound. Just off Princes Street at the east end, on the North Bridge under the North British Hotel, there is a plaque marking the site of Duncan and Flockhart's premises in 1847, when the chemists provided chloroform for Simpson.

At the west end of Princes Street in the gardens on the south side of the street is the statue of James Simpson. This was paid for by public subscription after his death, was sculpted by William Brodie and cast in bronze in London. When it was unshipped in Leith an arm came off, but in 1873 it was unveiled with due ceremony by Lady Galloway before a distinguished gathering. It is not set off to advantage by its leafy surroundings but it has a certain attraction. There is an irony in that it overlooks James Syme's grave in St John's churchyard just to the west, Syme dying a few weeks after Simpson.

Syme's town house, at the peak of his powers, was 9 Charlotte Square and after his death the house was lived in by his son-in-law, Joseph Lister. Three houses close to this on the north side of Charlotte Square are now owned by the National Trust and it is possible to visit number 7. Five rooms on three floors can be seen in number 7, called The Georgian House and these give a good understanding of what these houses were like, at least in the eighteenth century.

Moving out of Charlotte Square into Queen Street one comes to number 52 which was the home of James Simpson from 1845 until his death in 1872. The house now belongs to the Church of Scotland. They allow visitors to see the downstairs front room, known as the Chloroform Room, where the experiments of 1847 took place. The ground floor was, in later years used as a consulting room for poorer patients, usually seen by Simpson's assistants, with the well-to-do patients being seen by Simpson himself on the first floor. The family lived in the upper floors. The house must have seen some entertaining occasions during the 1840s, 50s and 60s. Apart from chloroform and other post-prandial inhalations, people came from all over the world to see Simpson, whose hospitality was well known.

There were always visitors, coming for breakfast, for lunch and even for dinner, although he tried to keep the evening meal a family affair. He eventually acquired in addition, a house in Trinity, to which he escaped at times for peace and quiet, but it was at 52 Queen Street that he died on 6 May 1870.

He was buried on 13 May and a contemporary account tells the story. 'The day was warm and bright and vast crowds thronged every street from his house to the grave on the southern slope of Warriston Cemetery, and on every side were heard ever and anon the lamentations of the poor, while most of the shops were closed and the bells of the churches tolled. The spectators were estimated at 100 000 and the most intense decorum prevailed. An idea of the length of the procession may be gathered from the fact that although it consisted of men marching in sections of four it took upwards of 33 minutes to pass a certain point'.

Warriston Cemetery is approached via Warriston Gardens which comes off Inverleith Row to the south of Heriot's sports ground. On entering the gates of the cemetery, there is a path leading almost due south off which several paths run to the east between lines of graves. Between the 4th and 5th paths from the gate, about 100 yards from the south running path, lies the Simpson family grave. The grave is marked by an obelisk engraved with the names and dates of Simpson's wife and children. Several feet in front of the obelisk on plain sandstone, with simple squared design is engraved 'Sir James Young Simpson, Bart MD DCC, born 1811 died 1870'. The grass grows high on either side and there is a feeling of quiet repose, with a sense of damp decay and perhaps unintentional neglect.

James Simpson spent his early years in Stockbridge. In his boyhood, and as a student, he lived with his brother, David Simpson, who was a baker and had a shop at 1 Raeburn Place on the corner of Dean Street. When he first began to practise as a physician he moved a few yards into town to a flat at 2 Deanhaugh Street. In 1840 he was living in 1 Dean Terrace, a little nearer to town and it was to this flat that he brought his wife, just before he gained the Professorship of Midwifery.

Closer into the centre of Edinburgh is 3 Great King Street, where Sir Robert Christison lived. Christison (1797–1882) was Professor of Medical Jurisprudence and then Materia Medica. Famous as a toxicologist, he chaired the committee which issued the first pharmacopoeia of Great Britain and Ireland and is well known for his pharmacological researches, amongst other things, on the Calabar bean.

Finally at 28 Heriot Row, is the house of Sir Douglas McLagan, born in 1812 and died here on 5 April 1900. He was Professor of Medical Jurisprudence from 1862 to 1897 and was in earlier life a noted wit and raconteur.

He wrote many poems or lays for medical dinners or occasions and these were published in 1850 as *Nugae Canorae Medicae — Lays by the Poet Laureate of the New Town Dispensary*.

In conclusion, though it may appear that one three or four storey Georgian building looks much like another from the outside, the people and the events that existed within and without the houses should make this an interesting tour.

NOTES ON ACCESS TO SITES

1. Old and New Hospitals/Surgeon's Square.

From South Bridge, walk east down Infirmary Street and through the gates into High School Yards. The Old Surgical Hospital is facing you. At the right of the building there is a passageway. On the south side of this is the New Surgical Hospital. Through the passageway is the old Surgeon's Square with the old Surgeon's Hall on the South side. There seems to be open access to all this area, although not to the buildings.

2. Alexander Monro's Grave, Greyfriars Kirkyard.

From the southwest corner of the Kirk take the path running almost due south. The Monros' grave is about 50 yards down on the right. The Kirkyard is open from roughly 8 am to 4 pm daily.

3. The Georgian House, 7 Charlotte Square.

The National Trust for Scotland own this property which is open 10 am to 4.30 pm (2.00 pm–5.00 pm Sundays). There is a charge for admission.

4. Simpson's House, 52 Queen Street.

The Church of Scotland own this building which is open for small numbers of visitors during office hours to see the Chloroform Room on the ground floor.

5. Warriston Cemetery.

By bus 23 or 27 from the Princes Street end of Hanover Street to Warriston Gardens (Inverleith Row). The cemetery is at the east end of Warriston Gardens. Entering through the gates there is a path running south with paths running east off this between lines of graves. The Simpson grave is between the fourth and fifth paths about 100 yards from the south running path and is marked by an obelisk and a plain sandstone inscription.

The family of Joseph Thomas Clover (1825–1882)

Aileen K Adams

Original presentations Edinburgh 1989 and Epsom 1990

Following the death of John Snow in 1858, Joseph Thomas Clover became the leading anaesthetist in England. The main biographical facts of his life are well-known [1,2,3]. This account of his family and domestic life has resulted from the generosity of some of his descendants. When I first met them they had little knowledge of their ancestor's role in the development of anaesthesia, partly no doubt, because his children had little memory of their father. He had married late and when he died his eldest child was only 9 years old.

My interest began whilst I was Dean of the Faculty of Anaesthetists of the Royal College of Surgeons of England, now the Royal College of Anaesthetists. My desk faced a portrait of the young and handsome Clover aged about eighteen, painted by his uncle, a previous Joseph Clover. This was loaned to the Royal College of Surgeons in 1949 by Clover's son Martin. In 1987 Professor Sir Robert Macintosh donated to the Faculty a number of items which had belonged to Clover. These were his diplomas and certificates, together with a tantalus of four decanters which Macintosh had had in his own home for some 35 years. I wanted to know more. In his Clover lecture of 1952, Macintosh, then Nuffield Professor at Oxford, had described how he first became acquainted with members of the Clover family [4], and he now elaborated this story. He told me he searched the *Medical Directory* and wrote to the only Clover in it, finding to his delight that this general practitioner was Martin, Clover's son. Their acquaintanceship blossomed, and both Martin in Worcestershire and his sister Mary in Cambridge were pleased to talk about the distinguished father of whom their personal memories were so sparse. Later another Clover, his great-grandson Anthony, whilst an undergraduate at Christ Church, had dined in Pembroke with the Nuffield Professor, but thereafter they lost contact.

Taking up the search, I tracked down Mr Anthony Clover in Luxembourg. Although he had researched the family history extensively, he had not appreciated the distinguished role his great-grandfather had played in the history of anaesthesia. He believed him to have made his name as a surgeon, which indeed he originally was — he had become FRCS in 1850 before changing to anaesthesia. Nor did Anthony know that as head of the family he was the owner of the painting in the Royal College of Surgeons. Later I met Miss Dorothea Clover, grand-daughter, and she shared with me memories of her grandmother.

SOURCES OF MATERIAL

Clover's son Martin and his daughter Mary both gave Macintosh many of their father's papers, diaries, pieces of apparatus and personal possessions. These were first kept in Oxford in the Nuffield Department of Anaesthetics but have since been widely dispersed. A few remain there, but the bulk of the papers and diaries were transferred to the Woodward Biomedical Library of the University of British Columbia in Vancouver, and have been described by Thomas [5]. Small collections of documents are held in the Wellcome Institute for the History of Medicine and in the Royal College of Anaesthetists, others will be referred to later. Mr Anthony Clover has a large collection of personal letters written by Clover to his wife.

FAMILY LIFE IN VICTORIAN SOCIETY

In 1869 Joseph Clover married Mary Anne Hall, the daughter of a Cambridge don, who on his marriage became Canon of St Paul's Cathedral and Professor of Mathematics at King's College, London. Some letters written by Clover to his fiancée are in Macintosh's collection. One, written light-heartedly, nevertheless reveals something of his perfectionist nature: 'I like to see good housekeeping — as I like to see good painting and hear good music, in a word the best of everything is good enough for me — but I am not an epicure'.

Clover married at the age of 44; he had five children in quick succession and died whilst they were still young. Therefore, there is little family memory of him, either as a father or as a man. He was heavily involved in his profession as an anaesthetist in London and worked immensely hard, in spite of the fact that he was never physically robust and suffered a succession of illnesses. The Clovers moved amongst a highly intellectual coterie, including Ruskin, Burne-Jones, the Terry family and Isambard Kingdom Brunel. It seems clear that they were at ease in this society. Gray in his Clover lecture [6] pointed out that Clover's notebooks included drawings of considerable artistic merit, as well as quotations showing him to be well-read in classical literature.

He was obviously careful with money. He retained among his papers the record of his income and expenditure as a student, as well as many letters referring to his fees as an anaesthetist, while another letter barely conceals a degree of pride in having renegotiated the marriage settlement from his father-in-law, to the Clovers' advantage. An interesting feature of his papers is that they are written in two different styles of handwriting — an untidy cursive script and a neater, more legible copperplate. The cursive style seems certainly to be in Clover's own hand for it matches his letters. Previous authors had noted these differences and wondered whether some writings had been copied by someone else. This seems unlikely, as the manuscripts in both styles are working papers with subsequent corrections to their texts. It is known that Clover could write in both styles. At the age of 13 he won a certificate for copperplate when a pupil at the Grey Friars School in Norwich. Perhaps he reverted to this for his more permanent records, such as financial accounts and lecture notes.

His wife Mary appears to have been well known as a socialite, and she was a talented artist. She was largely responsible for bringing up the children. Often they were in Norfolk while Clover was busy in London. Mary outlived her husband by 47 years. In later life she was described by her grand-daughter as having looked, dressed and behaved rather like Queen Victoria.

CLOVER'S CHILDREN

The firstborn died in infancy. Martin, the next son was born on 23 December 1873. He went to Shrewsbury, one of the first five 'public schools' recognized under the

Act of Parliament of 1882. There he did well both scholastically and athletically; he rowed the College boat, was treasurer of the Boat Club, played first eleven soccer, and went on to medical school. He qualified from University College Hospital in 1900 and settled into general practice in Kermsey, Worcestershire. It was whilst practising here that he and Macintosh met. He seems to have been a quiet, diffident man. When asked if he had thought of becoming an anaesthetist he replied he had certainly not, 'I could never have lived up to my father's reputation'. Martin died in 1959 and his only child Nancy never married.

The second son Harry was born on Christmas Eve 1874. He seems to have been a clever boy, who started well but failed to live up to his early promise. He was a scholar at Winchester where he is depicted as physically strong and good looking, and where he kept wicket for the College cricket team. He left a year early and won an open scholarship to Cambridge, obtained his BA and joined the army in 1900, serving in the Boer War and earning a medal with three clasps. In 1906 he became a barrister in the Inner Temple, married and had a son John. However he does not seem to have been cut out for professional life, preferring to live on his private income and winning competitions at bridge and chess. On the outbreak of war in 1914 he rejoined the army, but he was soon discharged, drinking heavily and with his marriage in ruins. His contribution to anaesthesia was as begetter of John Hugh Peterson Clover, the father of Anthony who is the present head of the family.

The third son Alan was born in 1875. Like his eldest brother he went to Shrewsbury and he too did well. He was a good cricketer and cross country runner, who went on to Cambridge and became an Anglican priest. He continued to be keen on cricket and also took to writing poetry. Sadly, he later developed mental illness and eventually died in a mental hospital. Before the onset of this illness, he married into a Bristol family and had two children. The eldest, always known as Joey, was a very talented musician who took up a post in Cape Town. He served in the South African Army in the Second World War, was taken prisoner at Tobruk, and was shot dead during his third escape attempt. The second child, Dorothea still lives in Bristol, where she remains active and interested in family affairs. In 1985 she kindly donated some Clover memorabilia to the Monica Britten Memorial Hall of Medical History at Frenchay Hospital, Bristol. She was for long the possessor of a portrait of Ellen Terry at the age of 15 painted by Clover's wife, and this she has donated to the Old Vic Theatre Museum in Bristol.

Thus all three of Clover's sons seem to have inherited something of their father's outstanding intellectual capabilities, as well as being fine athletes, though only the eldest pursued a conventional career. It was Clover's fourth child, his daughter Mary, who displayed not only intellectual talents but also much of her father's pioneering spirit and immense capacity for work.

Mary was born on 14 October 1876, and was only 6 when he died, but she was obviously proud of her father. This is clear from her letters to Macintosh, whilst her archive in Girton College, Cambridge includes a number of newspaper cuttings about him. Mary went to Notting Hill High School, and thence up to Girton to read mathematics, graduating in 1898. She remained in Cambridge all her life, not as a scholar but as an academic administrator of the greatest capability, serving Girton as secretary for 30 years. Plainly she was 'a ball of fire'. Her obituary reads: 'Working with Miss Clover was a lively experience. She throve on crises, and I sometimes suspected that she was postponing some urgent matter until the eleventh hour in order to have the excitement and challenge of a last minute rush' [7]. When she became secretary, Mary inherited a huge debt incurred when the College extended its buildings, overspending by £24000, a huge amount which had to be found somehow. She received an offer of half this sum provided the College raised the rest within one year. She hurled herself into the task with relish, saying 'we've got the moon, now we go for the sun'. She went round demanding, cajoling, threatening and persuading, and the money was raised on time.

During World War I, Mary was administrator of a military hospital in Cambridge. She liked wearing the Red Cross uniform because 'it saved such a lot of trouble about clothes'. For many years she was the very active treasurer of the Women's University Settlement in Southwark, one of the earliest examples of social work in London. Her paperwork shows her to have been meticulously accurate, even obsessive. Later she was one of the first women in Cambridge to own and drive a motor car, a yellow bullnosed Morris, she called Phyllis, which she kept on the road until well into World War II.

Like many perfectionists, 'Great-Aunt Mary' was not always popular with her family, who did not invariably appreciate her tendency to organize their affairs. Nevertheless she always helped out in crises, for example becoming John Hugh's guardian when Harry died young, and looking after Alan's family when he became mentally ill. Through Macintosh, the anaesthetists in Cambridge came to know Mary in her old age. He heard she had become frail and disabled, and asked the then senior anaesthetist Harold Youngman to visit her, to show that the specialty had not forgotten the surviving child of a pioneer anaesthetist. As a token of appreciation, she gave Youngman some sheets of lecture notes and case histories written by Clover, which are now in the Department of Anaesthesia at Addenbrooke's Hospital. Mary died in 1965 aged 89 [8].

COMMEMORATION

Clover died at the height of his career aged 57. Many tributes were paid to him in obituaries [9–12]. His widow had four children from 9 to 6 to educate. Her husband left £27932 14s 2d, a substantial sum which provided well for the family. All the children went to university, and all four have benefited our specialty by passing on to us directly or indirectly, memories and possessions of their distinguished father.

Clover is commemorated by the Royal College of Anaesthetists in its biennial Clover Lecture first delivered in 1948. Together with John Snow, he has been adopted as supporter of the Royal College's Arms, granted in 1989. Two plaques have been erected in his memory. One in the Market Place at Aylsham in Norfolk on the site of his birthplace, was unveiled on 6 May 1992 in the presence of Clover's great-great-grandson James, then a medical student. The other, a green plaque at 3 Cavendish Place on the site of his London home, was unveiled on 2 March 1994 by Miss Dorothea Clover, in the presence of both Anthony and his son James Clover.

ACKNOWLEDGEMENTS

Mr Anthony D Clover has generously transferred the loan of the portrait to the Royal College of Anaesthetists where it is now housed. I am greatly indebted to him for the generous way in which he has shared his knowledge of the family, derived from the personal letters in his possession, and to Miss Dorothea Clover for her recollections.

Lady Ann Macintosh has kindly allowed me access to Clover's letters which remain in her care following the transfer of her late husband's collection to the Wellcome Institute for the History of Medicine.

Mr Neville Ripley MBE, previously of Penlon Ltd, was given by Sir Robert Macintosh some photographs and apparatus belonging to Clover. Mr Ripley has most generously donated these to the Royal College of Anaesthetists.

REFERENCES

(1) Marston AD. A short survey of the life and work of Joseph Clover. *The Medical Press* 1946; **CCXVI**: 455–8.
(2) Marston AD. The life and achievements of Joseph Thomas Clover. *Annals Royal Coll Surg Eng* 1949; **4**: 267–80.
(3) Woollam CHM. Joseph T Clover (1825–1882). *Current Anaesth Crit Care* 1994; **5**: 53–61.
(4) Macintosh RRM. MSS of Clover Lecture 19 March 1952. Contemporary Medical Archives Centre, Wellcome Institute for the History of Medicine. PP/RRM. D1/19.
(5) Thomas KB. The Clover/Snow Collection. *Anaesthesia* 1972; **27**: 436–49.
(6) Gray TC. The disintegration of the nervous system. *Annals Royal Coll Surg Eng* 1954; **15**: 402–19.
(7) Peace KM. Obituary: Mary Clover. *Girton Review* 1965; Easter Term: 34–37. Girton College, Cambridge.
(8) Adams AK. Letter to the editor. *Anaesthesia* 1973; **28**: 213.
(9) Obituary: JT Clover. *Lancet* 1882; **Oct 7**: 597.
(10) Obituary: JT Clover. *Brit J Dent Sci* 1882; **LXXV**: 1021–3.
(11) Obituary: JT Clover. *J Brit Dental Assoc* 1882; **III**: 555–7.
(12) Browne B. Royal Society of Medicine: Section of Anaesthetics. *Lancet* 1913; **Mar 22**: 824–5.

Thomas Skinner

Phillida Frost

Original presentation Edinburgh 1989

The Logo of the History of Anaesthesia Society shows a Bellamy Gardner mask—
one of the many varieties of the open or ether mask. The Schimmelbusch is the
type most familiar to anaesthetists. It was described in 1890 and used in Wales up
to the mid 1960s. But 30 years before Schimmelbusch's modification, the wire-
framed mask had been invented by a Scottish obstetrician then working in
Liverpool. It is Thomas Skinner to whom we owe the concept of the open mask,
yet his name is virtually unknown.

Skinner was born in Edinburgh in 1825, the third son of Robert Skinner. His
elder brother William, known as Baillie Skinner, was later Town Clerk of
Edinburgh. Thomas was originally destined for a business career and entered an
office, but in 1849 he enrolled at Edinburgh University and the Royal College of
Surgeons as a medical student. He qualified in 1853, having been awarded the
Gold Medal in Midwifery. This was presented by Sir James Young Simpson, then
Professor of Medicine and Midwifery, who had described the effects of chloroform
in 1847. After qualification, Skinner left Edinburgh for Lochmaben, Dumfries,
until 1855 when he returned as private assistant to Simpson, living in his home at
52 Queen Street.

He took the MD St Andrews by examination in October 1857, and soon
afterwards moved to Liverpool where he set up practice as an obstetrician and
gynaecologist. He must have been a formidable figure in the city—assistant to
Simpson, gold medal winner and an MD. Soon he was active in many societies, as
early as March 1858, he read a paper before the Liverpool Medical & Surgical
Society defending the use of chloroform in natural labour. This was later
published with a dedication to Simpson [1]. At the Liverpool Medical Institute he
actively supported a resolution debarring from membership those who practised
homeopathy.

ANAESTHESIA—SKINNER'S 'FRAME'

Skinner published numerous papers, some reporting cases he had encountered in
Lochmaben. In May 1862, he read a paper before the Obstetric Society of London
entitled 'Anaesthesia in midwifery—with new apparatus for its safer and more
economical induction by chloroform' [2]. After a lengthy support of the use of
chloroform in labour, he described the new apparatus. The idea came to him he
said, on hearing of Simpson's administration of the agent by dropping it on a
cambric handkerchief cupped in the palm of the hand. There were problems with
not being able to see precisely where the drug was being dropped, and also in
protecting the eyes. He claimed that his apparatus solved both these difficulties.

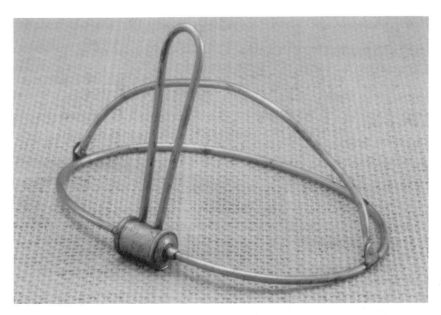

Figure 1 *Skinner's Mask, courtesy the Association of Anaesthetists of Great Britain and Ireland, and Department of Medical Illustration, St Bartholomew's Hospital*

He described a wire frame 'like a fencing mask but covering only the lower half of the face and covered with a layer of domette. For convenience it has a moveable handle and is otherwise made up so that it can be carried in the pocket or hat'. He also described a drop bottle which at one inversion delivered 'no more than 30 minims and no less than 10'. There is an illustration from which it is very difficult to visualize the mask, and the information that Messrs Maw of Aldersgate undertook to produce it at a cost of 11s, including a case.

It seems certain that this simple apparatus was widely used. In Berlin at the Bethanien Hospital it was used for chloroform anaesthesia for 20 years, when it was superseded by the Junkers bottle. When in 1891 Dudley Buxton investigated the use of chloroform and its associated mortality, he noted that Skinner's frame was the apparatus most commonly used [3]. The mask was recommended in Probyn Williams' textbook of 1909, and appeared in a catalogue as late as 1938, priced 7s 6d.

In 1873 Skinner wrote to the *British Medical Journal* deploring the use of inhalers with a common mouthpiece, pointing out that with his apparatus a clean cover could be used each time [4]. He did not believe that ether would ever supplant chloroform but as there were patients to whom it may have been safer to administer ether, he had adapted his inhaler to suit etherization as well. 'I shall soon give a detailed account of it and where it can be obtained'. No account of this modification has been discovered.

In 1890 the International Congress of Medicine met in Berlin and stressed the safety of ether anaesthesia over chloroform. In the same year, Kurt Schimmelbusch, then assistant to Von Bergman, a pioneer of aseptic surgery, described his open mask [5]. It is very like the Skinner frame. A drip tray was added by Rosthorn in 1897 [5], and by Kirchoff at about the same time [5], the Schimmelbusch mask eventually appearing in its familiar form.

A CHANGED CAREER

The story of the remainder of Skinner's life is surprising. In the early 1870s a flu-like illness left him with almost complete insomnia. This was helped by several years of travel. In America, he met a Dr Berridge of Philadelphia, a practising homeopath who prescribed sulphur for Skinner. The patient was so impressed that he became an active homeopath. In 1875 he resigned from the Liverpool Medical Institute as required by the statute which in 1858 he had supported. He gave up his obstetric practice and with another Englishman and two Americans he founded the *Anglo–American Journal of Homeopathy*, which survived for several years. In 1881, he moved to London where he soon had a large consulting practice with rooms in York Place, and a large house in Beckenham, Kent.

He remained very active, travelling to Scotland for the shooting, fishing and golf. In 1906, he moved to Inverness Terrace in London where a few months later he slipped on a banana skin and fell. He did not appear to have suffered any injury, but two weeks later developed abdominal pain, vomiting and melaena, and died within 48 hours. He was aged 81. No obituary appeared in the *British Medical Journal* or *The Lancet*, but the obituary in *The Homeopathic World* occupied no less than 23 pages [6]. Skinner, with two of his associates, were accounted 'the three liveliest minds in homeopathy in this country'. His invention of the open mask received the briefest of mentions.

In his lifetime Thomas Skinner was widely respected, firstly as an obstetrician, then as a homeopath. But undoubtedly his greatest contribution to medicine was the simple frame which in its many modifications was to be widely used for 100 years. The names of those who described modifications of his original frame are still well known. Thomas Skinner should also be remembered by anaesthetists, whose profession, to paraphrase Johnson on Oliver Goldsmith, he may 'merely have touched but which he certainly adorned'.

REFERENCES

(1) Skinner T. *Liverpool Medico-Chirurgical J* 1859; 1–8
(2) Skinner T. Anaesthesia in midwifery, with new apparatus for its safer and more economical induction by chloroform. *Br Med J* 1862; ii: 110.
(3) Report of the *Lancet* Commission. *Lancet* 1893; 1: 629–38.
(4) Skinner T. Anaesthetics and inhalers. *British Medical Journal* 1873; i: 353
(5) Duncum B. *The development of inhalational anaesthesia*. London: Oxford University Press, 1947; 251–2.
(6) Obituary. *The Homeopathic World* 1906; 498–521.

The Leicestershire life of Benjamin Ward Richardson

Sally E Garner

Original presentation Leicester 1988

Benjamin Ward Richardson was born in Somerby, a village to the east of Leicester, on 31 October 1828. He was the only son of Benjamin Richardson and his wife, Mary Ward. His mother died when he was a boy, but her early training exerted a permanent influence on his career. At an early age, he was placed under the care of a neighbouring clergyman, the Reverend Young Nutt, at Burrough School, Burrough-on-the-Hill. The young Richardson was very fortunate. His chosen mentor was a man of great learning who fostered the boy's love of physical and natural science, and entered thoroughly into the project of training him for the medical profession.

At the age of 13, Richardson's general education ceased and he was apprenticed to a local surgeon, Henry Hudson, in Somerby. Again he was fortunate. Mr Hudson was another enthusiast for science whose hobby was electrical experimentation. He was able to teach his apprentice much which in the future would prove of great use to him as a researcher and inventor. In 1845 Richardson entered Anderson's College, Glasgow, where in addition to his regular medical studies, he attended the lectures of Robert Knox the anatomist. His studies were interrupted when in 1847 he fell victim to a severe attack of 'famine fever'(probably typhus). This he contracted while attending a home delivery as a pupil at St Andrew's Laying-in Hospital, Glasgow. For the benefit of his health, the medical student was advised to return to England, where he became for a period, assistant to Mr Thomas Browne of Saffron Walden, Essex. During this time, the Reverend Nutt invited Richardson to visit Leicestershire to lecture and demonstrate in his old school. While at Somerby, he naturally called on his old master, surgeon Henry Hudson. Hudson gave Richardson a letter of introduction to his older brother, Edward Dudley Hudson, and later Richardson was to refer to this as the turning point in his life. The elder Hudson was also a surgeon who lived and practised at Narborough, some two dozen miles distant, on the other side of Leicester. It was a large and hard practice since Narborough was a poor area, with a large population of stocking weavers, this being the local cottage industry. Richardson was easily persuaded to leave Essex and become assistant to the elder Mr Hudson. Here he acquired a great deal of practical experience, but one episode was of particular significance. This was an attempt at resuscitation which, he said, 'from the moment of it, has been on my mind and has led me to many researches and beliefs that in its absence might never have been thought of'. Certainly he documented it very fully.

ATTEMPTED RESUSCITATION

The son of a local innkeeper, who was thought to have been lost in Australia, unexpectedly returned home. A feast was quickly arranged and the news spread

149

far and wide. At the celebration everything was going well, with plenty of food and drink, when two men were seen leaving the festivities, one of them looking extremely pale. After a little while, one man hurriedly returned saying his friend had collapsed in a paddock. There was a rush to render aid. The sick man was carried into a stable, and a doctor was summoned. That was Richardson. The facts presented to him were that a man of 35 years, a carpenter with a voracious appetite, had eaten hugely, until he had to leave the table from satiety, and had fallen to the ground. Upon examination, the man was stone dead. He was extremely cold, with the air outside very cold, no covering upon him, and they were not able to light a fire in the stable. In Richardson's own words: 'I therefore turned up my coat sleeves and commenced vigorously to set up artificial respiration, getting a man to help me who took my place and who, being strong, was an efficient aid. He kept this up for half an hour and some thinking that the man's feet were getting warmer and that his bloated face was more natural, he kept steadily vigorous. At last it seemed as if he choked and it was found that it was not so easy to squeeze out the air from his chest as if there was something in the way that stopped the breathing, so with my penknife I freely opened the trachea or windpipe with a quill that was at hand, cleared the windpipe, pushing up an obstruction into a space above and removing what could be removed. To my wonder, the artificial respiration began to take effect, the feet became warmer, and at last the man swung around his head and breathed of his own accord and looked as though he was struggling into life. He moved his hands and, letting him alone for a few minutes, he astonished everyone by the signs of life he manifested. Soon, however, he became choked up again from the stomach and all our efforts failed to restore breathing and in the end I had to ride home leaving a lifeless body, but duly accredited for many a long day afterwards with having raised a dead man back to life'. During the inquest there were some questions regarding the time the young man was laid in very cold circumstances prior to his breathing being restored. Richardson records that the fact a man could lie seemingly dead for nearly 2 hours in a very cold atmosphere, and then show signs of recovery with artificial respiration was new to him and momentous.

Shortly after these dramatic events, the young Richardson went back to Glasgow to complete his curriculum. Once qualified, he moved to the London area, and the start of a brilliant career. Reanimation, and particularly the effect of cold on resuscitation, were to feature largely in his researches. Some of his experiments were ingenious, and deserve to be better known.

RESEARCH ON REANIMATION

On electrical stimulation of respiration: 'By inserting a fine needle, insulated except at the point, into the larynx of an animal and the other needle into the diaphragm, and by regulating the shocks by means of a metronome . . . the most perfect appearance of natural respiration may be sustained . . .'.

On electrical stimulation of the circulation: 'In one experiment the negative pole from the battery was passed along the inferior vena cava to the right side of the heart and the opposite pole, armed with a sponge at its extremity, was placed over the heart externally. Sufficient action was excited to produce pulmonic current by contraction of the right ventricle . . .'. Surely he is here describing a pacemaker.

On 'artificial circulation' (his own terminology): Richardson also experimented with mechanical methods of restoring circulation, reasoning that with a syringe, blood could be artificially drawn through the lungs, to be oxygenated by simultaneous artificial respiration, and pumped on through the arterial circuit. Of course difficulties arose with coagulation, but on one occasion he did manage to get some circulation to produce muscular action, and for a brief period, all external phenomena of life.

On cardiac perfusion: 'By means of a machine which can be worked either by hand or by electromagnetism, I have been able . . . to introduce blood heated to 90°F into the coronary arteries of a dog by a rhythmic shock, and at the same rate as the stroke of the heart of the animal previous to its death . . . one hour and five minutes after complete death of the animal, its heart, perfectly still, cold and partially rigid, relaxed and exhibited for 20 minutes, active muscular motion, both atrial and ventricular . . . '.

Experiments such as these, together with his work on the effect of hypothermia, and his double-action bellows, mark Richardson as a man very much ahead of his time, and a true 'Victorian revivalist'. However, the great man never forgot his early training and experiences in Leicestershire. In *Vita Medica* [1] he is quite explicit—'I have held always in remembrance the case of the man I was called to near Narborough'.

REFERENCE

(1) Richardson BW. *Vita medica: chapters of medical life and work*. London: Longmans Green and Co, 1897.

R Lawson Tait — his influence on anaesthetic practice

ET Mathews

Original presentation Southend 1988

Robert Lawson Tait, the Birmingham surgeon, was described by William Mayo as the father of modern abdominal surgery. He was one of the most dynamic personalities of the Victorian period. According to his obituary in the *British Medical Journal* 'he showed a want of respect for age and authority which was remarkable, even in Birmingham . . . he was aggressive and unconventional . . . an original thinker who was never afraid to back his own opinions and fight for them for all he was worth' [1]. In a relatively short life — he died at 54 — he wrote some 328 papers and 270 letters on medical subjects, including many related to anaesthesia.

Tait's birth in 1845 in Edinburgh was unregistered. He was believed by some to be the natural son of James Young Simpson. He was educated at Heriot's Academy and Edinburgh University, and whilst a student he became a pupil of Simpson, living in his house and acting as his assistant. Simpson made a great impression on him, particularly by his work on chloroform, and Tait's interest in anaesthesia began at this time.

In 1867, Tait left Edinburgh for Wakefield. While there he published his first paper on anaesthesia, and another on the treatment of tetanus [2]. He used woorali, and this was one of the earliest reports in England on the therapeutic use of curare.

BIRMINGHAM, ANAESTHESIA AND CONTROVERSY

Lawson Tait moved to Birmingham in October 1870. This was an interesting time to arrive, at the beginning of the Chamberlain era in local politics. The town council led by Joseph Chamberlain took over the private companies supplying water, gas and sewage drainage. Tait liked the mood of change in the town. He stayed, later to become himself a councillor, and serve with great distinction on the public health committee.

Soon after his arrival, Tait unsuccessfully applied for a post as surgeon at the Birmingham General Hospital. He then joined Arthur Chamberlain, a brother of Joseph, in a campaign to establish a Women's Hospital. In less than a year they had succeeded; Tait was appointed to the staff, and rapidly established a national and international reputation and surgical practice.

Tait expressed a particular dread of deaths under anaesthesia. If he believed death threatened, he would close the abdomen, leaving the operation incomplete [3]. He was influenced by Benjamin Ward Richardson to change from sulphuric ether to methylene ether, believing it to be safer. However it was with methylene ether that Tait was to have his first death under anaesthesia. This was in June 1873, and he published an account of it with a commentary by Richardson [4]. His anaesthetist at the time was Dr Louisa Catherine Fanny Atkins, a very interesting woman. She was said to be a woman of great spirit, highly connected by birth, and educated in France. She left home as a young girl, went to India and married a Captain Atkins, many years her senior. When he died within a few years, she decided to train in medicine. She went to Zurich, one of the few schools then open to women, where she graduated MD in 1872. Although this degree was not acceptable for registration in England, Tait accepted her. He strongly believed in the right of women to practise medicine, and in 1874 published a paper of some 13 pages, setting forth his views on the medical education of women [5]. Dr Atkins achieved registration when the Irish College opened its doors to women in 1878.

For his essay on diseases of the ovary and their treatment, Tait was awarded the Hastings Gold Medal of the British Medical Association in 1873 [6]. This work included six pages on anaesthesia, which included much sound advice — for example the importance of an empty stomach, the removal of false teeth, and the lateral position for patients who vomit. He also stressed that 'even with an anaesthetic as safe as ether, it is absolutely necessary that the whole of the administrator's attention should be engrossed with it'.

Later in 1873, Tait came into serious conflict with the editor of the *British Medical Journal*. He organized a conversazione on anaesthesia at his house in Birmingham, inviting representatives of the three London weekly medical papers. The *British Medical Journal* refused his invitation, the editor attacking Tait over his arrangements for this meeting. He declared in the journal that 'such a meeting may degenerate into offensive and invidious public advertisement' and that it was a professionally objectionable exercise [7]. Tait replied that it was his intention to provide an occasion for Dr Benjamin Ward Richardson and Dr Norris to acquaint the profession with the results of their studies [8]. He also pointed out that the lay press were not invited and that the *British Medical Journal* had published accounts of many similar meetings. As usual, the editor had the last word, implying that Tait would get away with it on this occasion, but that he had been warned [9].

In 1876, Tait drew attention to the undesirable effects of inhaling cold anaesthetic gases. His apparatus for administering warm ether vapour was described in *The Practitioner* [10] and *The Lancet* [11]. In Sykes' *Essays on the First Hundred Years of Anaesthesia* this apparatus is subject to much ridicule, [12] but *The Practitioner* report of its successful use is not mentioned, nor the paper by Coste and Chaplin 60 years later which showed how difficult it was to explode or even ignite ether vapour produced in this way [13]. It is not my aim to defend Tait's apparatus, but to stress that he reported the importance of breathing warm gases as early as 1876. As with his advocacy of open ether, it was only after some years that his use of warmed gases was followed by others. A 1987 report [14] from Philadelphia claims the use of warmed gases produced a 31% reduction in recovery-room time following even short anaesthetics, the authors making no reference to Tait's original contribution in this field. The omission is not unexpected. Sir Francis Shipway [15] wrote of Lawson Tait's contributions to anaesthetic practice: '. . . these discoveries have been assumed to have originated in America. . . . It is fairly obvious that these (Tait's) are the first published accounts of open ether and of warmed ether. It is curious that they have been so long neglected' [15].

ANAESTHETIC STAFF

Tait's private practice was extensive. On occasion he attracted fees up to £1000. For this practice he engaged Dr Ann Elizabeth Clark. Dr Clark was born in 1844 at Street in Somerset, of a Quaker family. She trained in Edinburgh along with Miss Sophia Jex Blake and other female pioneers until 1874, when the school was closed to women. She then went to the new School of Medicine for Women in London, then to Switzerland to obtain a degree, the MD Berne; then later to Ireland to get the licence of the Irish College and thus her name on the Medical Register. In 1883 she became a Member of the Royal College of Physicians of Ireland. Dr Clark gave anaesthetics for Tait for many years, and overseas surgeons who came to watch him operate noted the expertise of his female physician anaesthetist [16]. Dr Clark wrote on tetanus and incontinence, but I have not traced any papers by her on anaesthetics. Tait reported that she used ether/chloroform mixtures in a Clover's inhaler very successfully. Other observers commented that she did not use the rebreathing bag with this apparatus.

In his hospital practice anaesthesia was administered by a nurse—for many years this was Sister Emily Nowers. In June 1895 Dr Mary Sturge, MD London, was appointed as anaesthetist to the Women's Hospital. The Medical Staff Committee reported enthusiastically: 'This addition is a source of satisfaction to the Board as, although they have every reason to be satisfied with the care the anaesthetics have been administered by Sister Emily, they have always held the opinion that anaesthetics ought only to be administered by a fully qualified practitioner' [17]. The Management Committee was also in favour, but from a different viewpoint: 'This appointment relieved the sister in charge of a very trying duty, and enabled her to give more time to the housekeeping. The new arrangement has resulted in an important saving in the housekeeping . . .'. The accounts show that the anaesthetist was paid £22 10s for the part she worked of the first year.

At the annual meeting in 1897, the medical staff reported that the position of the anaesthetist on the staff had been questioned. To regularize the situation they proposed a formal resolution that the anaesthetist be included in the membership of the staff. This was strongly attacked by Arthur Chamberlain and Lawson Tait [18]. Chamberlain opposed it on the grounds that the anaesthetist was paid and also had very little to offer; Tait endorsed these remarks, and did not consider that the anaesthetist—who must necessarily be a junior—should be put on the same level as the surgeons and himself. The proposal was withdrawn.

A BAD ANAESTHETIC, A GOOD RESULT

Despite these withering comments on anaesthetists, Tait, in the same year, did provide a more positive influence on the development of the specialty. This was indirect, and he was probably never aware of it. He had an operation for urethral calculus, the surgeon being Gilbert Barling, then a young man but later to become Sir Gilbert. The anaesthetist had qualified the previous year in Aberdeen. Now Tait was not the ideal build for an anaesthetic. Contemporaries described him as a short, stout man with a magnificent head, thick bull neck, corpulent body, podgy legs and small hands and feet; or as another saw him, the body of Bacchus and the head of Jove.

The anaesthetic was ether. Barling's account reads: 'Just as the perineal incision was made, I noticed that the patient was breathing badly. I saw he was black in the face and no air was entering the chest. The sight was an alarming one and to add to the trouble the anaesthetist dropped his tray and bolted from the room . . . I had visions of a coroner's inquest at which I, as a junior surgeon just beginning to get on his feet, would appear in the public's eye as the person who had killed Tait, the best known surgeon in Europe and America' [19]. I believe this incident was beneficial to our speciality, it being no coincidence that the same year Barling urged the promising young Dr McCardie to specialize in anaesthesia [20]. McCardie is regarded by Bryn Thomas and others, as the first provincial anaesthetist to devote himself exclusively to the specialty [21]. As to the young anaesthetist from Aberdeen, I have found no evidence that he was given any career advice following this episode, but I have been able to trace his subsequent career. He took up psychiatry and became the superintendent of a private mental hospital of which he was also the licensee.

CONCLUSION

The rapid decline in Tait's professional standing, and his financial failure about this time has not, as yet, been blamed on the hypoxic episode. He had many problems. He was involved in a libel action, was in dispute with the Medical Defence Union, participated in the Darwin controversy (he strongly supported Darwin), and in the anti-vivisection movement. He was the subject of slanderous allegations about his private life which were almost certainly untrue — and he had his urinary problems. After his many original contributions to surgery and anaesthesia, Tait's end was sad. He had to sell his yacht on the Solent, his houseboat on the Avon, his steam launch on the Severn, his country houses in the New Forest and at Cropthorne, and his fishing cottage at King's Bromley. He was forced to give up his private hospital, dispense with his staff, and sell his treasured collection of curios. He died in 1899 at his house in Llandudno. Following cremation in Liverpool, the ashes were returned to Llandudno. But later his widow had the urn buried in Edinburgh, in Warriston cemetery very near to the grave of the Simpson family. After Mrs Tait's death the stone on their grave was inscribed with the enigmatic tribute: 'She hath done what she could'.

REFERENCES

(1) Obituary. *Br Med J* 1899; **1**: 1561–4.

(2) Tait L. On the treatment of tetanus by woorali, calabar bean and chloral hydrate. *Lancet* 1870; **2**: 466.

(3) Tait L. Abstract of an address on one thousand abdominal sections. *Br Med J* 1885; **1**: 218–20.

(4) Tait L. Death under the administration of methylene ether, first fatal case recorded. *Medical Times and Gazette* 1873; **2**: 3.

(5) Tait L. On the medical education of women. *Birmingham Med Rev* 1874; **3**: 81–94.

(6) Tait L. *The pathology and treatment of diseases of the ovaries*, 4th ed. Birmingham & New York: Cornish Brothers & William Wood, 1883: 262–8.

(7) Notes to correspondents. *Br Med J* 1873; **2**: 563.

(8) Notes to correspondents. *Br Med J* 1873; **2**: 592.

(9) Notes to correspondents. *Br Med J* 1873; **2**: 622.

(10) Tait L. Note on a new method of administering ether vapour. *The Practitioner* 1876; **16**: 206–9.

(11) Tait L. New inventions — New ether inhaler. *Lancet* 1876; **1**: 721.

(12) Sykes WS. *Essays on the first hundred years of anaesthesia. Vol 1.* Edinburgh: Livingstone, 1960: 15–18.

(13) Coste JH, Chaplin CA. An investigation into the risks of fire or explosion in operating theatres. *Br J Anaesth* 1937; **14**: 115–29.

(14) Conahan III TJ, Williams GD, Apfelbaum Jl, Lecky JH. Airway heating reduces recovery time (cost) in outpatients. *Anesthesiology* 1987; **67**: 128–30.

(15) Shipway FE. Anaesthesia by warmed ether. *Br Med J* 1917; **1**: 826.

(16) Vander Veer A. Some personal observations on the work of Lawson Tait. *Am J Obstet Dis Women Child* 1885; **XVIII**: 673–88.

(17) Birmingham and Midland Hospital for Women. *Annual Report* 1896.

(18) Birmingham and Midland Hospital for Women. *Annual Report* 1897.

(19) Barling G. Reminiscences of Lawson Tait. *Birmingham Med Rev* 1931; **6**: 137–42.

(20) Barling G. Obituary, WJ McCardie. *Br Med J* 1939; **1**: 419.

(21) Thomas KB. *The development of anaesthetic apparatus.* London: Blackwell, 1975: 256.

Three lady anaesthetists of 1893

Elizabeth Gibbs

Original presentation Southend 1988

In 1988, with Dr Aileen Adams as Dean of the Faculty of Anaesthetists, it was interesting to reflect that just over 100 years previously, women had been unable to qualify in medicine in the United Kingdom. The Medical Register, first published in 1859, was designed for the protection of the public against unqualified practitioners. The requirement for registration was a degree in medicine awarded by any British university, or equivalent body. In 1859 only one woman's name appeared on the Register. Another was added in 1866, five more in 1877, and by 1893 there were 135 women on the Register.

The problems women faced to qualify in medicine were two-fold. At first, the British universities refused to admit women to their examinations. In 1862 the London University Senate decided that 'as women were neither a class nor a denomination' the University had no power to admit them [1]. However in 1876 the Irish College of Physicians and the Queen's University of Ireland admitted five women to their examinations, which accounts for the 1877 additions to the Register of the General Medical Council. In January 1878, the London University Senate laid before Convocation a new charter admitting women to all degrees of the University, and other examining bodies followed later.

The second problem these pioneering women faced was gaining access to clinical training. In 1874, the London School of Medicine for Women was founded, but it was not until 1877 that clinical access to the Royal Free Hospital was negotiated for their 17 students. This eased the way for women to qualify as doctors, as reflected in the Medical Register figures.

Once qualified, the women faced a further problem in that there were few hospitals where they could gain postgraduate experience. In London, hospitals specializing in women and children which accepted women as medical officers, included the Belgrave Children's Hospital and the New Hospital for Women. The latter was founded in 1866 and staffed entirely by women.

A further problem was that very few women doctors belonged to medical societies. Even the British Medical Association refused to accept female members until 1892. It is somewhat surprising therefore that in 1893, with 135 women's names on the Register, no fewer than three applied to become members of the new Society of Anaesthetists.

THE SOCIETY OF ANAESTHETISTS

This society was founded in London in 1893—the first anaesthetic society in the world. Its aims were to encouage the study of anaesthetics, and to promote and encourage friendly relations among members. At the second meeting of the provisional committee in June 1893, letters were read from the three women asking to be permitted to join the Society [2]. The Secretary of the provisional committee was instructed to reply that the committee had no power to decide as to the eligibility of the women for membership of the Society. It is obvious that the men of the provisional committee were not against women, they had just not thought about them. At their next meeting, just before the first General Meeting, the Secretary reported he had received notice from Dr Dudley Buxton of an amendment to Rule 4 of the proposed Society. This was to omit the words 'medical men' and to substitute in their place 'medical practitioners'. This was approved by the General Meeting, and in 1894 Mrs Frances Dickinson-Berry became the first woman member of the Society whose membership then numbered 40.

MRS FRANCES M DICKINSON-BERRY

Miss Frances Dickinson was born in 1857, the daughter of a barrister and Member of Parliament for Stroud. She was educated at home until she was 16, and then went to the Continent with her sister, where she acquired fluency in several languages. She also studied art, in which she retained an interest throughout her life. On returning to England, she studied for a year at Bedford College, matriculating in 1884. The next year at the age of 28, she began study at the London School of Medicine for Women. It was recorded at the time that she was distinguished among her fellow students for her personal charm and good taste in dress.

In 1889 she qualified MB at the University of London and became house surgeon at the Belgrave Hospital for Children. There she achieved the first of her many press reports. *The Evening News & Post* in 1890 noted 'A lady doctor at a coroner's court'. Miss Dickinson, a registered medical practitioner had given evidence after the death of a child, and the coroner had remarked that it was the first time he had had a female doctor in his court. Following her Belgrave post, she became Resident Medical Officer at the New Hospital for Women, and she married James (later Sir James) Berry, a surgeon at the Royal Free Hospital. In 1893, when she applied for membership of the Society of Anaesthetists, she was Anaesthetist at the Alexandra Hospital for Diseases of the Hip in Children, and Assistant Physician at the New Hospital for Women. She continued her appointment at the Alexandra Hospital, when in 1906 she also became Staff Anaesthetist at the Royal Free, and she retained both posts until retirement in 1920.

Dr Dickinson-Berry was active in fields other than anaesthesia. In 1894 she surveyed the statistics of the London School of Medicine for Women between 1874 and 1888. The results, reported in the *St James' Gazette* of 14 March 1894, showed that 159 women had qualified, nine had died and 28 had relinquished their profession. She retained her interest in the position and status of women in medicine, serving as Honorary Secretary and as President of the Women's Medical Federation. As secretary, she wrote to *The Times* [3] deprecating the policies of Glasgow Corporation and the St Pancras Borough Council in refusing to employ medical women whose husbands were in employment [3]. She had articles published in the *British Medical Journal* and in *The Lancet*. For some time she was Assistant Medical Officer to the Education Committee of London County Council.

Another interest was the advancement of medical education for Serbian women. She and her husband took many active holidays on the Continent, including visits to Serbia. When the Royal Free Hospital established a Red Cross unit in Serbia in 1915, the hospital journal reported '. . . the chief surgeon of the new War Hospital will have with him his wife. While in Serbia she will occupy the post of physician and anaesthetist to the institution of which her husband has charge'. This team were not in Serbia for long. Initially, they mainly dealt with an outbreak of typhus. Their work was more improving sanitation than treating war injuries of which there were very few at the time. The area was then occupied by the Hungarians, who were courteous, but insisted the team move, with their help, to Odessa to carry on their work. On her return to England, Dr Dickinson-Berry became Honorary Secretary of a committee set up to establish scholarships for Serbian women to train in Britain and then return home to practise medicine. In her will she left £1000 to this Fund. She died after a short illness in 1934.

MRS CAROLINE KEITH

The second lady applicant for membership of the Society of Anaesthetists was proposed by Mrs Dickinson-Berry and Dr Dudley Buxton, and elected in 1894, at which time she was anaesthetist to the New Hospital for Women. Caroline Keith had been born in Alsace. As a young woman, speaking only French, she married a Scot, one Surgeon Captain Keith. They came to England where she learnt to speak English and where she had a son. When the army posted her husband to India, he entreated her to enter the London School of Medicine and to qualify as a doctor, 'so she could secure her independence in case of need'. This she did, and qualified in Scotland (a fairly common occurrence then) in 1888. By 1891, her entry in the *Medical Directory* shows her as an anaesthetist at the New Hospital for Women, a post she retained until her retirement in 1912.

Anaesthesia was not her full-time occupation. Caroline Keith was also interested in, and good at, obstetrics. For 5 years, from 1894 to 1899 she was Lecturer in Midwifery at Clapham Maternity Hospital. During this time she also became Anaesthetist at the Chelsea Hospital for Women. She was obviously capable, well-liked and successful, but in 1912 in the prime of her life, she retired. She died in Southsea in 1925.

MISS EVELINE A CARGILL

The third female applicant to the Society is a more shadowy figure. Eveline Cargill first appears in the *Medical Directory* in 1891. She qualified in Scotland in 1889, but her medical school was again the London School of Medicine for Women. In 1891 she obtained an MD in Brussels (again a fairly common occurrence at that time). Two years later she was working as a medical officer at the Portobello Road Provident Dispensary for Women and Children. About this time she also became Assistant Anaesthetist at the New Hospital for Women. Her membership was proposed by Dr Dudley Buxton and Mrs Caroline Keith, in January 1895, but about this time she ceased to be an anaesthetist, becoming instead an Inspector of the Waifs and Strays Society. By 1900 she had given this up and had moved to Cheltenham. There she presumably was in medical practice, since from 1909 to 1916 she was Medical Inspector at the Ladies College, and is not recorded as having retired until 1920. She obviously kept her interest in anaesthesia as she attended meetings of the Society until 1898, and in 1907 was still a fully paid-up member, at half a guinea a year. She died during the 1930s.

CONCLUSION

These three women are of considerable interest to us. They came from different backgrounds, and their careers took differing forms, but they obviously knew each other and had a common interest in anaesthesia. All three must have been determined women to qualify when they did. At a time when there was prejudice against women doctors for renouncing their femininity, they were sufficiently professional and ladylike to gain the support and encouragement of male colleagues. In applying for membership of the new specialist anaesthetics Society, and being accepted, they established the right of women in our specialty to be regarded as equals, and they led the way for women throughout the medical profession.

REFERENCES

(1) Bell EHCM. *Storming the citadel: The rise of the woman doctor*. London: Constable, 1953: 57.
(2) Minutes of Provisional Committee of the Society of Anaesthetists, 1 June 1893. (Minutes held in the Library of the Royal Society of Medicine).
(3) Letter to *The Times* 14 April 1920.

The sad case of Dr Axham

J Alfred Lee

Original presentation Southend-on-Sea 1988

In June 1922, just before I was due to start as a medical student in Newcastle, I was astonished to read in the King's Birthday Honours List, the name of Herbert Barker, who had been recommended for a knighthood by the Prime Minister, David Lloyd George. The honour was for services to manipulative surgery. A furious row broke out in the medical and lay press, and I can still remember the controversy which made such an impression on me.

SIR HERBERT BARKER

Herbert Barker was an individual of outstanding personality and professional skill as a manipulative surgeon, a term which he claimed to have invented. He was unqualified and unregistered as a doctor. He was born in Southport in 1869 and eventually enlisted as an apprentice to his cousin, John Atkinson, who was a well known bone setter in London's West End (one is reminded of Sir Robert James and Hugh Owen Thomas and their forebears in Liverpool).

His early career was unsuccessful but in 1904 his cousin died and Barker inherited the practice, eventually settling in Park Lane. He was then 35 years old. Success came rapidly and his patients soon included many well known people in the world of politics, entertainment, sport, the arts, high society (including the King's son, the Duke of Kent), HG Wells, Bernard Shaw and Augustus John who was reputed to have said that if he (Barker) would rattle his bones he would paint his portrait free. This portrait can now be seen in the National Portrait Gallery in London. Barker was especially renowned for relieving by manipulation such conditions as internal derangement of the knee joint, metatarsalgia, sacroiliac strain, hallux rigidus and stiff neck. Soon Barker realized that he needed someone to anaesthetize his patients during manipulations and invited a neighbouring doctor—Dr Frederick Axham—to watch him at work. Axham was greatly impressed with what he saw and agreed to become Barker's anaesthetist. They worked together happily from 1906 to 1911, when Axham was 70 years old. Axham knew full well what he was doing but decided that it was his medical duty to continue to prevent Barker's patients from suffering pain from his manipulations.

An important event in the story was a well publicized law case in which an increasingly well known Barker, who attracted much envy and dislike from the London surgical fraternity, was sued by a former patient who blamed his treatment for the subsequent amputation of his leg. This caused a great deal of publicity in the press and drew attention to Axham's involvement as an anaesthetist. Soon afterwards the Medical Defence Union was on his trail.

In medicine, as in many other aspects of human contact, emotions set the ball rolling, and it seems possible that antipathy to the unorthodox Barker—the man who was not a member of the club, who had not joined the union, who was an outsider—rather than any feelings against the harmless Axham, resulted in a complaint being made by the Medical Defence Union to the General Medical Council against Frederick Axham. The idea was to hit Barker through Axham and to cause a serious problem to Barker which would ruin his lucrative practice. It was Barker's success which led to Axham's downfall.

CROSSED OFF THE REGISTER

How many anaesthetists have been crossed off the Medical Register for giving anaesthetics to patients undergoing painful manipulations by an unqualified and unregistered bonesetter? It is thought that it is only Axham who has this doubtful distinction.

In 1911, Axham was a GP who also held the post of Medical Officer to the Workhouse of the Westminster Board of Guardians in Poland Street, W1, and as part of his duties it may be supposed that he had to give anaesthetics for what we would now call 'minor surgery' and for dental extractions. Nitrous oxide, ether, and chloroform given by the open drop method would have been the agents used. In an abstract from the Minutes of the *Westminster Guardian* on May 23 1911, the day before Axham was crossed off the Medical Register, it is stated: '. . . that there be recorded an expression of the Board's high appreciation of the devoted services of Dr FW Axham as Medical Officer of the Workhouse of the Union from 1886 to 1911 in attending and alleviating the suffering of the sick poor under his charge in the institution, that during his long and faithful service his duties were discharged with the utmost punctility and exemplary proficiency and he leaves the Board's service with the unanimous wish of the guardians that he may long enjoy a well deserved retirement'. This was no mean testimonial for a man accused of professional misdoing.

The Medical Defence Union reported Dr Axham to the General Medical Council and he was required to appear before its disciplinary sub-committee on 24 May 1911. Axham was accompanied by his friend, the Reverend JL Walton, Vicar of All Saints' Church, Southend-on-Sea. Neither barrister nor solicitor accompanied the accused doctor, and he addressed the Council on his own behalf.

On being asked if he was prepared to dissociate himself from Barker, Axham answered 'no'. The chairman of the sub-committee was John McAllister, the well known Glasgow physician. He was then the President of the General Medical Council and on this occasion was accompanied by 34 of its members. The complainants were the Medical Defence Union, represented by Dr Bateman, their General Secretary. The charge formulated by the Council's solicitors was 'That you have knowingly and willingly on various occasions assisted one Herbert Atkinson Barker, an unregistered person practising in a department of surgery, in carrying on such practice by administering anaesthetics on his behalf to patients coming to him for treatment and that in relation thereto you have been guilty of infamous professional conduct'. Dr Axham answered questions put to him through the chair, the room was cleared and the Council deliberated in camera. Later the chairman returned, and announced the judgement of the Council as follows: 'I have to inform you that the Council have judged you to have been guilty of infamous conduct in a professional respect and have directed the Registrar to erase your name from the Medical Register'. There was, of course, no appeal from this verdict. A little while later Sir Edward Marshall Hall, the famous barrister, encouraged Axham to sue the General Medical Council and said that if he would do this he would defend Axham without professional fee, but Axham did not take up the offer.

The decision was widely criticized in the press and over the years there was much agitation that the verdict should be reversed. Axham had given nearly 50 years of service to the medical profession without a blot on his name or reputation. The General Medical Council (since 1951 officially named the General Council for Medical Education and Registration) was established by the Medical Act of 1858 under which a formal medical register was set up so that the public could differentiate between properly educated medical men and women and the large number of unorthodox healers or quacks who were practising. The Council was empowered to erase from the Register the name of any practitioner convicted of a criminal offence or judged to have been guilty of infamous conduct in a professional respect. Deregistration means that if he continued to work he would be at risk of being prosecuted for criminal neglect, if a patient had died he would not have been able to sign a death certificate, prescriptions for scheduled drugs cannot be dispensed by a chemist nor could he call in a legally qualified consultant if he was in trouble.

Poor Dr Axham had lost his appointment as Medical Officer to the Poland Street Workhouse and could no longer earn any sort of living by the practice of medicine. He lived with his wife in genteel poverty until 1926 when he died in a very decrepit state, aged 86. His last words, according to his widow were: 'I forgive them, as I hope to be forgiven'. His funeral took place in Mitcham in Surrey.

ANAESTHESIA AFTER DR AXHAM

When Dr Axham was prevented from anaesthetizing Barker's patients by the removal of his name from the Medical Register there was no problem about his replacement. According to Barker, many registered doctors contacted him offering their services as anaesthetists. This was partly because of the bad press that the removal of Axham's name had attracted, and it was thought that the General Medical Council would not be so foolish as to repeat the unwise action. One practitioner who frequently worked with Barker was Dr Frank Colley of Hove whose brother was a fashionable Harley Street physician. In after years Colley wrote enthusiastically about the quality of Sir Herbert's therapeutic work and about his outstanding qualities as a healer. The fact that Dr Colley was regularly anaestheizing Barker's patients was well known in London medical circles and nobody did anything about it. Officially registered dentists only made their appearance in the early 1920s and it is difficult to believe that the patients of some of the many unregistered dentists did not receive nitrous oxide, if nothing more potent, from registered medical practitioners before this time. Perhaps we should also remember that the first man to give ether in public, WT Morton in 1846, was not a qualified doctor, nor were Mr Robinson, nor Mr Squire, the first to follow Morton's example in England.

PROFESSIONAL RECOGNITION

This story would have been almost forgotten if it had not been for a U turn in the attitude of the medical profession to the skills of Barker, since 1922, Sir Herbert.

Orthopaedic surgeons in London became increasingly aware of Barker's success and they envied his prestige and wealth. The British Orthopaedic Association decided to break with tradition and invited him to give a demonstration which took place at St Thomas' Hospital in July 1936. Lord Moynihan, then the doyen of the surgical profession and a famous President of the Royal College of Surgeons, was a warm supporter of Barker and advised him to see the patients first to select those he might be able to help. Over 100 surgeons attended including Lord Moynihan, Sir William Arbuthnot Lane, Mr TP MacMurray of Liverpool and the young Archibald MacIndoe. The final irony of the story is that Dr Zebulon Mennell, anaesthetist to St Thomas' Hospital and due to become the President, and later Treasurer of the Association of Anaesthetists of Great Britain and Ireland, was asked officially to give anaesthetics for Barker's manipulations. For his services he was thanked by the company of distinguished surgeons and no criticism of his activity was heard, either officially or unofficially. The demonstration was impressive and a film was taken so that Barker's methods could be studied by those who were interested.

As he left the auditorium Barker, thinking of his old friend Dr Axham, said: "Gentlemen, are you not now guilty of unprofessional conduct?" Favourable reports of this event appeared in the medical and lay press—*The Lancet*, *The Times* and *The Observer*. It was reported as a landmark in surgical history that at last the orthodox profession had allowed itself to learn from the unregistered, but justly famous, manipulative surgeon some of the tricks of the trade of unorthodox manipulative surgery.

THEN AND NOW

Two questions can now be asked: Was Dr Axham when he acted as anaesthetist to patients of Herbert Barker, not doing his duty as a member of a profession whose duty it is to ease pain and human suffering? Were the General Medical Council wise to prolong this ostracism? This body was accused, rightly or wrongly, of continuing the victimization of Dr Axham, so that any registered practitioner who would like to follow in his footsteps would be inhibited from doing so. I believe that now it is quite common for some of our anaesthetic colleagues to give instruction to chiropodists on the technique of injecting local analgesic drugs, but I do not know whether any of them are ever asked to give general anaesthetics. I do not know how they would react to such requests.

Sir Herbert Barker must have been a man of outstanding ability with a great gift for healing. Towards the end of his life, he was appointed as Honorary Consultant in Manipulative Surgery to Noble's Hospital in the Isle of Man, so he very nearly made it. He was much more than a fashionable bone setter. Our professional forebears could not stop him from practising but they were empowered, by the use of the General Medical Council's ability to erase a name from the Medical Register, to make it very difficult for him to provide his patients with reasonably safe anaesthesia during his manipulations. Of course, their action did nothing of the sort because he was still able to get registered doctors to give anaesthetics for him. Dr Axham's erasure in 1911, and even more the agitation by well known citizens to influence the Council to reinstate the old doctor towards the end of his life, both caused wide discussions 60 years ago. It is certain that many of Barker's supporters were not primarily campaigning for the recognition of unregistered practitioners and healers, but of orthodox surgeons to learn from Barker how to apply these skills so that the general public could receive the benefit. Even today, some of our orthopaedic colleagues still seem slow to apply manipulative skills and this is a pity. Non-registered osteopaths and chiropractors still thrive and would seem to benefit their patients, at least in some cases.

Today, there is a steady agitation for non-registered healers to be given facilities in our hospitals in the National Health Service, to ply their trade and exercise their skills. Already in the USA their battle has been won. In these libertarian times will we always be able to prevent this exclusion of the unorthodox manipulative practitioners, and if we do will it always be to the benefit of those patients whose skeletal disabilities cause them such suffering? It seems ridiculous that when an obscure GP gave anaesthetics for Barker in 1911 he was crossed off the Medical Register and yet, 25 years later when the President-elect of the Association of Anaesthetists rendered the same service to the famous Herbert Barker in public, he received both praise and warm thanks. Is this a just world?

ACKNOWLEDGEMENTS

I would like to pay tribute to Dr Barbara Duncum for some factual information and to Mr IF Lisle the Librarian of the Royal College of Surgeons of England for permission to consult the Barker papers deposited at the College.

Joseph Blomfield 1870–1948

DDC Howat

Original presentation Croydon 1989

I first met Joseph Blomfield when I was a clinical medical student at St George's Hospital during World War II. It was a small medical school in those days, only a skeleton crew of senior students remained at Hyde Park Corner, whilst others were evacuated to the West Middlesex Hospital in Isleworth. Dr Blomfield had bought a house there after retiring from the staff of St George's 10 years before, and had returned to work in the Emergency Medical Service at the West Middlesex for the duration. A pleasant elderly gentleman, he was very kind to the students, allowing us to give anaesthetics, usually open ether, under his direction. My most abiding memory of him is of looking through the oval window into the anaesthetic room and seeing a fellow student pouring ether on to a Schimmelbusch mask, while Jo Blomfield stood over him, a theatre cap perched on his head, a cup of tea in one hand and a lighted cigarette in the other. In those days there was little movement of air in the theatre suites, so relative safety was assured by the heaviness of ether vapour.

At that time I was quite unaware that he had played a significant role in the development of anaesthetics, and have only recently discovered that his life and work are well worth recording.

He was born in London in 1870, the son of Louis and Salie Blumfeld, changing his surname to Blomfield in 1916. After education at University College School, and Gonville and Caius College, Cambridge, he came to St George's in 1891 and immediately entered into the life of the medical school. He played three-quarter in the First XV, was frequently congratulated on his performance, and received a presentation cup. It is said that after the 1914–18 war, he turned out for the first game of the revived School team, and scored a try—at the age of 50. He always followed the fortunes of the Rugby Club and was its President from 1941 until his death. He was a prolific contributor to the *Hospital Gazette*, which was started soon after his arrival. After a proposal that it should appear ten times a year, he made the more realistic suggestion of once a term. His forte was the recital at students' and nurses' concerts of humorous poems, usually of his own composition, delivered with a dead-pan expression.

Blomfield qualified MB Cambridge in 1894, did various house jobs in St George's and elsewhere until 1896, but returned to the hospital as Assistant Anaesthetist the following year, when he obtained his MD. All this time he was writing in the *Gazette*, and was soon editing it. Between 1898 and 1905, Blomfield was also appointed anaesthetist to the Grosvenor Hospital for Women and Children, the Metropolitan Hospital and the National Dental Hospital (all now gone), and to St Mary's Hospital, where he worked for some years, and was a popular teacher.

PUBLICATIONS

In 1902, he published a small handbook of anaesthesia which ran to four editions, although it dealt only with nitrous oxide, chloroform and ether [1]. The reviews described it as being excellent for students, though rather conservative in outlook. The *Hospital Gazette* of that year has a photograph of Blomfield, with the other anaesthetists on the staff, who were Henry Menzies, Llewellyn Powell (later President of the Section of Anaesthetics), and the most senior — Frederic Hewitt.

Blomfield's publications were many. There were papers read before the Society of Anaesthetists, the predecessor of the Section of Anaesthetics, and before the Chelsea Clinical Society. He wrote on post-operative vomiting, caudal and spinal anaesthesia, the influence of narcotics on general anaesthesia and the ignition points of various anaesthetic vapours. His best known publication was with Sir Francis Shipway in 1929, on the use of rectal Avertin as a basal narcotic [2]. They advised its use in very nervous patients and some major procedures, particularly thyroidectomy for hyperthyroidism, but stressed that it should be used with care and in moderation*.

Blomfield wrote frequent letters to *The Lancet* and the *British Medical Journal* on a wide variety of subjects connected with anaesthesia, and there were few meetings he attended which did not hear his voice in discussion. His views tended to be conservative, but his comments were modest and full of common sense. His concern was particularly with the status of anaesthesia, and for its safety. In 1919, responding to a letter in *The Lancet* advocating the training of nurses as anaesthetists, Blomfield wrote that nurses 'will perforce remain rule-of-thumb administrators, often no doubt perfect in one particular method they have acquired' [3]. He added the pithy comment: 'They helped the war machine — they will be a brake on the progress of the car in peace'. In the same *Lancet*, a surgical nurse wrote that her experience had led her to realize that trivial operations could be associated with serious effects from the anaesthetic; that had she wished to be an anaesthetist, she would have become a doctor, not a nurse, and that a nurse administering an anaesthetic might reasonably feel she should receive the same fee as a doctor.

Of Alcock's temperature-compensated chloroform vaporizer, Blomfield stated it was a useful instrument to have in hospital, but of little use in teaching students, who would be unlikely to employ it. For private practice, where surgery was often performed in the patient's home, he was more scathing: 'If each anaesthetist could be supplied with a boy to work the bellows, or with an electric fan, or with a motor car to carry the boy, machine and the fan, conditions would be about ideal, and he would always take Dr Alcock's apparatus with him'. This, in spite of the fact that he was full of praise for the vaporizer [4].

---

*Avertin or tribromethanol was made available in solution in amylene hydrate, which had to be protected from heat and light. This was diluted to 2.5% in distilled water by the anaesthetist, who then tested it with a few drops of Congo Red, as it was liable to break down to dibromacetic aldehyde and hydrobromic acid. If the dye turned blue, the solution was discarded. When I was resident anaesthetist at St George's, toxic patients for thyroidectomy were operated first on the morning list. We made up the solution in a thermos flask last thing the night before, and delivered it to the ward with the Congo Red already in, giving the nurses instructions not to administer it unless the solution had remained pink. This gave us a few more precious minutes in bed in the morning.

On several occasions, Blomfield sounded a note of caution about the indiscriminate use of spinal anaesthesia, pointing out that the danger of general anaesthesia in cases of heart disease had been greatly exaggerated. He always stressed that the anaesthetist was more important than his apparatus. In 1939 he wrote: 'Anaesthetists are more prone to invention than judgement. Every anaesthetist (myself alas! excepted) has invented a bit of apparatus, or has modified someone else's bit' [5]. He was anxious that apparatus should be kept simple and compact. In 1944, when he was 74, he wrote that there were two great faults in the teaching of anaesthetics: a persistent mortality and ineffective teaching; there were not nearly enough experts to go round and medical schools should take notice [6]. His last paper was published in the *British Journal of Anaesthesia*. It was intended to be the first in a series on famous anaesthetists and was about his old chief, Frederic Hewitt [7]. On the following page appeared Blomfield's own obituary by RJ Minnitt.

In addition to the 1902 handbook, Blomfield wrote two major books which became well known. *Anaesthetics in Practice and Theory* appeared in 1922. Very well reviewed, it was possibly the last comprehensive book on anaesthesia by a single author. It mentions every anaesthetic agent available at the time, including hypnosis and electronarcosis. It has sections on resuscitation, shock, pain relief and on local anaesthesia, and concludes with chapters on medico-legal aspects and education. Of great interest is his description of the differing arrangements for hospital anaesthetists: 'At one we find the anaesthetists placed on a level with the other honorary officers of the hospital. They manage their own department and are not subject to annual election. At another the position is very different. The anaesthetists have a place on the staff of the medical school, but not on that of the hospital'. (This was the case at St George's at that time). 'At none, I believe, is there any stipulation as to the quality of degree which a candidate for the post of anaesthetist must hold. The more attractive the post . . . to the best type of student, the better, of course will be the men who hold these posts. And it is on (their) ability and enthusiasm . . . that progress in anaesthesia, the training of students, and consequently the public safety ultimately depend'. He quotes Frederic Hewitt on the unfortunate tendency of coroners to blame the anaesthetist for deaths on the operating table, and praises the Scottish system with the Procurator-Fiscal's investigation.

His second book was *St George's 1733–1933*, a definitive history published by the Medici Society in 1933 [9]. Much of the first part, as he admits, was transcribed from George C Peachey's history of the hospital, which was never completed. Peachey had published six parts, the first appearing in 1910, with the help and support of Clifford Dent, the surgeon. Unfortunately Dent died in 1912, when Peachey had only reached the year 1753. In discussing the history of anaesthesia at St George's, Blomfield noted that, in spite of John Snow's having worked in the hospital, a qualified doctor was not appointed to give anaesthetics until 1879, when WH Bennett (later Sir William Bennett, a well known surgeon) became 'chloroformist' on a salary of £20 a year.

COMMITTEES, STATUS AND SAFETY

The Society of Anaesthetists was founded in 1893. Blomfield first attended as a visitor to a meeting in 1898. He was elected a member the following year, became auditor in 1903, a Councillor in 1904 and secretary in 1905. As senior secretary, he represented the Society at the meeting of medical societies to consider their amalgamation. He proposed that the Society of Anaesthetists should be amalgamated with the Royal Society of Medicine, and this was approved in April 1908 [10]. The first meeting of the new Section of Anaesthetics took place in November 1908, with Richard Gill as President. Blomfield was elected President in 1912. The custom of the Presidential Address was not yet established, but Blomfield took part in discussions of all the papers, with a particular interest in the reactions of coroners to deaths under anaesthesia [11]. In 1916, he was made Editorial Representative, following Francis Shipway, and remained so continuously until 1947, when Geoffrey (Later Sir Geoffrey) Organe took over. He was much in demand as an editor, as we shall see.

In 1909, the British Association for the Advancement of Science formed an Anaesthetic Committee of its Section of Physiology, with the purpose of investigating various anaesthetic agents, and the possible diminution of deaths under anaesthesia. The chairman was AD Waller FRS, the secretary Frederic Hewitt, and the other members were JA Gardner, GA Buckmaster and Sir Frederick Treves. When Treves resigned, Blomfield was elected in his stead. During the next few years, this committee reported on the rate of uptake of chloroform by the blood, the percentage of ether obtainable by the open method, and on Waller's chloroform balance, which was tested in the Out Patient Department of St George's [12]. In its report of 1913, the committee resolved: 'that in view of the fact that numerous deaths continue to take place from anaesthetics administered by unregistered persons, the Committee appeals to the Council of the Association to represent to the Home Office and to the Privy Council the urgent need of legislation'. Unfortunately, the imminent world war put paid to that.

Throughout this time, Blomfield was speaking at major anaesthetic meetings, writing many letters to the medical press and contributing articles on anaesthesia to various surgical textbooks. From 1913 he was editor of the *Medical Annual*, a post he held until Langton Hewer took over in 1938.

During the 1914–18 war, he was anaesthetist to several officers' hospitals, including the famous King Edward VII Hospital for Officers, still called 'Sister Agnes' after its formidable first matron, Miss Keyser. She and Blomfield were great friends, and it is said that no anaesthetist was permitted to work there without his approval.

In the early 1920s there was concern about the purity of anaesthetic agents, particularly nitrous oxide, and about ensuring the manufacture of newer agents in Britain. A combined anaesthetic committee of the Royal Society of Medicine (RSM) and the Medical Research Council (MRC) was set up in 1924. The MRC members were all Fellows of the Royal Society — HH Dale, FG Donnan and MS Pembrey; those from the RSM were Blomfield, Shipway and Hadfield. Blomfield was appointed chairman, and Hadfield secretary. This committee investigated such matters as the ignition points of ethylene, dimethyl and divinyl ether, cyclopropane and acetylene, and did some work on Avertin and Evipan. Dr Ernest Landau, who took part in the trial of Evipan at St George's, told me that Blomfield never seemed very enthusiastic about it, and the report in the *British Medical Journal* on its clinical value was severely factual [13]. In later years the committee considered explosions, problems of respiratory exchange, and ether convulsions [14,15]. Blomfield resigned from the committee in 1945, when Nosworthy replaced him.

In January 1923, the first number of the *British Journal of Anaesthesia* appeared, under its American editor, HM Cohen, who practised in Manchester. Contributors included Gwathmey, Wesley Bourne, McKesson, Dudley Buxton, Langton Hewer and Joseph Blomfield, who described the use of Stovaine 2% with adrenaline 1:100 000 for sacral analgesia [16]. In January 1924, Blomfield wrote an editorial: 'Some remarks on post-operative lung trouble' [17]. Cohen died suddenly in August 1929, and no autumn number appeared. Blomfield was appointed editor, and he continued to edit the journal until the year of his death in 1948, when Falkner Hill and Cecil Gray took over.

His first editorial, on 'Machines and Men', discussed the danger of the anaesthetist becoming a technician rather than a doctor. It was a theme which recurred in several of his publications and lectures. He did not question the benefits of new apparatus and methods, but was concerned at the younger anaesthetists' lack of clinical observation and acumen. 'It is no use perfecting the gun', he said, 'if we neglect in any respects the training of the man who is to fire it'. In 1932, he returned to another favourite subject — the widespread tendency for deaths associated with operations to be attributed to the anaesthetist, particularly by coroners. He deplored the fact that there were no proper statistics of the circumstances under which patients died during or soon after operation. Detailed accounts of the drugs and methods employed during anaesthesia were needed. He advocated the establishment of a proper system of recording anaesthetics, with their immediate and late sequelae, and recommended that the newly-formed Association should find time to study this [19].

As editor of the *British Journal of Anaesthesia*, Blomfield was one of a provisional committee of ten elected to form the Association of Anaesthetists of Great Britain and Ireland. The Association came into being on 1 July 1932, and at the first Annual General Meeting in October, Featherstone was elected President and Blomfield Vice-President. The first Treasurer was Zebulon Mennell, and the first Secretary was Howard Jones. In 1934 Council asked Blomfield to discuss with Sir Bernard Spilsbury, then President of the Medico-Legal Society, the practice of coroners dealing with anaesthetic deaths. He submitted a paper on the subject to the next Council meeting, at which Magill also put forward his subcommittee's proposal for the new Diploma of Anaesthetics. Blomfield was involved in that too! He was one of the Association's representatives whose joint meeting with the President and Councillor representatives of the Royal College of Surgeons secured the agreement of the Conjoint Board to the holding of an examination.

Magill took on the negotiations about coroners' inquests in July, when Blomfield was nominated President. His term of office commenced in October 1935, at which meeting he reported there had been hard arguments to convince the Conjoint Board's Examining Body that teaching hospital anaesthetists of 10 years standing should be allowed to apply for the DA without examination. It was later agreed that this exemption should also apply to non-teaching hospitals of at least 100 beds. Blomfield and others turned down the suggestion that the *British Journal of Anaesthesia* become the organ of the Association, but offered its full help. In 1938, the last year of his very active Presidency, the colour coding of gas cylinders was agreed, the matter of discussions with the Central Midwives Board was raised, and even the possibility of reducing the subscription to the Association. Blomfield remained on the Council of the Association until 1943 [20].

PERSONAL LIFE

There is very little information about Joseph Blomfield the man, since nearly all his relatives are dead. He had connections with Fleet Street, for his sister Daisie had married Ralph Blumenfeld, the editor and later Chairman of the *Daily Express*.

Blomfield used to take parties of students to the paper's offices to see it being 'put to bed'. In 1912, he married Sheila Lehmann. Their son Derek was born in 1920. He became an actor, appearing in *The Lady's not for Burning* in 1948, and from 1957 to 1959 as Detective-Sergeant Trotter in *The Mousetrap*. He died in the 1960s. In 1933 Blomfield was married for the second time, to Miss Dorothy Kathleen Bell, a distinguished Secretary of the Genealogical Society. Mrs Blomfield was still alive in 1989, but in her nineties and in failing health.

I have already noted Blomfield's popularity as a student and young doctor. His genial personality and his command of English together with his thoughtful, somewhat conservative outlook made him much sought after for committees, lectures and as an editor. Mennell reported in his obituary of Blomfield: 'As an editorial contributor to our own columns, he was for many years a valued and entertaining colleague. In those relatively spacious times it was his habit to drop into the office after lunch, wearing a button-hole, smoking a cigar, and bearing a manuscript which could be deciphered only by the expert. (When he bought a typewriter the results were so remarkable that our printer begged him to return to the pen)' [21].

When Blomfield retired from St George's Hospital, his vigour was unimpaired; indeed, much of his valuable work was done after that date. He had a serious illness and operation in 1945 and, although he recovered, he was never as active again. He died on 11 November 1948, in his 79th year. There is no memorial, as his body was cremated.

Joseph Blomfield was not responsible for any great advances in the theory or practice of anaesthetics, yet he played an important part in raising the status of its practitioners from untrained chloroformists to qualified specialist anaesthetists. Although conservative in the drugs and methods he used, he recognized the real advances being made, but did not hesitate to point out their disadvantages. His obituary in *The Times* described him as 'an eminent anaesthetist who had taken a prominent part in the modern development of his specialty' [22].

ACKNOWLEDGEMENTS

My thanks to Dr TB Boulton; the late George Edwards; Robert Headley; EF Johnson; the late Ernest Landau; to Miss Brady, Librarian, St George's Hospital; Mr Jonathan Booth, Secretary, Green Room Club; Mr Anthony Camps, Director, Society of Genealogists; Mr Archibald Donaldson; Mr Palmer, Librarian, St Mary's Hospital; Mr Peacock, Librarian, University College Hospital; Mr Yeo, Archivist, St Bartholomew's Hospital; and The Head Archivist, Greater London Record Office.

REFERENCES

(1) Blomfield J. *Anaesthetics*. London: Baillière, Tindall and Cox, 1902.
(2) Blomfield J, Shipway F. The use of Avertin for anaesthesia. *Lancet* 1929; **1**: 546–9.
(3) Correspondence. *Lancet* 1919; **2**: 665–6.
(4) Zuck D. The Alcock chloroform vaporiser. *Anaesthesia* 1988; **43**: 972–80.
(5) Correspondence. *Br Med J* 1939; **1**: 1200.
(6) Correspondence. *Br Med J* 1944; **1**: 337.
(7) Blomfield J. Famous anaesthetists I. Sir Frederic Hewitt. *Br J Anaesth* 1948–9; **31**: 149–51.
(8) Blomfield J. *Anaesthetics in practice and theory*. London: Heinemann, 1922.

 (9) Blomfield J. *St George's 1733–1933*. London: Medici Society, 1933.
(10) Minutes of the Society of Anaesthetists, 1893–1908 (Held in the library of the Royal Society of Medicine).
(11) Minutes of the Section of Anaesthetics, and of the Council of the Section, Royal Society of Medicine, 1908–1948. (Held in the library of the Royal Society of Medicine).
(12) Reports of the Anaesthetic Committee to the Section of Physiology of the British Association for the Advancement of Science, 1909–1916 (Held in the library of the Royal Society of Medicine).
(13) A report on the clinical value of Evipan. *Br Med J* 1933; **2**: 63–4.
(14) Minutes of the Council of the Section of Anaesthetics, Royal Society of Medicine, May 1924, November 1938, 1945.
(15) Hadfield CF. The Joint Anaesthetics Committee: A retrospect of 11 years work. *Proc Royal Soc Med* 1935; **28**: 1133–44.
(16) Various authors. *Br J Anaesth* 1923; **1**: 1–108.
(17) Editorial. *Br J Anaesth* 1924; **3**: 128–30.
(18) Editorial. *Br J Anaesth* 1930; **7**: 97–8.
(19) Editorial. *Br J Anaesth* 1932; **10**: 1–2.
(20) Minutes of the Council of the Association of Anaesthetists of Great Britain and Ireland, 1932–1943.
(21) Obituary. *Lancet* 1948; **2**: 833–4.
(22) Obituary. *The Times*, 18 November 1948.

Hamer Hodges 1919–1961

RC Birt

Original presentation Southend 1988

Robert James Hamer Hodges, known as Jim, was born on 22 April 1919, the son of a Portsmouth GP. He attended Portsmouth Grammar School and read medicine at St Mary's, Paddington 1938–1944, winning the Kitchener Scholarship and qualifying Licentiate in Medicine and Surgery of the Society of Apothecaries in January 1944. There were several probable reasons why he chose LMSA. He was anxious to qualify as early as possible. While still a student, he had married a nurse during his war-time secondment to the Hammersmith Hospital. His father's practice was destroyed by bombs in 1941; his father then joined the army, dying in 1943. All in all, there was a lot of pressure on Hamer Hodges to qualify and start work as soon as possible. For the rest of his life, however, he regretted not taking a University degree. He was, of course, unable to present any of his research as a PhD thesis.

Once qualified, he returned to Portsmouth to take up house jobs, then moved back to London — to the Miller General Hospital, as Resident Surgical Officer, and to the Royal Marsden as Senior Resident Medical Officer. It was during this period he contracted pulmonary tuberculosis which was treated by thoracoplasty. He must have realized that this severely prejudiced his chances of a surgical career and with the help of Dr Cope, later consultant at University College Hospital, he obtained some experience in anaesthesia. In 1949 he was back in Portsmouth at Queen Alexandra Hospital as a Senior Surgical Officer, equivalent to a Senior Registrar. This year convinced him that he was no longer fit enough for general surgery and in 1950 he moved sideways, starting his career in anaesthesia as a Registrar. He spent only a year as a Registrar, becoming a Senior Hospital Medical Officer in 1951. He obtained the then two-part DA in 1952, and was elected FFARCS in 1954. In the same year he was appointed Consultant Anaesthetist to the Portsmouth group of hospitals, and Consultant to the Thoracic Surgical Unit of the Wessex region. This involved sessions at Southampton, which later moved to Portsmouth, and also sessions on the Isle of Wight.

It was at Ventnor on the Isle of Wight that the young GP Mike Tunstall, while attending an operation on one of his patients, met Hamer Hodges and become interested in anaesthesia. Hamer Hodges obtained a lot of the data for his papers on the action of suxamethonium from these lists, which one presumes were under less pressure than those at Portsmouth. Mike Tunstall left general practice, to work as a Registrar and later as Senior Registrar in anaesthesia at Portsmouth.

Hamer Hodges was also consultant to the Poliomyelitis Centre at Priorsdean Hospital, and to the Obstetric Unit at St Mary's, Portsmouth. This responsibility for obstetrics enabled him to have a 6 month period in America with Professor Robert Hingson, who published the first paper on the organization of obstetric anaesthesia in 1951 [1].

Hamer Hodges had already formulated his theories on the changes in end-plate response to suxamethonium, from his observations in carefully monitored clinical practice. In the US he met Francis Foldes who set up an animal experiment, which to Hamer Hodges was more a public trial of this theory than an experiment. Fortunately, all went well and the work was published [2]. On his return to Portsmouth, he turned his main energies to getting his messages across in the fields of obstetric and paediatric anaesthesia.

EARLY PAPERS

He published a group of miscellaneous papers. Replying to someone who thought there was little danger in a stomach tube entering the trachea [3], Hamer Hodges reported a patient who was given brandy by the ward sister, suffered intense pain in the chest and collapsed cyanosed. Pulmonary embolism was diagnosed until the chest X-ray showed the nasogastric tube to be in the right lower bronchus. The patient did not survive. Another paper detailed an incompatible blood transfusion in which anaesthesia did not mask the signs [4]. A further paper reported a series of multiple Stokes–Adams attacks during anaesthesia [5]. From Priorsdean came the description of a tracheotomy tube [6] which was still in use in 1961 when I was a Senior House Officer. This was a typical piece of British do-it-yourself. It was made from an endotracheal tube with the distal end cut square and chamfered. A single angle was slid onto the tube using KY jelly and this had to be a tight fit, but one could choose the length of both the intra and the extra tracheal portions of the tube. A latex collar was added. The finished tube was tailormade; you could have it cuffed or uncuffed, red rubber or plastic and, of course, in many different sizes. The last of this group of papers reported a case of gangrene of the forearm following intramuscular chlorpromazine [7].

MUSCLE RELAXANTS

Hamer Hodges produced 18 publications on muscle relaxants, ranging from letters to papers. One was an annotation on decamethonium [8]. One was a letter discussing the effects of suxamethonium in myasthenia gravis and hyper-thyroidism [9], five were concerned with pseudocholinesterase levels [10–14] eight with changes in end-plate sensitivity [2,15–21] and three with effects of oxytocin on the response to suxamethonium [22–24]. Hamer Hodges took up suxamethonium as it was coming into clinical practice; it was obviously his favourite relaxant and he very quickly observed the variations in its effects, at first investigating differences in pseudocholinesterase levels in healthy and diseased adults and children. It became clear to him that some variations in the actions of suxamethonium were not related to pseudocholinesterase and, as early as 1952, he had cases in which he reversed suxamethonium with neostigmine, concluding that the action of suxamethonium had changed to one which was curare-like. Most of these publications were letters, but there were major papers in the *British Journal of Anaesthesia* in 1955 [12] and *Anesthesia & Analgesia* in 1957 [2]. The paper he hoped to see in the *Journal of Pharmacology* was in the event published as an abstract [21]. Jenden, in 1951, was probably the first to report changes in end-plate response to decamethonium [22], but Hamer Hodges' papers carefully explained his concept that the change in the action of suxamethonium was due to a gradual alteration of the sensitivity/resistance relationship of the end-plate to depolarization, and made an important contribution to the understanding of the clinical use of suxamethonium. The articles on changes in end-plate sensitivity due to oxytocin refer mainly to long term pitocin drips. It is unlikely that the problem would arise in modern practice [23–25].

PAEDIATRIC ANAESTHESIA

In paediatric anaesthesia [26–28], Hamer Hodges felt it was unfortunate that so much attention was devoted to premedication. He endeavoured to obtain the intelligent cooperation of children and held a pre-anaesthesia class the day before surgery, explaining what was to happen. He used atropine or no premedication, and thiopentone for induction. All unnecessary people were kept out of the anaesthetic room and he insisted that a strict plan was adhered to. No-one was allowed to be out of position, the pre-anaesthesia class had to be followed to the letter. To keep the confidence of the child nothing unexpected was allowed to take place. There is a video* of the 20 minute film he made of this technique, which was first shown at the Association of Anaesthetists' meeting at Stratford in November, 1959.

OBSTETRIC ANAESTHESIA

Of his eight publications on obstetrics, two concerned chlorpromazine which Hamer Hodges felt should be restricted to very isolated instances — its use being contraindicated in general hospital obstetric practice [29,30]. It is interesting to note that Jeffrey Selwyn Crawford was a Senior Hospital Medical Officer in the Department whilst this work was in progress around 1957. Another letter discusses the problems of domiciliary midwifery for the non-specialist anaesthetist [31], while the five remaining papers outline the development of the Portsmouth standard technique. With later modifications, this formed the basis of current general anaesthesia for obstetrics. One paper described a record card devised for the study [32]. Another compared four different techniques in 264 patients [33]. These were: thiopentone, suxamethonium, intubation, intermittent positive-pressure ventillation, oxygen and nitrous oxide; this standard anaesthetic plus trichloroethylene; thiopentone, cyclopropane-oxygen, with intubation 'when indicated', and curare for all Caesarean sections; and nitrous oxide/oxygen/ether with or without thiopentone for induction. The standard thiopentone-suxamethonium-nitrous oxide technique was then used for a second group of 600 patients. The comparisons made were on the numbers of fully active infants delivered using each technique and, for Caesarean sections, the incidence of depressed infants overall and among those who had pre-operative fetal distress. The standard technique was better in all respects, and outstandingly better if there had been pre-operative fetal distress. This, and the clear, logical case put for the technique in typical Hamer Hodges fashion won widespread acceptance for the method, enhanced by a further paper in 1961 reviewing its use in 2000 cases during the 10 years 1952 to 1961 [34]. It is interesting to note that there was just one failed intubation in this series. In 1961, lecturing to a mixed medical audience

---

*Video loaned by Dr ME Tunstall and the Department of Medical Illustration, Aberdeen Royal Infirmary.

in Portsmouth, Hamer Hodges demonstrated a sharp drop in the Portsmouth perinatal mortality from well above to well below the national figures [35].

Before he died, Hamer Hodges had prepared two chapters for the *Recent Advances* series. These were revised by Mike Tunstall and published as one chapter in 1963 [36]. With financial help from the British Oxygen Company, Hamer Hodges made a film of his standard technique, which Dr Andrew Doughty has had copied on to video, so it too is available for viewing.

THE BACKGROUND TO THE STANDARD TECHNIQUE FOR OBSTETRICS

Early anaesthetic textbooks had, at best, a few paragraphs on obstetric anaesthesia. The anaesthetics were given by general practitioners, obstetric junior staff, and in the USA by nurses. Anaesthesia was a common event for normal delivery, although Caesarean section was rare. Maternal mortality was high, roughly 1 in 200 in 1928–29 [37]. Despite this, there were no deaths ascribed to anaesthesia for this period; the operator/anaesthetist was discouraged, not because of the risks of anaesthesia, but because of the danger of sepsis. In 1937 Charles Hall, an American GP, had one of his fit patients die from aspiration pneumonitis following a general anaesthetic for normal delivery [38]. Enquiring among his friends, he found 15 similar cases, five of which were fatal. Mendelson's 1946 study on rabbits set off further enquiries into obstetric anaesthesia [39].

One of the best early papers was from Lock in Carolina, who found the main causes of death to be aspiration of vomit, followed by spinal shock* [40]. The anaesthetics in use were firstly nitrous oxide and oxygen (even for sections, and at least 10% oxygen was recommended), and secondly, of course, ether. Whitacre in 1947 tried curare for Caesarean section — together with inhalation agents, with local anaesthesia and on its own [41]. Gray used 15 mg of curare with oxygen and cyclopropane, but he recommended not even inserting an airway in order to avoid vomiting [42]. Parker reported in the mid-1950s that general practitioners in Birmingham were safer with open ether than hospital doctors with oxygen, nitrous oxide and ether [43,44]. The Bart's anaesthetists were promptly told to use open ether [45].

There was considerable controversy about the advantages and disadvantages of intubation. Morton and Wylie suggested both headup tilt, and crash induction in 1951 [46]. Hingson, whom Hamer Hodges later visited, wrote on the organization of obstetric anaesthesia in 1951 [1]. Hamer Hodges' major contribution was to evolve a logical system from the chaos that existed, and to report on its use in over 2000 cases.

NEONATAL RESUSCITATION

As well as the chapter in *Recent Advances* [36], he had three publications on neonatal resuscitation [47–49]. The Portsmouth sterile disposable Magill/Cole type endotracheal tube is still in use today, now made by Portex. The condition of the neonate was fundamental to the Portsmouth technique. In the early 1950s and 1960s the anaesthetist was considered partly at least responsible for the neonate

---

*Hingson said the spinal shock was due to 'overwhelming and assassinating doses' [1].

and wholly responsible for its resuscitation at Portsmouth. Trainees were stationed at the head of the table with a very basic anaesthetic machine, delivering nitrous oxide in oxygen, with an ether bottle if required, and a clip-board and stop-watch to facilitate completing the record card. To the right was a neonatal resuscitation trolley. Hamer Hodges was a little embarrassed to find that 25% of neonates were intubated; the vast majority of cases were emergencies for fetal distress and all were lying flat on their backs, compromising the placental circulation.

POOR HEALTH

Despite his thoracoplasty in the 1940s, he remained a heavy smoker, but appeared to be in reasonable health until at least 1957. It is probable he had one, possibly two, myocardial infarcts between then and 1961. In 1961 he was very ill, although still working. He appeared to get angina walking downstairs, and it was thought at the time that he had constrictive pericarditis. At the Portsmouth conference in November 1961, he gave his lecture, and on the last day he spoke on neonatal resuscitation. He had helped to organize the meeting, so he must have been under a certain amount of stress. Nevertheless, his sister believes he was as well as usual at the dinner which rounded off the occasion. Later that night, Hamer Hodges suddenly died.

It would be nice to be able to say that Hamer Hodges' standard technique dramatically reduced maternal mortality due to anaesthesia, but as with so many Health Service statistics the figures we have are inappropriate. The maternal death rate was very high, and now is very much lower — from 4420 to 86 per million pregnancies [37,50]. Previously very light anaesthesia was common for vaginal delivery and Caesarean section was rare, the reverse is now the case. Irrespective of statistics, it is widely recognized that Hamer Hodges' short career in poor health did provide significant improvements to obstetric anaesthesia. Through his teaching, example and inspiration to many colleagues and trainees, his influence lives on.

ACKNOWLEDGEMENTS

I would like to thank Mike Tunstall, David Hamer Hodges and Margaret Crowley-Smith, Hamer Hodges' sister, for their help.

REFERENCES

(1) Hingson RA, Kellerman LM. Organization of obstetric anaesthesia on a twenty-four hour basis in a large and small hospital. *Anesthes* 1951; 12: 745-52.
(2) Foldes FF, Wnuck AL, Hodges RJH, Thesleff S, de Beer EJ. The mode of action of depolarizing relaxants. *Anesthes Analgesia Cur Res* 1957; 36: 23-7.
(3) Hodges RJH. Ryle's tube in trachea. *Br Med J* 1952; 1: 710–11.
(4) Hodges RJH. Incompatible transfusion under anaesthesia. *Lancet* 1952; i: 923–4.
(5) Hodges RJH, Witzeman RA, Leigh AM. Multiple Stokes–Adams episodes during anaesthesia. *Br Med J* 1957; 1: 625–6.
(6) Hodges RJH, Morley R, O'Driscoll WB, McDonald I. A tracheotomy tube for use in acute poliomyelitis. *Lancet* 1956; 1: 26.
(7) Hodges RJH. Gangrene of forearm after intramuscular chlorpromazine. *Br Med J* 1959; 2: 918–19.

(8) Hodges RJH. Decamethonium bromide. In: *New and non official remedies*. American Medical Association, Chicago: Lippincott, 1957: 503–504.

(9) Hodges RJH. Myasthenia gravis and hyperthyroidism. *Lancet* 1955; **2**: 1137–8.

(10) Hodges RJH. Therapeutic application of plasma cholinesterase. *Lancet* 1953; **1**: 143–4.

(11) Hodges RJH. Prolonged apnoea following succinyl-dicholine. *Lancet* 1953; **2**: 1210.

(12) Hodges RJH. The mechanisms concerned in the abnormal prolongation of effect following suxamethonium administration, with reference to the use of neostigmine. *Br J Anaesth* 1955; **27**: 484–91.

(13) Hodges RJH, Harkness J. Suxamethonium sensitivity in health and disease. *Br Med J* 1954; **2**: 18–22.

(14) Hodges RJH. Suxamethonium tolerance and pseudocholinesterase levels in children. In: International Anaesthetics Research Society, eds. *Proceedings of the World Congress of Anaesthesiologists, Scheveningen, The Netherlands*. Minneapolis: Burgess Publishing Company, 1955: 247–51.

(15) Hodges RJH, Foldes FF. Interaction of depolarising and non depolarising relaxants. *Lancet* 1956; **2**: 788.

(16) Hodges RJH. Neostigmine-resistant curarization. *Br Med J* 1956; **2**: 1240–1.

(17) Hodges RJH, Foldes FF. Dual action of suxamethonium chloride. *Br J Anaesth* 1956; **28**: 532–3.

(18) Hodges RJH, Foldes FF. Interaction of depolarising and non depolarising relaxants. *Lancet* 1957; **1**: 373.

(19) Hodges RJH. Relaxant technique. *Br Med J 1957;* 1: **648.**

(20) Hodges RJH. Reversal of suxamethonium paralysis with neostigmine. *Lancet* 1952; **2**: 100–1.

(21) Foldes FF, Wnuck AL, Hodges RJH, de Beer EJ. The interaction of depolarizing and non depolarizing neuromuscular blocking agents in dog and cat. *J Pharmacol* 1958; **122**: 145.

(22) Jenden DJ, Kamijo K, Taylor DB. The action of decamethonium (C10) on the isolated rabbit lumbrical muscle. *J Pharmacol* 1951; **103**: 348–9.

(23) Hodges RJH. Interaction of suxamethonium and oxytocin. *Br Med J* 1958; **1**: 1416–17.

(24) Hodges RJH, Bennett JR, Tunstall ME, Shanks ROF. Effects of oxytocin on the response to suxamethonium. *Br Med J* 1959; **1**: 413–16.

(25) Hodges RJH. Non depolarising neuromuscular blocking effects due to suxamethonium, following the infusion of oxytocic posterior pituitary extracts in obstetrics. *Acta Anaesth Scand* 1959; **supplementum II**: 25–6.

(26) Hodges RJH. Premedication of children for tonsillectomy. *Br Med J* 1955; **1**: 45.

(27) Hodges RJH. Tonsillectomy. *Br Med J* 1955; **2**: 434–5.

(28) Hodges RJH. Induction of anaesthesia in young children. *Lancet* 1960; **1**: 82–7.

(29) Hodges RJH, Foley JJ, Bennett JR. Forceps delivery. *Lancet* 1958; **1**: 103.

(30) Hodges RJH, Bennett JR. Some contraindications to the use of chlorpromazine (with particular reference to obstetric analgesia and anaesthesia). *J Obstet Gynaec British Empire* 1958; **66**: 91–8.

(31) Hodges RJH. Anaesthesia for domestic midwifery. *Br Med J* 1959; **1**: 1528.

(32) Hodges RJH. An obstetric anaesthetic record card. *Br J Anaesth* 1959; **31**: 32–4.

(33) Hodges RJH, Bennett JR, Tunstall ME, Knight RF. General anaesthesia for operative obstetrics with special reference to the use of thiopentone and suxamethonium. *Br J Anaesth* 1959; **31**: 152–62.

(34) Hodges RJH, Tunstall ME. The choice of anaesthesia and its influence on perinatal mortality in caesarean section (A review of the use of thiopentone and suxamethonium over the ten year period 1952–1961). *Br J Anaesth* 1961; **33**: 572–88.

(35) Hodges RJH. General anaesthesia for operative obstetrics in hospital practice. In: Barnett T, Foley JT, eds. *The obstetrician, anaesthetist and the paediatrician in the management of obstetric problems*. Oxford: Pergamon Press, 1963: 43–52.

(36) Hodges RJH, Tunstall ME. Obstetric anaesthesia and analgesia: resuscitation of the newborn. In: Hewer CL, ed. *Recent advances in anaesthesia and analgesia*, 9th ed. London: JA Churchill, 1963: 205–43.

(37) Ministry of Health. *Interim report of departmental committee on maternal mortality and morbidity*. HMSO, 1930.

(38) Hall CC. Aspiration pneumonitis an obstetric hazard. *JAMA* 1940; **114**: 728–33.

(39) Mendelson CL. The aspiration of stomach contents into the lungs during obstetric anaesthesia. *Am J Obstet Gynecol* 1946; **52**: 191-205.

(40) Lock FR, Griess FC. The anaesthetic hazards in obstetrics: North Carolina Maternal Welfare Study 1946-1948. *Am J Obstet Gynecol* 1955; **70**: 861–75.

(41) Whitacre RJ, Fisher AJ. Curare in caesarean section. *Anesth Analgesia* 1948: 164–7.

(42) Gray TC. d-Tubocurarine in caesarean section. *Br Med J* 1947; **1**: 444.

(43) Parker RB. Risks from the aspiration of vomit during obstetric anaesthesia. *Br Med J* 1954; **2**: 65–9.

(44) Parker RB. Maternal death from aspiration asphyxia. *Br Med J* 1956; **2**: 16–19.

(45) Atkinson RS. Personal communication.

(46) Morton HJV, Wylie WD. Anaesthetic deaths due to regurgitation or vomiting. *Anaesth* 1951; **6**: 190–205.

(47) Tunstall ME, Hodges RJH. A sterile disposable neonatal tracheal tube. *Lancet* 1961; **1**: 146.

(48) Hodges RJH,Tunstall ME, Knight RF. Endotracheal aspiration and oxygenation in resuscitation of the newborn. *Br J Anaesth* 1960; **32**: 9–15.

(49) Hodges RJH, Wilson EJ, Knight RF. Some factors associated with neonatal depression in operative obstetrics. *Br J Anaesth* 1960; **32**: 16–20.

(50) Department of Health. *Report on confidential enquiries into maternal deaths in England and Wales 1982–84*. London: HMSO, 1989: 140–1.

Sir Ivan Magill — a personal tribute

C Foster

Original presentation London 1987

Sir Ivan died at the age of 98 in November 1986 and his obituaries documented his long career and achievements. He was a charming Irishman, and fortunate to have been the right man in the right place at the right time. He was a keen and excellent fisherman — a very good illustration of his patience. His thoughtful approach to what he was doing, and his kind attitude to people led him to be inventive in both apparatus and techniques, for the benefit of his patients, who ranged from the lowest to the highest in the land. Sir Ivan very kindly sent St Thomas's Hospital Museum two of his original nasotracheal tubes, and a modified Doyen gag made in the 1920s with much bigger blades to ensure that it did not slip out of the mouth. He also donated a resuscitator which he made himself from an oxygen 'Sparklet', an ordinary M&IE paediatric bag and a plastic facepiece.

I first met Sir Ivan when he had retired from his private anaesthetic practice and had decided to give us some more of his anaesthetic kit. I was invited to his flat in Hallam Street where he had arranged his apparatus around the room. He offered me a drink. Unfortunately, because of his failing eyesight, he used the gin bottle instead of the sherry bottle. This was extremely disconcerting and I didn't quite know how to get out of the situation, but I plucked up courage and said, 'Sir, I am very sorry, this is actually gin and because I am driving I really don't think I can drink it all'. So we put it back in the bottle and I poured myself a sherry, and that actually seemed to cement the relationship.

There followed a fascinating viva and teaching session as we moved from one item to the next. Fortunately, he seemed to approve what I said. He gave me his dental apparatus and explained how it worked. After the viva was over, he gave me a cigar box containing little items — the hook he used to deliver gases to the mouth, when they weren't using an intratracheal technique; some endotracheal connections which came in different sizes; the original patterns were made of thick metal so the patient couldn't bite through them, a reminder of the problems of spasm, which was quite common in the days before relaxants, even in the hands of an expert anaesthetist. He didn't approve of anything which wasn't exactly to his original description, and would not take responsibility for such things. There was also a small lead plate to protect the upper teeth when he intubated and it still bears teeth marks. He used a right-angled rubber tube when he was working with Gillies, the plastic surgeon, to connect his oral endotracheal tube to the endotracheal connection, because he was not allowed to have sticky tape or any other method of tube fixation when Sir Harold was working on the face. This arrangement lay nicely and didn't need fixation.

Sir Ivan's thought for his patients is exemplified by the use he and Rowbottom made of tincture of lavender, and tincture of bitter lemons to disguise the smell of ether. Ellis had used oil of lemon and oil of nutmeg in 1866 for the same purpose.

We are fortunate that few patients nowadays have previously had an ether anaesthetic. Some of the problems were well described by Rowbottom and Magill to the Anaesthetic Section of the Royal Society of Medicine in 1921: 'A little ether accidently spilled in the ward is quite sufficient to put most of the inmates off their dinner; many men begin retching immediately they enter the anaesthetic room. Fear of operations was unknown, but fear of anaesthesia was universal, many flying officers reliving their crash whilst going under'. It is all to easy to forget the skills required before the discovery of thiopentone and the relaxants.

It was a great honour and pleasure to have met such a kind and caring man, with his wonderful Irish humour and prodigious memory — one of the great men who laid the foundations on which the new generation has built.

Tribute to Dr John Alfred Lee

RS Atkinson

Original presentation Edinburgh 1989

Alfred Lee died on 27 April 1989. He enjoyed a wonderful life, witnessing the evolution of anaesthetic practice from the days of the gauze mask to the present. He was interested in all these developments, even after retirement and right up to the last week of his life.

Alfred was interested in all branches of the speciality, but especially in regional analgesia, extradural block and the history of anaesthesia. He was the first

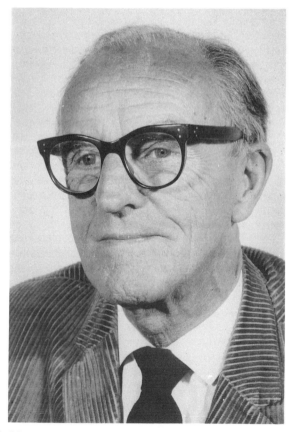

Figure 1 *J Alfred Lee*

President of the History of Anaesthesia Society. He is, however, best remembered as the author of the *Synopsis of Anaesthesia*, the first edition of which appeared in 1947 and the tenth in 1987. He contributed many articles to the literature on historical and biographical subjects and was the British editor of the *Proceedings of the First International Symposium on the History of Anaesthesia*.

He made contributions to all our national bodies. He was a member of the Board of Faculty and was awarded the Faculty Medal. He was President of the Association of Anaesthetists and before that Assistant Editor of *Anaesthesia* and Chairman of the Editorial Board. He was President of the Section of Anaesthetics of the Royal Society of Medicine in 1959. He also received the Hickman Medal. Foreign honours include the award of the first Carl Koller Medal of the European Society of Regional Anaesthesia on the occasion of the centenary of the first use of local analgesia in Vienna and the invitation to deliver the Gaston Labat Lecture to the American Society of Regional Anesthesia.

What of the man? He was acclaimed as a teacher, and took particular interest in overseas graduates. He was a loyal friend, respected for his wisdom, he was also known for his absolute integrity and for his humility.

We have lost a great man.

ORGANIZATION AND COMMUNICATIONS

Heraldry and anaesthesia

TB Boulton

Original presentation Croydon 1989

Heraldry (the art and science of personal identification) originated spontaneously in Europe and the British Isles for utilitarian reasons in the twelfth century. The heavily armoured knights of the period with their faces concealed by the visors of their helmets could not be easily identified as friend or foe. They therefore painted and embroidered distinguishing devices on their shields, clothes and flags.

These devices were very soon artistically formalized and used to identify individuals and their retainers, for opulent display at sporting tournaments of prowess in the martial arts, and on great ceremonial occasions such as coronations. They were also used on seals to authenticate and approve documents in an era in which the ability to write was given to few people, whatever their station in society. At first heraldic devices were adopted at the whim of the individuals, but very soon their use was rigorously controlled by Royal command to avoid duplication and, from then on, the right to bear arms was by means of a warrant issued on behalf of the Sovereign in the case of a new grant, or inherited by sons from their 'armigerous' fathers.

The use of heraldry on armour in war was comparatively short-lived, due to the introduction of the use of gunpowder in Europe in the early fourteenth century. This made heavy armour obsolete in the face of cannon balls. Despite this the main purposes for which heraldry originated survive to this day. Aircraft, tanks and warships carry flags and other identification marks, football and other sporting teams proudly display their unique emblems on their distinctively coloured shirts, seals are still used on state and other formal documents, and heraldic arms appear on banners and robes on state occasions and on notepaper, buildings and official vehicles. Nowadays, of course, grants of arms are made to corporate bodies as well as to individuals. Anyone can design or use a logo, or register a trade mark, but the right to bear heraldic arms is an honour bestowed only on eminent people or institutions by the Monarch under the Royal prerogative. This is exercised through the College of Arms, an organization founded in 1484 by Richard III. It is under the jurisdiction of the Earl Marshal and its function is to regularize and control the use of arms, and to avoid unauthorized usage. The officers of the

Essays on the history of anaesthesia, edited by A Marshall Barr, Thomas B Boulton and David J Wilkinson. 1996: International Congress and Symposium Series No. 213, published by Royal Society of Medicine Press Limited.

College of Arms are the Heralds, each with an ancient and resounding title, and it is they who originate the grants of arms [1].

The term 'coat of arms' is derived from the surcoat which was worn over armour to keep the wearer cool and to display his armorial bearings. Nowadays, it is usually applied to armorial bearings themselves. An 'Achievement of Arms' consists of the armorial bearings on the shield surrounded by various adjuncts which denote the interests and status of the person or institution which is entitled to the arms. The arms are always described ('blazoned') as one would an X-ray, the right (or 'dexter') side is on the left as you look at it from the front and the left or ('sinister') side is on the right. The convention arises as the description is from the point of view of the bearer of arms holding the shield from behind.

THE ARMS OF THE ASSOCIATION OF ANAESTHETISTS OF GREAT BRITAIN AND IRELAND

The Association of Anaesthetists was formed in 1932, at the instigation of the officers of the Section of Anaesthetics of the Royal Society of Medicine. It is an independent body founded to take care of those aspects of the life of anaesthetists, which we now designate as 'terms and conditions of service' and to promote the conduct of examinations, which the Section could not concern itself with under the terms of the Charter of the Royal Society of Medicine. The Section of Anaesthetics was itself derived from the original Society of Anaesthetists which joined other similar medical specialist societies to form the Royal Society of Medicine in 1909; neither the original Society of Anaesthetists nor the Section itself were armigerous bodies. It therefore seems that the arms of the Association of Anaesthetists were largely designed by the Heralds *de novo* incorporating appropriate medical and specialist anaesthetic symbols [2].

The blazon of the shield or escutcheon of the Association of Anaesthetists is defined as 'gules a rod of Aesculapius proper in chief two poppy heads' or, 'a red background with a rod of Aesculapius in its natural colours surmounted by two gold poppy heads'. The Aesculpian staff symbolizes the status of members of the Association as physicians, which nowadays can be taken to include their function in critical care medicine and the management of pain. The poppy heads represent morphia, one of the principal drugs used by the specialty.

The helmet is that of an esquire or gentleman (it has a closed visor and is turned to one side), in accordance with the professional standing of physician anaesthetists.

The crest is fixed on the top or 'skull' of the helmet. The whole coat of arms is sometimes referred to as 'the Crest'; however this is incorrect. The crest was a three dimensional object mounted on the helmet. It was originally made of metal, like the mascot on a Rolls Royce car, and its purpose was to distinguish the wearer when his visor was closed. A crest is frequently used on its own, as a badge or as a device—on a tie for example. The Association of Anaesthetists' crest consists of two mandrake plants—extract of mandrake roots was used traditionally as a soporific in surgery.

The 'mantling' or 'lambrequin' depicted as being a piece of cloth secured to the helmet under a wreath, is nowadays decorative and can be used to display symbolic colours. Originally it kept the hot sun off the metal helmet. A similar piece of cloth to protect the neck hangs from the back of the cap of the French Foreign Legionnaire. The mantling on the helmet of the Association is in the medical colour of red entwined with silver.

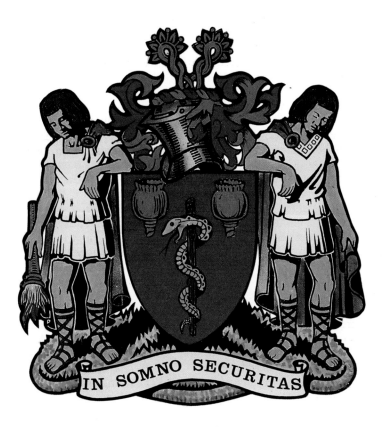

Figure 1   *Arms of the Association of Anaesthetists of Great Britain and Ireland*

The Supporters are on either side of the shield. Supporters are hardly ever granted to esquires and rarely to knights, but in recent years it has become customary to allow more eminent institutions to use them. In the case of the Association the choice had led to some criticism [2]. They are not drunken or sleeping anaesthetists, but Somnus the god of sleep on the dexter side, and his son Morpheus the god of pleasant dreams on the left or sinister side. The inverted torch of learning represents both the academic function of the Association and the diminished but surviving flame of life under anaesthesia.

The motto was originally a battle cry shouted by the armoured knight to rally his troops and frighten his enemies. It is now more usually a declaration of the more peaceful intentions of the individual or institution bearing arms!

'In somno securitas' is an appropriate but limited declaration for the Association of Anaesthetists. It does not cover local anaesthesia or the activities of the anaesthetists outside the operating theatre, but, of course, it must be borne in mind that technical general anaesthesia was practically the only *raison d'être* of anaesthetists at the time the grant of arms was made in 1945.

The arms were re-drawn by Peter Cull, the Medical Artist at St Bartholomew's Hospital, London, at the time of the 4th World Congress of Anaesthesiologists in

1968, and the new version was subsequently adopted on the cover of the journal *Anaesthesia* which was designed in the following year.

THE ARMS OF THE ROYAL COLLEGE OF ANAESTHETISTS

The College of Anaesthetists came into being in 1988 when a supplementary charter to the charter of the Royal College of Surgeons of England enabled its 'Faculty of Anaesthetists' to be designated as a College. The new College of Anaesthetists remained part of the Royal College of Surgeons of England.

The College of Arms at first were reluctant to grant arms to an organization which was not itself independently chartered but remained part of another body. The grant was eventually made to the Surgeons' College for the use of the College of Anaesthetists. Provision was also made in the warrant for the right to use the arms to pass absolutely to the College of Anaesthetists should it at any time itself receive its own Royal Charter and become independent as it did in 1991, becoming the Royal College of Anaesthetists.

The Faculty of Anaesthetists of the Royal College of Surgeons of England was founded in 1948 on the petition of the Association of Anaesthetists of Great Britain and Ireland. The objective at the time was to create a chartered academic and examining body for anaesthetists which would ensure that its Fellows would be able to assume the responsibilities of Consultants in the new British National Health Service. The arms of the Royal College of Anaesthetists has elements derived from the arms of its armigerous forebears (the Association of Anaesthetists of Great Britain and Ireland and through it the Royal Society of Medicine [2], and of the Royal College of Surgeons of England and, in turn, through it of the older Company of Surgeons) [3].

The shield of the Royal College of Anaesthetists therefore has a design which echoes that of the surgeons' College but is itself unique. Both the shield of the Royal College of Surgeons of England and that of its predecessor the Company of Surgeons displayed crosses on a silver (or white) field. The device on the surgical College shield is the red cross of St George of England but the one used on the shield of its predecessor, the Company of Surgeons, was a distinctive blue "engrailed" cross; this has now been adopted for use by the College of Anaesthetists. The bright blue colour, coincidentally and appropriately, mirrors the 'french' or 'electric' blue currently used to distinguish British nitrous oxide cylinders. The shield of the Royal College of Surgeons of England has a red band 'in chief', across the top of the shield. This has also been included on the new shield. The colours, red, white (silver) and blue also suggest that the College of Anaesthetists has jurisdiction throughout the United Kingdom, whereas the red and white of the surgeons' shield with its St George's cross, only represent England.

The charges on the shield have been carefully chosen. The golden morphia poppy heads or seed boxes, which come from the arms of the Association of Anaesthetists of Great Britain and Ireland are displayed 'in chief'; they represent general anaesthesia and analgesia. The knotted serpents in the first and fourth quadrants are taken from the surgeons' shield; snakes are traditionally associated with the power of healing. The novel cocaine leaves in the second and fourth quadrants represent local anaesthesia. The lion's 'face', at the centre or 'fez point', echoes the crouching lions of the surgeons' coat of arms and represent vigilance.

The helmet depicted by the College of Arms is that of an esquire or gentleman because the visor is closed. This reflects the status of British anaesthetists as

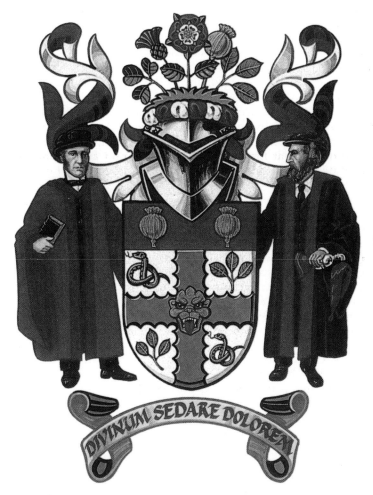

Figure 2 *Arms of the Royal College of Anaesthetists*

members of the medical profession. The helmet is, however, unusual as it faces forward, (affrontée), like that of a knight which usually has an open visor. An esquire's helmet is usually set in profile with a closed visor, as in the arms of the Royal Society of Medicine and the Association of Anaesthetists of Great Britain and Ireland.

The crest of the Royal College of Anaesthetists symbolizes general and local anaesthesia (the poppy head and cocaine leaves) and the geographical jurisdiction of the College (the Tudor rose of England and Wales, the thistle of Scotland, and the shamrock of Northern Ireland).

The mantling of the helmet is in red, green and white (silver); these are the principal colours of the arms of the Royal Society of Medicine.

The supporters of the arms of the Royal College of Anaesthetists are the pioneer British anaesthetists John Snow (1813–1858) and Joseph Thomas Clover (1825–1882). Snow is depicted as a Doctor of Medicine of the University of London and has his early treatise *On the Inhalation of Ether in Surgical Operations* in his hand,

and Clover holds his famous portable ether inhaler and is dressed in the robes of the Royal College of Surgeons of England. The dress of the supporters emphasizes that Snow was primarily a physician and that Clover was originally a surgeon. This again follows a tradition; the arms of the surgeons' College are supported by Machaon and Podalirus, the legendary surgeon and physician at the siege of Troy, and those of the Royal Society of Medicine by the twin medical and surgical saints Cosmos and Damian.

The motto 'Divinum sedare dolorem' (It is divine—or praiseworthy—to alleviate pain) was chosen by the College Council with great care. It reflects the primary function of the specialty of anaesthetists of the treatment of chronic as well as acute pain. It is also easily translated by those who are not familiar with the Latin tongue.

CONCLUSION

The Royal College of Anaesthetists is a new institution born out of compromise and representing the endeavours of many anaesthetists, most of whom are also members of the Association of Anaesthetists of Great Britain and Ireland. Heraldry is an ancient science but it is right and proper that the institutions representing the younger science of anaesthesia should be dignified by Coats of Arms.

REFERENCES

(1) Lynch-Robinson C, Lynch-Robinson A. *Intelligible heraldry*. London: Macdonald, 1948.
(2) Boulton TB. Arms and the anaesthetist. *Anaesthesia* 1973; **29**: 627–8.
(3) Rees AJM. The armorial bearings of the Royal College of Surgeons of England. *Coat of Arms* 1967; **9**: 298.

History of the Society for the Advancement of Anaesthesia in Dentistry

P Sykes

Original presentation London 1987

The history of dental anaesthesia in the United Kingdom and the history of the Society for the Advancement of Anaesthesia in Dentistry are inextricably bound together. The acronym SAAD is probably known to every dentist in Great Britain, but only a few were involved in its inception because the Society started as a very small organization indeed.

By the time that John Snow put the seal of respectability upon anaesthesia by administering chloroform to Queen Victoria, nitrous oxide anaesthesia was firmly established in dental practice. When it later became discredited for use in general surgery, nitrous oxide continued to be used where it had started, in dentistry. Although a few anaesthetists, including Clover, did give chloroform for dentistry, the development of anaesthesia in Great Britain, generally speaking, followed two separate, if parallel lines. Anaesthetists who routinely exhibited open ether or chloroform in theatres, would use nitrous oxide when they attended a dental practice. This differentiation persisted, and still applied when I was a student.

At Guy's Hospital, in 1950, we were taught the technique which has been called 'elegant strangulation', and I could never understand why. When 100% nitrous oxide, leather straps, the restraining influence of members of the Guy's rugby team and ethyl chloride sprayed on to the mouth pack, had all failed to subdue a 20 stone brewer's drayman from the Borough, the anaesthetic registrar would be called in to give a quick shot of thiopentone—and peace reigned immediately. Why should not peace reign all the time I wondered. The motto of Guy's Hospital is *dare quam accipere*, which you will have translated instantly as 'it is better to give than to receive'. It struck me at the time that this should also be the motto of the dental anaesthetist.

INTRAVENOUS ANAESTHESIA FOR DENTISTRY

With this background, early in 1955 a group of professional gentlemen gathered at 53 Wimpole Street, London, the practice house of Mr Stanley Drummond-Jackson, who had been using intravenous anaesthetic agents for dentistry since the 1930s. During the war he had been seconded as anaesthetist to a Field Ambulance Unit of the Parachute Regiment, and had broken his neck jumping with the Red Berets. Re-establishing his practice after the war, he felt that the time was ripe to spread his passionate conviction that intravenous anaesthesia was the only true way. The others in the group were dentists and anaesthetists, and their intention was to form a study club.

For some years, the use of intravenous agents was strongly opposed by large sections of the medical profession, just as general anaesthesia itself had been back in the 1850s. So when it was proposed that intravenous anaesthetics should be used in dentistry, it can be imagined how this was greeted by the profession which had largely opposed their use by anaesthetists. Yet administering general anaesthesia was an officially required part of the dentist's work. For some peculiar reason, the blue, anoxic, jactitating patient was thought to be in less danger from the 'black gas' than was the pink, peaceful recipient of an intravenous barbiturate. So when the Wimpole Street group started their study club, they did so with a distinct feeling of adventure and of living dangerously. At least one anaesthetist member, the Australian Dr Donald Blatchley, whose wife was one of Drummond-Jackson's patients, joined the club because he thought that if other dentists were going to use intravenous drugs, they'd better learn how to do so properly!

By 1957, the study club had met on a number of occasions, and had decided to expand its aims and form a Society—the Society for the Advancement of Anaesthesia in Dentistry (SAAD). The Society had drawn up a draft Constitution. (The Constitution was actually drawn up by the then Lord Chancellor of England: Drummond-Jackson made shameless use of his patients!). The new Society was due to hold its inaugural meeting in October 1957, the speaker being Dr WS McConnell, Head of Anaesthesia at Guy's and a partner with Sir Robert Macintosh in the famous 'Mayfair Gas Company'.

However, some time before this meeting was due, Drummond-Jackson learned that Dr Harold Krogh of Washington, an experienced and much-respected dental anaesthetist, would be passing through London on his way to Rome, where he was to be reporter on anaesthetics at that year's Congress. Krogh agreed to speak to the Society, and on 15 August 1957, an audience of 42 heard what was in effect the very first lecture given to SAAD. One of Dr Krogh's phrases became the Society's watchword—'the team goes into action at the first altered breath'. Another—'a good way to make friends of an anesthetist is to ask him what any particular drug is doing in the body at that exact moment'—I have never had the courage to test out.

By the end of its first year the Society had 43 members, and by the end of the next 90. In March 1958, they heard Dr John Buxton in a lecture on 'Training the Dental Anaesthetist', say 'Every anaesthetist should become so adept in the use of the intravenous barbiturates such as thiopentone that this method of induction would eventually become the normal procedure and not the exceptional method practised by the minority, as at present'. That was said less than 40 years ago!

TRAINING COURSES

The demand for information and for training was increasing, and it became evident that some form of teaching would have to be undertaken. Six of the senior members were formed into a sub-committee on education, and they produced a syllabus for an intensive 3-day weekend course, restricted to experienced practitioners who wished to update their knowledge. There were five lecturers: Blatchley, Buxton, and Hudson, who were consultant anaesthetists, with Mandiwall and Drummond-Jackson, both dentists, between them covering a wide range of subjects. There were to be eight participants on each course, so the staff/student ratio was pretty impressive. These courses were held in the basement of 53 Wimpole Street, Drummond-Jackson's practice, which had been adapted for the purpose. The projection room was the partitioned arched alcove of an old wine cellar, and the lecture room was made by lining the cellar with oak panelling which had come from the board room of St Mary's Hospital. The first course was scheduled for October 1959 with one a month thereafter until February 1960. It was anticipated that five courses would probably be sufficient to cope with the demand—a total of 40 people. In hindsight, this was a most remarkable misjudgement.

The technique originally taught was a single shot of thiopentone or hexobarbitone, the drug and the dosage being chosen to allow sufficient operating time. It was recognized that incremental dosage would produce summation and so take the patient unpredictably and possibly dangerously deep. Although hexobarbitone (Cyclonal) took longer to wear off, it was often preferred, because the patients woke with a tremendous feeling of euphoria.

The first courses were heavily over-subscribed and the number of members was increased from eight to ten, and from ten to twelve. There were in addition four scientific meetings a year, the digested reports of the presentations and discussion being circulated. February 1960 saw publication of the first of the *Librarian's News-sheets*. In the years to come, these were to form a powerful, if idiosyncratic, expression of the Society's views, which was hardly surprising since the librarian was the powerful and idiosyncratic Stanley Drummond-Jackson. The news-sheets led directly to publication of the first *SAAD Handbook* the 6th edition of which I produced after Drummond-Jackson's death. At the time, they were the most authoritative books on the subject available to the dental anaesthetist.

The first news-sheet in 1960 noted a prize of 200 guineas offered by the Association of Anaesthetists of Great Britain & Ireland for 'The best essay based upon new and original work related to the subject of general anaesthesia for dental surgery'. With the addition of sedation, this is essentially the same subject-matter for which SAAD has three times awarded prizes totalling £1000 in memory of Stanley Drummond-Jackson. The same news-sheet also noted that Eli Lilly & Co of Indianapolis had produced a new intravenous anaesthetic agent called methohexital sodium. The paragraph carried this sentence, 'It is probable that this drug will herald a greater advance in dental induction anaesthesia on the ambulant patient than in any other branch of anaesthesia'. Not even the writer himself could possibly have foreseen how amply his prophecy was to be fulfilled.

It was soon recognized by a number of dentist administrators that with methohexitone (the UK name) the operating time could be extended by intermittent incremental dosage. After testing to produce an assuredly safe method, this was adopted as the Society's principal technique. At this time the National Health Service was very new, dentists were struggling against an unparalleled backlog of need, many of these new patients were extremely fearful yet needed vast amounts of restorative work, and none of our present sedative drugs existed. Whether it was regarded as light anaesthesia or deep sedation (or even, if you were clever enough, light sedation) there is no doubt that it was a successful technique. Whatever its theoretical dangers, incremental methohexitone in dentistry proved in practice to have an unmatched safety record. It led directly to the use of total intravenous anaesthesia by anaesthetists, but not until the furore had died down over its initial introduction by dentists.

Those early days were filled with innovation and a sense of enquiring discovery. There was a constant flow of new inventions, particularly in instruments and materials, in order to keep pace with the changing techniques. Patients were still seated upright in the conventional dental chairs, so do-it-yourself adaptations abounded; the more successful to be followed by commercial versions. There were many notes in the news-sheets: about the explosiveness of divinyl ether when mixed with oxygen (patients were advised not to smoke after the anaesthetic); about the mortality rate of dental anaesthesia in Britain, which Victor Goldman gave as 1:80 000 from 1952–1957, while in 1980 it was, according to Coplans & Curson, at the very most 1:260 000; on the use of alcohol as premedication (often seeming more valuable for the administrator than for the patient); and on the use of rectally-administered thiopentone. This latter was advised, amongst other cases, for the difficult child. One speaker gave the case of a boy who vociferously refused all treatment. Eventually, his trousers were forcibly removed and a thiopentone suppository inserted. Whereupon he calmed down immediately, and in a very hurt tone of voice said, 'Well! That was NOT a very nice thing to do, I must say!'

The demand for places on the training courses increased rapidly. The size of the courses went from the eight students of 1959 to 24, and the number per year from four to six. The waiting list continued to grow and the content of the course was continually altered and updated. In 1963, Drummond-Jackson conceived the idea of an updating meeting for past course members. This was organized at very short notice, held at the Royal Society of Medicine in London, and attracted almost half of all the past course members. The first day was devoted to question panels and table demonstrations, and culminated in a dinner at the Café Royal (because Charles Forte, who owned it, was a patient of Drummond-Jackson).

This 2-day meeting was so successful that it led immediately to the idea of a more open and general instructional meeting, a 'Two-Day Tutorial', to be held in July 1964. University College was chosen as a venue—it had a lecture theatre which seated 250, and another room which could be converted into a clinical demonstration theatre from which closed-circuit television could be screened in the lecture room. The meeting was booked to capacity.

The success of this larger tutorial gave Drummond-Jackson the idea which was to make his and the Society's name better-known than he could possibly have imagined. If the Society could cope with 250 people for a 2-day seminar (which in the event became nearly 3 days anyway), why not take similar numbers on a fully structured 3-day mass teaching course? The waiting list then stood at about 240. In July 1966 the first of the so-called 'Jumbo' courses took place. The first speaker was John Buxton, Consultant Anaesthetist at Guy's, who opened every course thereafter until his retirement from the Society.

Venepuncture practice was compulsory and was organized in teams of four so that each member both gave and received two venepunctures. If any team was short of numbers, the demonstrators had to sit in and take what was coming to them. After some trials with closed-circuit television, clinical demonstrations became settled into what was called 'the four-ring circus'. This was a sort of non-musical chairs, where four different techniques were demonstrated simultaneously and all the viewers changed seats when the bell rang. We never did find a really satisfactory solution to the problem of good clinical demonstrations in all our years at University College, but the courses themselves acquired a legendary reputation for efficient organization, even if subject to instant extemporization. During one summer course when the air conditioning failed, D-J sent out on the spur of the moment for 200 ice creams, to be issued all round, on the house.

The list of speakers during the years reads like an honour roll-call of the greats in dental sedation and anaesthesia: Massey Dawkins; Professor Dundee; Victor Goldman; Sir Robert Macintosh; Sir Ivan Magill; Professor Mushin; the Americans Joel Berns; Professor Niels Jorgensen; Harry Langa of relative analgesia fame; Professor Monheim; Sylvan Shane; Darryl Beach, who converted us to the supine position, and many more.

In 1969, the teaching staff on the SAAD courses consisted of Professor Sir Robert Macintosh, of Oxford; Donald Blatchley, Consultant at Atkinson Morley's Hospital; John Buxton; James Bourne, Consultant at St. Thomas's; Maurice Hudson, Consultant at University College Hospital; Henry Mandiwall, Consultant Oral Surgeon, West Middlesex Hospital, and Drummond-Jackson himself. There were in addition, 24 group tutors and demonstrators, all either dental or medical general practitioners.

By this time, so many overseas dentists had participated in the courses that Drummond-Jackson was well-known abroad, and in 1969 he was invited to Temple University, Philadelphia, to start the first of their courses in dental anaesthesia. In 1971 he went to Hong Kong, Australia and New Zealand. As a result of SAAD's teaching, its sister Society in the US adopted the name. There is also an Italian SAAD and daughter Societies in Australia, Ireland and New Zealand.

LIBEL ACTION

Sadly, 1971 was the last peaceful year for Drummond-Jackson, because in 1972 a libel action came to court which made British legal history. In 1969, Professor John Robinson of Birmingham University Anaesthetics Department, together with other anaesthetists and a dentist, had published in the *British Medical Journal* and the *British Dental Journal* the results of a series of trials they had conducted into the use of methohexitone in conservative dentistry. By SAAD's standards, where ultra-light anaesthesia and minimum dosage were the rule, the times taken were excessive and the dosages massive. When their paper appeared, I was so appalled by the technique that they had used that I wrote immediately to the journals to condemn the investigation. Several consultant anaesthetists did the same.

To add what Drummond-Jackson considered insult to injury, the investigators referred to their method as the 'Drummond-Jackson technique'. He was so incensed that he took both the authors and the *British Medical Journal* to court for libel. The case came to Court in March 1972 and ended in November at the judge's insistence, having become the longest libel case in British legal history to date. The costs were already astronomical, Drummond-Jackson's case had not yet been fully presented and the defendents' case had not been heard at all! There was an agreed compromise, by which each party whitewashed the other, and each side bore its own costs. The defendants' costs were covered by their Defence Societies, but Drummond-Jackson's came from his own pocket and swallowed up the savings of a lifetime. His pride had cost him dearly. Although this had been a personal case, it made a great mark on the Society, because of the animosity which it engendered. Things did go on much as before, but the effect on Drummond-Jackson was profound. In 1974 he had his first heart attack. He appeared to recover, and became even more energetic than before. He was elected President of SAAD in April 1975, but in December he died of his second coronary. The two newest members of SAAD Council suddenly found themselves pitchforked into positions of responsibility; myself as Course Organizer and Editor of *SAAD Digest*, Gerry Holden as President.

THE MODERN ERA

Naturally, things have changed, not only because of changing faces and personalities, but with changing circumstances. The Robin Brook Centre at St Bartholomew's Hospital is now the site for the theoretical part of our courses. New drugs having made possible effective sedation instead of anaesthesia, SAAD now teaches only dental sedation, and basic and advanced cardiopulmonary resuscitation. True to the Society's tradition of excellence, the latter subjects are taught by senior consultant anaesthetists who are members of both the British and European Resuscitation Councils.

The Society has always moved with the times, but its philosophy has remained constant. Certainly its first 20 years owed almost everything to the remarkable man Stanley Drummond-Jackson. The path of the Society has not always been easy; indeed, at times it has not been an acceptable Society to belong to, but it continues to be in the forefront of developments in dental sedation in Great Britain. SAAD occupies a leading place among dental anaesthesiology Societies world-wide, having established a foundation upon which others have discovered that they, too, could build.

The Scottish Society of Anaesthetists

AW Raffan

Original presentation Edinburgh 1989

Early in 1914, a group of Scottish general practitioners, all interested in and practising anaesthesia, decided to meet for discussion. Fourteen were invited to a dinner at the Balmoral Hotel, Princes Street, Edinburgh on 20 February 1914.

FOUNDATION

Eleven doctors attended—McAllum, Gibbs, Jones, Ross and Torrance Thomson of Edinburgh; Boyd, Fairlie, Lamb and Napier of Glasgow; Johnston of Aberdeen and Mills of Dundee. After dinner, they resolved unanimously to form a society to be called The Scottish Society of Anaesthetists, with the objective of promoting the study of the science and practice of anaesthetics, the proper teaching thereof, and the conservation and advancement of the interests of anaesthetists. Ordinary membership was to be restricted to members of the medical profession practising the specialty of anaesthetics.

The first regular meeting was held in the Guild Hall, Edinburgh on 18 April 1914. Drs Home Henderson of Glasgow, and Ogston and Robertson of Aberdeen who had sent apologies for the dinner meeting, were admitted to Founder Membership. Dr McAllum had been elected first President, and he gave an address entitled 'False Anaesthesia' [1]. He was a keen and expert chloroformist and a leading exponent in paediatric anaesthesia [2]. Sadly he died shortly afterwards.

The distractions of World War I might well have destroyed this fledgling society, for it was $5\frac{1}{2}$ years before the second regular meeting was held—in November 1919 under the Presidency of Dr Boyd. Dr Johnston reported the death of another Founder Member, James Robertson, who had been killed in action in March 1918 when serving as Officer Commanding the 2/1 Field Ambulance of the Highland Division.

In 1920 the Annual Meeting was held in Aberdeen when Torrance Thomson was President. The Vice-President, John Johnston, read a paper on 'The importance of carbon dioxide in relation to general anaesthesia'. At this meeting Ross MacKenzie of Aberdeen became a member. Johnston became President in November, and was re-elected a year later, when he spoke on 'Pre-anaesthetic intoxication'.

In April 1922 Alexander Ogston read his paper 'Notes on the administration of ether by the per-halation method'. He claimed that by using his adaptation of the Bellamy–Gardner mask he found no difficulty in inducing even a powerful subject with 'straight' ether [3]. The simple addition of the chimney served to trap the expired ether vapour, thereby increasing the concentration and speeding the induction by the partial retention of expired carbon dioxide. This mask was so popular with the house physicians who had to give the emergency anaesthetics in those days, that they invariably armed themselves with one when they went further afield.

CHLOROFORM AND ETHER

The controversy about the use of chloroform raged throughout this period. I quote Dr Lamb of Glasgow: 'We had to fight against the belief and teaching of Sir William Macewen and all other Scottish surgeons that chloroform was the one and only anaesthetic, even though the death rate on the table was very high, an average of 50 annually in Glasgow Royal Infirmary. The vested interest of the general practitioners for whom the fee for the administration of chloroform was a valued perquisite, also had to be overcome. We went through all the stages of mixing chloroform and ether, ether with Clover's inhaler, later preceded by nitrous oxide or ethyl chloride' [4]. When Arthur Mills was President in 1923 his address was 'The present position of chloroform'. He was an outspoken critic, no doubt because so many anaesthetics were being given by the casual anaesthetist. The choice of chloroform by the tyro was obvious. It was non-irritant and quick to produce relaxation which satisfied the surgeon, and he could easily say '. . . the operation was successful, but the patient died'. Dr Mills stressed the teaching of open ether to his students. At a meeting of the Society in the 1950s he recalled; 'When I went to France in the First World War, I left all my juniors with the instruction that open ether, slow as it may be, should be the routine . . .' Demonstrating slowly dropping ether on the mask, he would tell them, 'This do ye in remembrance of Mills'.

In 1924 the question of admitting women as members was raised, not without some opposition, but the proposition was agreed—by a majority of three. In the following year, the first woman was elected, Dr EJ Swan. In 1926 the Society were hosts to the Associated Anesthetists of the United States and Canada, represented by Mary Batsford of San Francisco; Wade Elphingstone of Pittsburg; Hammard of White Plains, New York; McMechan of Avon Lake, Ohio; McKesson and Schuey of Toledo and Wesley Bourne of Montreal. Ross MacKenzie gave a lantern lecture and demonstration on carbon dioxide in nitrous oxide and oxygen anaesthesia. 'Re-breathing', he claimed, '. . . conserved the body heat, retained the expired carbon dioxide, and delayed the onset of surgical shock'. Torrance Thomson demonstrated ethyl chloride and ether with the Ogston mask, and the President, Dr Stuart Ross spoke on 'The provision of an anaesthetic service'. He set out to prove the need for increasing the supply of skilled anaesthetists, and that special instruction should be given to resident housemen immediately on taking office. No hospital had the right to offer a service of skilled anaesthetists for a few hours only in the day, since a 24 hour service alone could reduce the mortality rate. Referring to the rising death rate, he noted, 'The increased boldness and activity of the surgeons meant the tax upon the anaesthetist's skill was greater than ever before' [5].

Dr Ogston, President in 1927, continued the theme of better training. In Aberdeen the students had to attend a minimum of four lectures, and administer a minimum of 12 anaesthetics. 'Not a very satisfactory state', he suggested, 'but improvement seemed impossible because the curriculum is so overloaded with subjects that most students find it difficult to give much time to anaesthetics; they are usually attending a clinic in a subject in which they have to face examination' [6].

In May 1928 Dr Barras was elected President, but sadly he was killed in a car accident just 2 months later. The Vice-President, Ross MacKenzie took over and discussed 'Post-anaesthetic sickness'. Much later, in the first edition of the *Scottish Society of Anaesthetist's Newsletter*, MacKenzie recalled the early days. Of the 'founders and pillars of our society', 'Stuart Ross was a robust man, an administrator and the author of an excellent book on practical anaesthetics; Fairlie was a man of refined character with great ability and vision. He was the perfect anaesthetist and had the complete confidence of the surgeons of Glasgow. Torrance Thomson was the scientific anaesthetist and observer. He was a philosopher and appeared to scorn the mundane things of everyday life. Napier was the genial, cynical, highly efficient secretary'. He went on to discuss delicate situations in his practice in Aberdeen. 'On occasions, I was reminded that the anaesthetist had no patients and that any suggestion I made regarding pre- or post-anaesthetic treatment would require to be sanctioned by the surgeon in charge and might be vetoed by him. It was a very hard, sometimes humiliating road . . .' One must appreciate his difficulties, common to others in his position, for he was the first doctor in Aberdeen to forsake general practice and concentrate on anaesthetics, rendering himself dependent financially on surgical private practice, his hospital work being honorary. It was Ross MacKenzie who eventually persuaded the Governors to appoint the first resident anaesthetist in 1937.

NEW TECHNIQUES

In Dundee in 1930 Torrance Thomson entertained his audience with 'Random reflections'. At this time anaesthetists were uneasy about the traditional methods of saturating patients with ether or chloroform, and with the cooperation of the surgeons were attempting 'balanced anaesthesia' as described by McKesson. Crile had advocated such a combination of agents in 1920, and Lundy had coined the term in 1926 for his combination of premedication, general anaesthesia and local analgesia. 'What we are searching for,' said Torrance Thomson, 'is a method immediately safe, with adequate operating facilities and free from postoperative ill effects. Surgeons have become accustomed to the flaccid abdomen of deep etherisation in which they can roam freely without troubling much about the effects of their stimuli; but now, with nitrous oxide, oxygen anaesthesia, if it is to have a fair chance in abdominal surgery, the surgeon must in the first place reduce his demands regarding relaxation. Secondly he must remember he has a narrow zone of anaesthesia on which to draw, any extra stimulus may bring the patient outside this zone. There is still', he continued, 'a belief outside Scotland, that chloroform is with us the anaesthetic of choice, comparable with the belief that we all wear kilts, subsist on haggis, porridge and whisky. It is true that most of us make a modest use of these commodities and it is true that we make a moderate use of chloroform, but in inhalation techniques ether predominates, and it is probable that in time ether will be superseded . . . in the meantime we should welcome any adjuvant which lessens the quantity of ether used' [7].

In 1931 the first female President, Dr Winifred Wood, addressed the Society on 'Pre-medication, with special reference to rectal ether' a method she had studied under Gwathmey in America. In 1936 John Johnston of Aberdeen became President for the third time, a unique honour. He spoke on intravenous evipan sodium, the question of dosage demanding close attention. He described 'biological dosage: twice the sleep dose for a short operation, three times for a longer one'. The speed of injection was important: 'If sleep is slow to come, pause before continuing' [8]. Anaesthetists in those days, preoccupied with the clear and definite signs of ether anaesthesia as described by Guedel, were extremely worried at using a drug with no such signs. I am indebted to Dr Johnston for leaving me copies of the early minutes of our Society, and many other records and memorabilia.*

ANOTHER GAP—AND PERSONAL REFLECTIONS

With the advent of war in 1939, the Society went into limbo once again, this time for 11 years. The gap gives the opportunity for a few personal reflections.

During the 1930s, techniques and even status improved, but fees did not. It was a heavy responsibility to give up general practice and rely on anaesthetics for a living. Anaesthetists of my vintage form the last link with the pre-war days when we moved from open ether with ethyl chloride, and very occasionally chloroform, to nitrous oxide, oxygen, and ether, and spinal anaesthesia. My interest in the specialty, like that of many others, was born of necessity when as housemen we were expected to cope with night emergencies. When I worked in Eastbourne, I saw at first hand Dr Bodkin Adams, who was in general practice with an appointment as visiting anaesthetist. Even to my young eyes he was a most undesirable character; reasonably proficient, no doubt, but his real skill lay in persuading elderly lady patients to alter their wills in his favour. I had a close interest when in 1957, he was charged with murder, and narrowly escaped hanging. It was not his activities which inspired me to take up anaesthetics.

I became the second resident anaesthetist in Aberdeen in 1938–9 under the guidance of Ross MacKenzie. Perhaps for me the greatest adventure in those days was to anaesthetize for a partial thyroidectomy. Pre-operative assessment was minimal, as was the preparation for surgery, and the patients tended to be in a highly toxic state. As our surgeon, Gordon Bruce, was a skilled operator, Surgeon to the Royal Household and a close fishing friend of Thomas (later Sir Thomas) Dunhill, and the physician Stanley (later Sir Stanley) Davidson, we felt we were in the forefront of this pioneering surgery. We followed the well-known method of 'stealing the thyroid'. The surgeons did not favour the endotracheal tube and so the face mask devised by Hewer was used.

Of World War II, Sir Donald Douglas observed when speaking to our Society in 1975, 'The average anaesthetist entered the war as a purveyor of sleep but ended it as a skilled physician of trauma' [9]. My own experience varied from general surgery with Richard Handley, and on occasion Sir Heneage Ogilvie; urology with Ogier Ward; ophthalmology with Hyla Stallard—who became very appreciative of continuous thiopentone; maxillo-facial surgery with Michael Oldfield and Reginald (now Sir Reginald) Murley, where one had to master blind nasal intubation; and finally to Field Surgical Units with Tom Brownlee, Rodney (later Lord) Smith, and John Fairbank, where one became familiar with the Oxford Ether Vaporiser, and worked closely with Gladwin Buttles' Field Transfusion Units.

---

*In 1915 a young midshipman from *HMS Collingwood* was landed in Aberdeen with appendicitis. Professor (later Sir) John Marnoch operated and John Johnston gave the anaesthetic. The patient was Prince Albert, later to be anaesthetized by another President of our Society, John Gillies, when he had become King George VI.

Then back to civilian life as a resident anaesthetist, once more with a much reduced salary, attending courses in Oxford, London and the Thoracic Unit of George Mason at Shotley Bridge, to learn the intricacies of thoracic anaesthesia from Joan Miller. All of this fitted me to obtain an Honorary Appointment in 1946, but with no hospital salary apart from that of the municipal hospitals and the Red Cross Sanitorium. With the National Health Service at last came the security and equality which our founders had fought for.

THE MODERN ERA

The Scottish Society of Anaesthetists was reconstituted in 1950, with the annual meetings allocated to convenient places of neutrality—Dunblane, Gleneagles, St Andrews, Pitlochry, Aviemore. The rebirth was largely due to the efforts of Dr Pinkerton of Glasgow and John Gillies of Edinburgh. No history of the Society would be complete without special reference to these two anaesthetists.

HH Pinkerton, like all the others of the time, started in general practice before specializing in anaesthetics. By the end of the war he was well established in the Western Infirmary in Glasgow and in private practice. Those returning from the war saw him as a mentor of the highest esteem; a natural teacher, he enjoyed the opportunity to train, and set about developing a department of anaesthesia. This was no easy task, but eventually the Board agreed and he was appointed Consultant in Charge. He was a man of infinite charm, and quietly persuasive, who became President of the revitalized Society in 1951, and also President of the Association of Anaesthetists.

John Gillies won a Military Cross for gallantry while serving in the infantry in World War I. From general practice in Yorkshire, he came under the influence of John Hunter and Ivan Magill, when he went south to learn more of his chosen specialty. In 1932 he left London to take an appointment at the Children's Hospital in Edinburgh, with an honorarium of £50 per annum. He was dependent on the goodwill of the surgeons for private work which meant 'rushing from nursing home to hospital to nursing home, lumbered with heavy equipment. A pressurised, competitive existence' [10]. Having been appointed President-in-waiting in 1939, he at last took up office in 1950. As President of the Anaesthetic Section of the Royal Society of Medicine in 1951, he gave his famous address on 'Physiological trespass'.

The rejuvenated Society expanded rapidly in members and in enthusiasm. As well as the Annual General Meeting, a Scientific Meeting and a Registrar's Meeting and Prize have been developed. Since 1977 a Memorial Lecture has been endowed by his family in honour of John Gillies, to 'reflect his interest in the young anaesthetist and his special concern for safe clinical anaesthesia' [11]. The first Gillies Memorial Lecture was delivered by Professor (later Sir) Gordon Robson [12]. He observed that when the Beveridge Committee was taking evidence for its Report which resulted in the National Health Service, John Gillies was an active member of the Council of the Association of Anaesthetists. The Association requested the Council of the College of Surgeons to set up a Faculty Joint Committee, and Gillies, along with Marston, Low, Bernard Johnson, Edwards and Murtagh represented the anaesthetists.

Other stalwarts of the modern Society include AC Forrester, the first Professor of Anaestheics in Scotland, a charming quiet enthusiast for everything concerned with anaesthesia and with the Scottish Society; JD Robertson, Professor in Edinburgh, and President in our Jubilee year of 1964, when he made a plea for our specialty in the undergraduate course; Professor Donald (now Sir Donald) Campbell, the first resident Scot to be appointed Dean of the Faculty; and Malcolm Shaw, who was the backbone of the Society in those post-war years. He was Secretary and Treasurer from 1957 to 1963, and President for 1969. In 1960 he created the *Newsletter*, which he edited until 1967.

The Society has made successful overseas trips, to Scandinavia in 1965 and to Poland in 1970. Our young Polish courier, in his final speech announced, 'You Scots and we Poles have much in common, we both have our Big Brother watching over us.' When asked to explain he said, 'We have the Russians, you have the English'. Shrugging off the English oppression, our Society has continued to flourish both socially and scientifically. We have led the way in such matters as reviewing and reporting deaths under anaesthesia. When our founders met in 1914 they had a dream—to promote the study and the teaching of anaesthetics and the status of the anaesthetist. In less than the lifetime of some of us, their dream has been fulfilled. No longer, in the words of Sir Donald Douglas, is the anaesthetist a mere 'purveyor of sleep'.

REFERENCES

(1) Minutes. Scottish Society of Anaesthetists. 1914.
(2) Hovell BC. *Newsletter, Scottish Society of Anaesthetists*, 1966; **7**: 6.
(3) Minnitt RJ, Gillies J. *Textbook of anaesthetics*. Edinburgh: Livingstone, 1945: 165.
(4) Wright D. *Newsletter, Scottish Society of Anaesthetists*, 1984: 25.
(5) Minutes. Scottish Society of Anaesthetists, 1926.
(6) Minutes. Scottish Society of Anaesthetists, 1927.
(7) Minutes. Scottish Society of Anaesthetists, 1930.
(8) Minutes, Scottish Society of Anaesthetists, 1936.
(9) Douglas D. *Newsletter, Scottish Society of Anaesthetists* 1975: 16.
(10) Gillies J. *Newsletter, Scottish Society of Anaesthetists*, 1972: 13.
(11) Lawson J. *Newsletter, Scottish Society of Anaesthetists*, 1977: 18.
(12) Robson G. *Newsletter, Scottish Society of Anaesthetists*, 1978: 19.

A Leicester dentist — Robert Marston

I McLellan

Original presentation Leicester 1988

Robert Marston, the son of a Leicester pharmacist, was born in 1853. He became a dentist, unqualified prior to the Dental Act of 1878, and had a fairly large practice. He was an inventive man, working on dental ceramics, dental baking ovens, signalling devices for railways, and shoe making equipment — but it was in the field of anaesthesia that he came to the attention of both the general public and the anaesthetists of the day.

MARSTON AND ANAESTHESIA

He developed an anaesthetic machine, basing it on a Clover bag, putting chloroform liquid into an iron tank and pumping in air so it vaporized under pressure. This meant that he had an enormous volume available for anaesthesia. He also used very concentrated chloroform vapour and diluted it with a variable orifice air entrainment system using the Venturi principle, thereby delivering a known concentration of chloroform to the patient. The machine was very cumbersome and stationary. The model later developed in a number of ways, one of which can be seen in the British Dental Association museum in Wimpole Street. He developed a portable type with bag and bellows and, later, a nitrous oxide reservoir. Marston used his apparatus for up to an hour on each patient, an unusual event at that time. He later turned his talents to manufacturing nitrous oxide.

Marston was a good Victorian. He was a strong minded individual; some people would even have called him cantankerous. Several attempts were made to introduce laws in the early twentieth century to restrict the administration of anaesthesia to medical practitioners only. He fought this idea over 25 years, challenging the views of people such as Sir Frederic Hewitt and Dr Dudley Buxton. Marston believed that the operator/anaesthetist was wrong. In his book [1], he stated that the anaesthetist should be one dentist and the operator another (all four of his sons were dentists and worked in the practice with him). This book was a small volume produced in 1899, and included space at the back for individual case records and tables for air entrainment so that the dilution of chloroform vapour could be calculated.

He was deeply concerned with safety, both in controlling the concentration of chloroform vapour as exemplified in his apparatus, and in the training of medical and dental practitioners about anaesthesia. He distributed his views on legislation controlling anaesthesia throughout the country at his own expense, spending enormous amounts of effort, time and money. He even went so far as to write to

Ministers of the Crown, because he believed that a great wrong was being done to the dental profession.

INHALATION OF A TOOTH. NEGLIGENT OR NOT?

With this background, from 11–13 June 1912, an event took place in a court of law in Leicester, which was to have a profound effect on British anaesthesia. An action was brought by a lady's companion, Miss Ethel May Geary aged 25, claiming damages for bronchial pneumonia following the inhalation of a tooth or abscess material during anaesthesia for dental surgery. The plaintiff claimed that she suffered from pneumonia and lost £100 in wages, a large sum. She had gone to the dentist the previous August, and was anaesthetized by Robert Marston. He had by now antagonized local medical opinion; someone must have provided the impetus for this action. A lady's companion in 1912 was unlikely to sue a locally successful businessman and a very respected dentist. There was also conflict between medical practitioners in Leicester. This became quite obvious at the trial when the medical administrators of anaesthesia at the Leicester Royal Infirmary testified for the plaintiff while those from what is now the Leicester General Hospital, for the defendant. Marston lost the case and bitterly resented it and within days had appealed against the verdict. This appeal was held in the following year and Marston won. By this time, it had become a crusade for him and in winning he entailed costs of £11 000 (£403 000 today, or just under $750 000).

The effect of losing the case was immense. He started to transfer the practice and his various interests to his daughters and sons. He felt he was professionally stressed and he was certainly financially strained, even though an appeal fund was started. He sold his factory which was making dental apparatus as well as nitrous oxide and appeared to withdraw from practice, except for occasionally writing and protecting the dentist's right to practise anaesthesia.

ARCHIBALD DANIEL MARSTON

In 1891 a young man was born, who went to Guy's Hospital in 1909 to train as a dentist. After completing this he decided he wanted to read medicine. He qualified in dentistry in 1913 and medicine in 1915. After some surgical training, including gaining his Fellowship, he wished to become an anaesthetist and was appointed as such to Guy's Hospital in 1919, eventually becoming the Head of Department. He became involved with the provision of qualifications in anaesthetic practice and was with the first group who started the Diploma of Anaesthesia. This man was Archibald Daniel Marston, the nephew of Robert Marston, who was also brought up in Leicester.

It is my opinion that the enormous trauma his family had undergone affected him greatly, and for this reason he became involved with the setting up of standards and qualifications. I understand from other sources that during the formation of the National Health Service, Archie Marston was one of the strongest protagonists forcing the Ministry of Health of the time to make anaesthetists and surgeons of equal grading within the NHS.

What happened to Robert Marston's family? Three became qualified dentists, one practised unqualified. The most famous is Alvin Theophilus Marston, his son who became a learned geologist and became the silent member of the Leakey team in Olduvai Gorge.

Robert Marston, one way or another, had an enormous background influence on what anaesthetists are doing today.

REFERENCE

(1) Marston R. *The anaesthetist's pocket book compendium*. Leicester: Marston and Parr, 1899.

The Victorian anaesthetists at the Middlesex Hospital

OP Dinnick

Original presentation Croydon 1989

JOHN TOMES

The first person credited with administering anaesthetics at the hospital was the 'surgeon-dentist' John Tomes. He was the first Middlesex graduate to be appointed to the senior staff, and later became Sir John, the doyen of English dentistry [1]. On 25 January 1847 Tomes gave his first anaesthetic for a general surgical operation—a long and difficult lithotomy. But part of the credit for this achievement must be attributed to another great man, Jacob Bell, the founder of the Pharmaceutical Society and editor of its journal. Although Tomes was nominally the anaesthetist, the ether inhaler was 'invented by Mr Bell, Chemist, of Oxford Street, who was present and assisted Mr Tomes in its application' [2].

JACOB BELL, CHLORIC ETHER AND CHLOROFORM

Bell had described his inhaler 12 days previously [3], but the contemporary accounts do not say why Tomes chose it from the many others then available. The implication is that the two men had previously worked together, as it is unlikely that Tomes would choose an unknown assistant for his first anaesthetic for a major procedure. The anaesthetic for the lithotomy was undoubtedly sulphuric ether, but they had some experience of chloric ether. By then Tomes had already given some dental anaesthetics—not all successful [4]—using 'sulphuric and sometimes chloric ether' [5] and only a few days later, on 1 February, Bell reported that 'chloric ether had been tried in some cases with success' [6] but he did not say whether he had conducted the trial or where it had been performed. Not until Simpson announced in November his use of chloroform, did the editor of the *London Medical Gazette* reveal that Bell's trial in January had been made at the Middlesex [7].

Much later Alfred Coleman wrote 'Mr Bell employed it (chloric ether) at the Middlesex Hospital where several dental operations were performed under its agency' [8]. The surgeon could only have been Tomes, who described how 'Mr Bell brought to the hospital a little chloric ether that its effect might be tested' [9]. Unfortunately he did not record the date. His concluding remark that 'I did not again use this drug' suggests that this incident occurred before 25 January, as his diary made no later reference to chloric ether. Moreover, for his early dental cases Tomes had also administered chloric and sulphuric ether together [10]—a combination also used repeatedly by Bell [11].

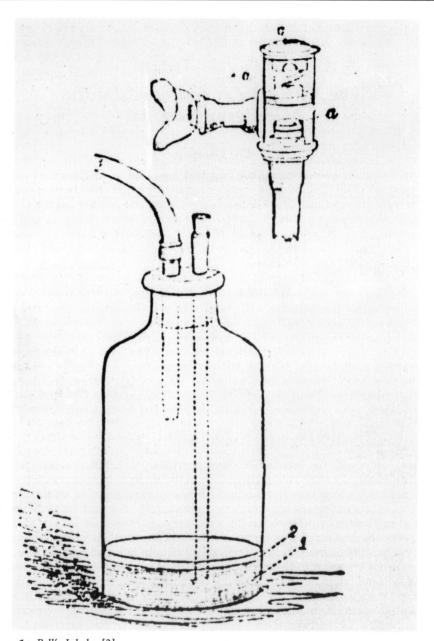

Figure 1 *Bell's Inhaler [3]*
'The glass mouth-piece could be removed and washed as easily as a cup or a wine glass'. The unidirectional valves were glass discs offering 'trifling resistance' and were enclosed in a glass case. 'Instead of a sponge a little water (1) was introduced into the bottle with the ether (2) through which the bubbles of air passed from the lower end of the glass tube . . .'

Even though some of the evidence is circumstantial, it would seem that Bell's January trial of chloric ether was made on those early dental patients of Tomes, and while there are no records at the hospital to prove this assumption, there is a compelling reason for believing it to be correct. When I wrote on Tomes [1], I could find no evidence that Bell had any connection with the hospital, other than that his firm was a subscribing governor, and had supplied the ether used on 25 January. But I have since discovered from the Board minutes that both men were present at the Weekly Board Meeting on 19 January, and that Bell was a member of the Medical Committee (though Tomes was not) from February 1846 until the end of 1848 [12]. That advisory committee did not then consist solely of physicians and surgeons, and Bell as an expert pharmacist (then known as a chemist and druggist) was well qualified to serve on it, especially as he had also studied anatomy and physics.

Bell's close association with the Middlesex dispels the uncertainty perpetuated by Snow's much quoted comment that Bell '. . . had tried chloric ether in the beginning of 1847' [13], without mentioning that this trial had been made at the Middlesex. The reference Snow quoted was the London Medical Gazette [7] which we have noted did give this information. Snow also referred to trials later in the year at the Middlesex and St Bartholomew's. The former I have been unable to confirm; the latter, made at Bell's suggestion by his pupil Furnell, is well known [14].

Before January 1847 there was no mention of chloric ether or of chloroform in any English pharmacopoeia. The composition of the former was uncertain and variable while both drugs had many confusing synonyms [15–19]. In 1845 Pereira showed that the product then known as chloric ether differed from the one originally so named, but he did not entirely clarify the distinction between it and chloroform — or simplify the nomenclature [20]. However, in January 1847 Bell would have known what his colleague Redwood would publish in February — that 'chloric ether was chloroform in 6–8 parts of spirit' [21]. When Simpson reported his use of chloroform, Pereira wrote to Bell '. . . he (Simpson) does not seem to be aware that chloroform in solution is bought and sold. I have told him that you have used chloric ether and referred him to the Pharmaceutical Journal Vol 6, p 357. Of couse you will have a notice on the subject in the next number of the Journal' [22]. Bell's 'notice' included the unequivocal comment that 'Dr Simpson re-introduced the same drug in more concentrated form' [11]. Bell predicted that chloroform would be extensively used, and in January 1848 his firm produced a simple wicker mask containing a sponge for giving chloroform [23]. This would seem to be his last contribution to practical anaesthesia, apart from his professional interest in the preparation of pure chloroform.

One apparent contradiction remains to be explained. The London Medical Gazette [7], Coleman [8], Snow [13] and Pereira [22] all implied that Bell had personally administered the chloric ether in the January trial, and indeed, it is likely that he did. Yet Tomes claimed that distinction. As the dental surgeon, he would have regarded the anaesthetic as an adjunct to his treatment, and therefore that he was responsible for it. (He would not be the last surgeon to invoke that argument). Bell was not a clinician and did not contest the claim. The two men remained friends, and Bell later assisted in the formation of the Odontological Society of which Tomes was a founder [8].

Jacob Bell's outstanding achievement was his creation of the Pharmaceutical Society, with its School of Pharmacy and its journal. This was part of his life-long campaign to further the interests and professional status of pharmacists, for which purpose he entered Parliament in 1850. He was a Fellow of the Linnean, Chemical and Zoological Societies, the Society of Arts, and an honorary member of several foreign societies. Quaker and philanthropist, he was a patron of the arts and left his own collection to the nation. When he died in 1859 aged 49, 'nearly all the chemists in the country closed their shops' [24]. He is remembered by anaesthetists for his reports of the Pharmaceutical Society meetings, his inhaler, described as having the merit of efficiency, compactness and elegance' [25] (though apparently used only at the Middlesex), and especially for his trial of chloric ether.

SEPTIMUS SIBLEY

In 1853 the hospital created the new post of Registrar (later Medical Registrar) at £50 a year with 'the specific duty of administering chloroform', though without the title of chloroformist. The man appointed was Septimus Sibley (1831–1893) who had qualified from University College Hospital and the Middlesex with the Gold Medal in Surgery and the Silver Medal in Medicine. He had been a house surgeon for a year.

Sibley had the misfortune to have a death on the table (number 41 in Snow's book [26]). The patient was a stout and florid man of 65, the oldest in Snow's series. After 10 minutes of uneventful anaesthesia there was a violent spasm which continued for 3 minutes, before the pulse became irregular and ceased. The post mortem revealed an enlarged heart in which 'fat formed three quarters of the thickness of the wall of the ventricle'. To me, this was not a typical chloroform death, but is suggestive of gastric regurgitation followed by death from the hypoxic strain on the diseased heart. Sibley's resuscitative efforts were exemplary—mouth to mouth ventilation within a few seconds and galvanism within 2 minutes. ('Electric shocks to the thorax' had been used at the Middlesex in 1794 on an apparently dead woman who had fallen from a 'one pair of stairs window'. Her health was reportedly restored [27].)

In 1857 Sibley became FRCS and was appointed Lecturer in Pathological Anatomy for the medical school and Visiting Apothecary to the hospital. He wrote several papers (not concerning anaesthesia), and a description of the hospital's response to the cholera epidemic in Soho in 1854, when Florence Nightingale came to assist the overwhelmed nursing staff. Sibley was acting Resident Medical Officer when 120 cases of 'cholera' and at least the same number with 'diarrhoea' were admitted in three days [28].

Sibley later had a distinguished career in general practice, and was a member of council of the British Medical Association, and President of its Metropolitan Counties Branch. He was also chairman of the managing committee of the Dental Hospital of London, Vice-President of the New Sydenham Society, and was the first general practitioner to sit on the Council of the Royal College of Surgeons. With Tomes and Bell, he is commemorated in the *Dictionary of National Biography* [29,30].

JOHN MURRAY

In 1867, the hospital appointed its first staff member with the title of Chloroformist as well as Medical Registrar. John Murray had attended classes in the Faculty of Arts at Aberdeen University for two years, before studying medicine there, and in Edinburgh, Paris, Vienna and Berlin—and at the Middlesex, where he qualified MRCS and became house physician in 1865. He proceeded to MD Aberdeen in 1867, and MRCP in 1870.

Murray was among the first to employ nitrous oxide for dental patients after the American TW Evans had demonstrated its use in 1868. This technique had aroused considerable controversy, several authorities maintaining that the apparent anaesthetic effect of the gas was simply due to deprivation of oxygen [31]. Murray, together with John (later Sir John) Sanderson FRS, then Assistant Physician and Lecturer in Physiology at the hospital, soon put the hypothesis to the test. He administered pure nitrogen to six dental patients at the Middlesex and showed that to produce insensibility with nitrogen took 3–4 times longer than it did with nitrous oxide, while recovery was slightly prolonged [32]. Sanderson confirmed these differences with some animal experiments [33] and Murray gave a further demonstration of nitrogen inhalation at a British Medical Association Meeting in Oxford [34].

Murray designed a neat folding chloroform mask which, with a $1\frac{1}{2}$ ounce bottle of chloroform, fitted into a small case which could be carried in a breast pocket [35]. However, a few years later, quoting numerous authorities — mainly in France and the US — he supported the view that ether was safer than chloroform [36].

This remarkable young man abounded with energy. He was an active member of the London Pathological and Clinical Societies, and served as President of the Middlesex Hospital Medical Society. He was the honorary secretary of the Volunteer Medical Association, and after barely 18 months as Chloroformist at the Middlesex, he worked with the Red Cross Society around Sedan in the Franco–Prussian War. He progressed from hospital reporter, to become a sub editor of the *British Medical Journal* and 'as a large contributor to its columns was closely identified with its utterances on most of the questions of the day'. As a prominent member of the British Medical Association, he led a number of campaigns to improve conditions in several hospitals. In 1871 he was appointed Assistant Physician to the Hospital for Sick Children at Great Ormond Street, and shortly afterwards to a similar position at the Middlesex. He was also Lecturer in Pathology in the Medical School, of which he became Dean in 1873. Tragically, he died in October of the same year, after an illness of less than a week. He was just 29 years of age.

The manner of John Murray's death is of some interest to anaesthetists. He had 'hospital sore throat' — tonsillitis, oedema of the larynx and respiratory obstruction. His attending colleagues called in Morell Mackenzie, who proposed to scarify the epiglottis. He went to his nearby home to collect his instruments, prudently including those for tracheotomy, which proved on his return to be necessary immediately. Respiration was restored, but Murray died two days later.

Murray's obituaries were glowing testimonies to his character, ability and friendliness [37,38]. He is remembered at the Middlesex by a portrait bust [39] and an eponymous annual prize endowed jointly by the Medical School and the University of Aberdeen.

EVERITT NORTON

In October 1870 the Middlesex appointed the first of its graduates to follow a career in anaesthesia — George Everitt Norton, who had been a house surgeon and resident obstetric physician at the hospital. He was among the first to report experiences with ether after its virtues had been forcefully advocated in 1872 by the American visitor Jeffries [40] and the *British Medical Journal* [41]. In December he wrote [42], 'I have for the last month administered ether in hospital (though in his first five cases he was assisted by Murray [43]) and in private practice, in place of chloroform in all those cases in which it has seemed possible'. He felt it was too soon to give an opinion on the superiority of ether. Five weeks later, he concluded that 'ether does not appear to have any advantages over chloroform unless it be proved safer' [44]. He first followed Jeffries' method, using a towel and sponge, but because 'the theatre became full of ether, and the amount used very large' he thereafter used an inhaler. This was a compact device in which the inspired air passed over five metal shelves covered with flannel saturated with ether, which was intermittently replenished from a small reservoir [42]. This inhaler proved unsatisfactory, because it was difficult to tell when the flannel became dry (and presumably also because it got too cold), so it was soon replaced. The new and better model [45] was based on a Wolf's bottle which was surrounded by a water bath at 70°F, as with the later 'Boyle's bottle' the inspired vapour could be either drawn from above the surface of the ether or bubbled through it. Norton was ahead of his time in another way: 'I have now fixed to the expiratory valve of the inhaler a long India-rubber tube which conveys the expired ether to the floor. This prevents the operator and assistants from being annoyed by the vapour' [44].

By 1876 he had concluded that ether was safer than chloroform, and it was his choice, using the same inhaler, for normal adults. He preferred chloroform for elderly bronchitics and children, and for obstetrics, eye operations and procedures round the mouth. Nitrous oxide he reserved for dental operations [46]. He reported unhappy experiences with bichloride of methylene [47] and with bromide of ethyl [48]. The former had been used for 'small operations' for a year, and a brewer's drayman died under its influence, galvanism to the phrenic nerves failing to revive him; the latter caused excessive vomiting and did not always produce relaxation.

Norton was also anaesthetist to the National Dental and St Saviour's Hospitals and surgeon to the Royal Humane Society. He had previously been a keen volunteer, Surgeon-Major to the West London Rifles, and also Surgeon to the Western General Dispensary. He was a member of the British Medical Association and of the Harveian Society, and a founder member of the Society of Anaesthetists, serving on its first Council. His stature was reflected in his telegraphic address, 'Anaesthetic London'. Norton died in 1906, still working, and 'held in high esteem by his colleagues' [49].

FURTHER APPOINTMENTS

In 1885 a second chloroformist appointment was established. With one exception, I shall deal very briefly with the holders of that post. WE Dixon, A McCausland and AL Bright did not pursue a career in anaesthesia, but H Davis and TGS Burns did so with distinction, both later becoming founder members of the Society of Anaesthetists and serving on its Council. Henry Davis held the post in 1885–6, and also had anaesthetic appointments at the Dental Hospital of London and at St Mary's, where he later became a distinguished consultant. Theodore Burns was appointed in 1892 having previously been Assistant Administrator of Anaesthetics at St Bartholomew's Hospital. When Norton died, he became the senior anaesthetist until 1919 when he resigned. He served on the Council of the Anaesthetic Section of the Royal Society of Medicine, and as a captain in the Royal Army Medical Corps.

A third anaesthetist was appointed in 1899. This was HP Noble, a Middlesex man who had qualified with honours. He was also anaesthetist to the Metropolitan, Paddington Green Children's and the National Dental Hospitals. He continued at the Middlesex until ill-health brought premature retirement in 1914. He too was a member of the Society of Anaesthetists, and later served on the Council of the Anaesthetic Section of the Royal Society of Medicine.

CHARLES SHEPPARD

Charles E Sheppard was Chloroformist for little over a year until his death in June 1891, at the age of 35. He had a brilliant early career at St Thomas's, where he gained many prizes and qualified in 1879 with honours in both medicine and surgery. Two years later, he proceeded MD with the Gold Medal, and also became FRCS, after which he was appointed Resident Assistant Physician and Medical Registrar at his *alma mater*. This double appointment (afterwards split into two posts) was particularly arduous, and this, together with a family bereavement, led to a breakdown in his health. He gave up medicine for several years, before returning to clinical appointments at St Thomas's, the Children's Hospital and the National Hospital for Paralysis. It was only then that he took up anaesthesia, having enjoyed his earlier experience in this field as a houseman, and he did so with determination and success. He became anaesthetist to Guy's Dental School, the National Orthopaedic Hospital, the Victoria Hospital for Children and the Dental Department of St Thomas's, as well as to the Middlesex.

He was described as a man with an encyclopaedic knowledge of literature, and of many other subjects outside medicine, and had an extensive collection of old books. He made a particular study of Scottish poetry and compiled a glossary of Robert Burns' work. He was an accomplished musician who built an organ and could play to concert standard on many instruments. Happiest when playing music, he was a retiring man, who 'had many friends and no enemies' [50].

Sheppard made an important modification to nitrous oxide cylinders which were to be used lying horizontal on the floor. This was unsatisfactory because liquid nitrous oxide was often delivered and this, together with excessive cooling, resulted in interruption of the gas supply. Sheppard persuaded Barth and Co, the manufacturers, to fit a draw-off tube inside the cylinder neck, with its inner end bent up so that its orifice was above the level of the liquid [51]. Cylinders thus modified were in regular use for the next 60 years. He also described a device to enable Clover's inhaler to be used with the patient in the prone position. The concept was delightfully simple, and is now in universal use (though no longer with a Clover) — an angle-piece which fitted between the face mask and the inhaler. His paper was more than just a description of the angle-piece, as he discussed the physiological changes and practical problems occurring with the prone patient, and gave a sound rationale for using ether rather than chloroform in these circumstances [52].

Charles Sheppard's other contribution to anaesthetics was indirect — an unpublished collection of 'most carefully recorded notes of 2350 administrations', gracefully acknowledged by Frederick Hewitt in the preface to his textbook [53]. Hewitt referred to 'all the valuable observations' made by his friend Sheppard 'upon the pupil under chloroform and upon many other points connected with the effects of anaesthetics', and ended, 'I have incorporated these observations with my own'. Sheppard's contribution to this influential book should not be forgotten.

ACKNOWLEDGEMENTS

I am grateful to Miss K Arnold-Foster, Museum Officer of the Royal Pharmaceutical Society of Great Britain and to Mr SWF Holloway, Senior Lecturer in the Faculty of Social Science, University of Leicester, for their help concerning Jacob Bell, and to the late Mr WR Winterton FRCS, FRCOG, formerly Archivist at the Middlesex Hospital.

REFERENCES

(1) Dinnick OP. John Tomes—Anaesthetist 1846. In Atkinson RS, Boulton TB, eds. *The history of anaesthesia* (International Congress and Symposium Series 134). London: Royal Society of Medicine Services Ltd, 1989: 505–10.
(2) Anonymous. Painless operations at the Middlesex Hospital, London. *London Med Gazette* (NS) 1847; **4**: 219.
(3) Meeting report. *Pharmaceut J* 1846–47; **6**: 355.
(4) Obituary: Sir John Tomes. *Nature* 1895; **52**: 396.
(5) Obituary: Sir John Tomes. *Br Dent J* 1895; **16**: 462.
(6) Editor's footnote. *Pharmaceut J* 1846–47; **6**: 357.
(7) Editor's footnote. *London Med Gazette* (NS) 1847; **5**: 939.
(8) Coleman A. On anaesthesia with special reference to operations in dental surgery. *Trans Odontological Soc* 1862; **3**: 152–70.
(9) Tomes J. *Dental physiology and surgery*. London: John W Parker, 1848: 349–50.
(10) Obituary: Sir John Tomes. *Br Med J* 1895; **2**: 396.
(11) Anonymous (Bell J). *Pharmaceut J* 1847–48; **7**: 277–9.
(12) List of Governors and Subscribers of the Middlesex Hospital with an Abstract of Receipts and Expenditures for 1848 (Annual Report). London: James Truscott, 1849–50: 15.
(13) Snow J. *On chloroform and other anaesthetics*. London: John Churchill, 1858: 20.
(14) Sykes WS. *Essays on the first hundred years of anaesthesia*. Edinburgh: E & S Livingstone, 1961; **2**: 168–77.
(15) Ure J. On the nature and properties of a liquid sold under the name of terchloride of carbon. *Pharmaceut J* 1843–44; **3**: 170–2.
(16) Redwood T. On the preparation of ethers. *Pharmaceut J* 1843–44; **3**: 369–71.
(17) Correspondence (reply). Chloric ether. *Pharmaceut J* 1843–44; **3**: 458.
(18) Anonymous. Notes on Mr Redwood's lecture. *Pharmaceut J* 1843–44; **3**: 490–5.
(19) Dinnick OP. Jacob Bell and his trial of chloric ether at the Middlesex Hospital. *Pharmacy in History* 1991; **33**: 70–75.
(20) Pereira J. Historical notice of the chloride of formyle commonly called chloric ether or tetrachloride of carbon. *Pharmaceut J* 1845–46; **5**: 412–4.
(21) Redwood T. *Gray's supplement to the pharmacopoeia*. London: Longmans, 1847: 633.
(22) Cloughly CP, Burnby JGL, Earles MP, eds. *My dear Mr Bell: Letters from Dr Jonathan Pereira to Mr Jacob Bell, London 1844–1953*. Edinburgh: American Institute of the History of Pharmacy, Madison, British Society for the History of Pharmacy, 1987: 35.
(23) J Bell & Co. Chloroform inhaler. *Pharmaceut J* 1847–48; **7**: 341, 422.
(24) Smith GB. Jacob Bell. In: *Dictionary of national biography*. London: Smith Elder & Co, 1885; **4**: 162.
(25) Meeting report. *Med Times* 1847; **16**: 306.
(26) Snow J. *On chloroform and other anaesthetics*. London: John Churchill, 1858: 180–2.
(27) Perman E. Successful cardiac resuscitation in the 18th century? *Br Med J* 1979; **2**: 1770
(28) Sibley S. Report on cholera epidemic. *Middlesex Hospital Weekly Board Minutes*, October 1854. Summarized in: Winterton WR. The Soho cholera epidemic of 1854. *History of Medicine* 1980; **8**: 11–20.
(29) Obituary. Septimus Sibley. *Br Med J* 1893; **1**: 671.
(30) Carlyle EI. Septimus Sibley. In: *Dictionary of national biography*. London: Smith Elder & Co, 1887; **52**: 185.
(31) Duncum B. *The development of inhalational anaesthesia*. London: Oxford University Press, 1947: 279–84.
(32) Anonymous. The administration of nitrogen as an anaesthetic at the Middlesex Hospital. *Br Med J* 1868; **1**: 593.

(33) Meeting report. *Trans Odontological Soc* 1869 (NS); **1**: 53–54.
(34) Editorial. *Br J Dent Sci* 1868; **11**: 414.
(35) Anonymous. Chloroform inhaler of Dr Murray. *Medical Times Gazette* 1868; **1**: 540.
(36) Reports. Reprint of article by Murray J. in the London Medical Record of 7 May, 1873. *Br Med J* 1875; **2**: 781.
(37) In Memorium. John Murray. *Br Med J* 1873; **2**: 476.
(38) Obituary. John Murray. *Lancet* 1873; **2**: 57–58.
(39) Anonymous. Memorial bust of the late John Murray. *Br Med J* 1878; **2**: 118.
(40) Jeffries J. Ether in ophthalmic surgery. *Lancet* 1872; **2**: 241–2.
(41) Editorials. *Br Med J* 1872; **2**: 449–502, 554–6, 583.
(42) Norton GE. The administration of ether. *Br Med J* 1872; **2**: 629–30.
(43) Reports on medical and surgical practice. *Br Med J* 1872; **2**: 550.
(44) Norton GE. Report on the administration of ether in hospitals. *Br Med J* 1873; **1**: 35.
(45) Anonymous. A new ether inhaler. *Br Med J* 1872; **1**: 353.
(46) Norton GE. Report on chloroform and ether as anaesthetics. *Br Med J* 1876; **1**: 12–13.
(47) Norton GE. Death during the administration of bichloride of methylene. *Br Med J* 1872; **2**: 449.
(48) Norton GE. Bromide of ethyl as an anaesthetic. *Br Med J* 1880; **1**: 735.
(49) Obituary. G Everitt Norton. *Br Med J* 1906; **2**: 1523.
(50) Obituary. Charles E Sheppard. *Br Med J* 1891; **2**: 104–5.
(51) Sheppard CE. Difficulties with the use of nitrous oxide bottles in horizontal position. *Lancet* 1891; **1**: 424.
(52) Sheppard CE. The administration of ether in operations requiring the prone or lateral positions. *Br Med J* 1891; **2**: 68–70.
(53) Hewitt FW. *Anaesthetics and their administration*. London: Charles Griffin and Co, 1893: viii.

Memories of anaesthesia in Croydon (1938–1952)

Ruth E Mansfield

Original presentation Croydon 1989

Before the war anaesthetics at Croydon General Hospital, at the Oakfield Lodge site in London Road, were given by honorary staff, and most emergencies looked after by house physicians. Honorary staff were usually in general practice for a livelihood, although there was a private ward in the hospital and a private nursing home in the town. Croydon General Hospital was rather like a converted country house, with wards, outpatients departments, two theatres and two very small anaesthetic rooms, the latter being equipped with Boyle's machines, endotracheal tubes, laryngoscopes and the basic drugs then available.

The Mayday, known originally as the Croydon Union Infirmary had 643 beds and was in Mayday Road, with Queen's for geriatrics nearby and St Mary's for normal maternity cases. At Mayday the anaesthetics were given by physicians like Dr Spearing, or by the house physicians — whether they knew anything about it or not. Dr Spearing told me a revealing story. One of the house physicians, was giving an anaesthetic for Dr Tamlin who suddenly exclaimed 'This patient is dead'. 'No, he is not', the houseman assured him, 'he is still warm'. Fortunately Dr Spearing was able to take over and resuscitate the patient.

WAR AND THE MAYDAY

In 1939, with the outbreak of World War II, the Emergency Medical Service (EMS) was set up. Our sector was administered by King's College Hospital from a mental hospital at Horton, Epsom, with Mr John Hunter in charge. Volunteers were asked to work in the EMS and I was appointed to anaesthetize casualties at the Mayday Hospital.

In an interview with the Medical Superintendent I was told that he would send for me when needed! I assumed this would be when casualties arrived. On asking about equipment, I was shown a few bottles and masks in a cupboard and a gas and oxygen machine that the orderly, who was called Watson, warned me never worked and that the surgeon, Mr Walsh, had told him to throw down the stairs. This he had refused to do unless he had the order in writing!

When the Blitz started in earnest in 1940, Mr Swinton had been appointed Surgeon Superintendent, and better equipment such as a Boyle's machine, laryngoscope and rubber tracheal tubes were available. Watson stored the rubber endotracheal tubes in a biscuit tin to keep their shape, and labelled them 'Mrs Mansfield's tubes for Incubating'. The top floor theatre was abandoned for the gynaecological theatre on the ground floor. The gynaecology cases had their surgery in the Maternity Block. Two receiving wards, 3 and 7, were organized for the assessment, resuscitation and premedication of air raid casualties. We soon realized that in the severely shocked cases we were asked to anaesthetize, intravenous premedication was safer and more effective than the intramuscular route, because of slow absorption. The day rooms off these wards were used as dormitories by staff on call and were sandbagged outside in an attempt to provide protection during air raids.

We saw the first dogfight over Croydon airport from home, and were soon called on duty. In that raid, 64 people were killed and many injured [1].

In September 1940, there were so many casualties it seemed best to sleep-in on call, and as the schools were closed, my family went to a cottage we had on the North Wales coast. After a month they rang and asked if I could join them for a weekend. An Australian, Dr Taylor, offered to stand in for me and I travelled by night train with my father to join them.

On my return, I found that a bomb had fallen down the lift shaft opposite Ward 7, keeping the blast inside the building, the effect of which was increased by the sandbagging on the outside. The telephonist who was sleeping in the bed next to mine was killed. Dr Taylor on the other side of the day room had a radial artery severed by glass and two nurses in the damaged Ward 7 were also injured. This was not the only bomb to fall on the hospital.

BOMBS ON CROYDON

Numerous incendiary bombs were dropped on Croydon's hospitals. Twenty-six were extinguished on the night of 11 January 1941, including one which was initially unnoticed in the Chapel. In April 1941, a bomb fell on the Maternity isolation block, fortunately empty at the time, but a woman in labour had a ruptured abdomen from flying glass. This unusual obstetric emergency was difficult to treat as all theatres were out of order due to a power cut. Many other casualties had arrived and there were only torches and hurricane lamps in the receiving ward.

The geriatric hospital, Queen's, was hit in 1941, and again in 1944 by a landmine. I will never forget that night, nor one particular casualty who remained unrecognized because she was covered by debris. She was noisy, as she had cerebral irritation, and had been scalped as well as suffering a fractured pelvis, left arm and both legs. By the evening, after morphia, she was quiet and could be recognized as the Queen's Hospital night sister. With a drip in the one visible vein, and endotracheal oxygen, two surgeons stitched her scalp with 90 stitches and dealt with the fractures.

In 1944, the doodlebugs fell thick and fast on Croydon, dropping short of London. From June to August, 485 casualties were admitted and 248 outpatients treated, so Mayday was virtually a casualty clearing station. Patients were transferred as soon as possible to sector headquarters at Epsom, which had been reserved for D-Day wounded until it was felt to be too dangerous for them and they were taken from the beaches straight to Scotland. I was told to go to Horton leaving Dr Spearing to cope at Mayday.

I was involved in one of the transferred cases, a woman with shrapnel in the mediastinum. It had been arranged that whoever was on duty, regardless of specialization should cope. The senior gynaecologist was on duty and removed the foreign body with a pair of Volsellum forceps in a split second. He was so pleased. 'What a fuss these chest surgeons make', he observed!

During the war, oxygen cylinders were fitted with 'Endurance' reducing valves and on one occasion when a small boy was waiting for his anaesthetic the oxygen was turned on vigorously and a flame 3–4 feet long appeared. We pushed the boy out into the corridor while we sprayed the cylinder and the anaesthetic machine with a CO_2 fire extinguisher. The boy, most impressed, enquired 'if that was usual before going to sleep'.

During this time, regular lists at Mayday, Croydon General and other hospitals continued so we were kept busy. In such stressful times the atmosphere was so friendly and co-operative that 'on' and 'off' duty was often disregarded when staff were urgently required.

Working single handed, one was glad of a theatre orderly such as Watson, an ex-naval sick-bay attendant, who often entertained us with his naval stories. I quote one. He noticed the rum disappearing faster than it should, so decided to fix the culprit by putting a few drops of croton oil, a potent laxative, in the bottle. Shortly after, he was horrified when the Captain looked as if he was going to die!

Mr Rufus Thomas was in charge of the gynaecological and midwifery departments when I first went to Mayday. He did all his cases under spinal analgesia with 2 ml of 1/200 Nupercaine then positioning the patient in steep Trendelenberg. I was asked to anaesthetize any problem cases, and used a general anaesthetic technique on principle. Writing up his method, Mr Thomas stated that its chief advantage was that an anaesthetist was not required!

THE POST-WAR MAYDAY HOSPITAL

After the war and with the introduction of the NHS in 1948, surgical and anaesthetic staff increased. General surgery returned to the top floor, gynaecology and midwifery remained at the north end of the long corridor, with orthopaedics at the south end, making staffing of both nursing and anaesthesia difficult. Perhaps it would have helped if we had been issued with bicycles! I remember Mr Swinton asking for a single theatre block in the 1940s, but it took another 40 years for the excellent theatre complex and intensive care unit to materialize.

The tonsil and adenoid sessions took place three times a week in children's Ward 3. Using two tables and a screen, Mr Swinton guillotined the tonsils, helped by a team of part-time nurses and the ubiquitous orderly Watson. Dr Spearing anaesthetized with alcohol, chloroform, ether in a 'Top Hat'; his record was 14 cases in 28 minutes. My method was with N_2O, O_2 through 5 ml Vinesthene in a Goldman inhaler, my fastest being 12 cases in 20 minutes. The child was turned on the side for adenoids and Watson carried them out to the recovery room. It was surprising that with this old fashioned method that there was so little bleeding.

In the early 1950s, there was a polio epidemic in Croydon. I remember one teenager with respiratory paralysis being ventilated in an old type tank ventilator, who developed a respiratory infection needing suction. We decided to bronchoscope him, but found we could not extend his head sufficiently to do this, so had to take him out of the ventilator for the procedure. The ventilator had to be hand pumped for 24 hours when there was a power cut.

As surgery grew, both at Mayday and Croydon General, the anaesthetic staff had to increase further in number, and drugs, equipment and monitoring became more sophisticated. I hope they have not forgotten how important it still is to watch the patient's colour, pulse and blood pressure and remember how much patients appreciate pre- and post-operative visits.

REFERENCE

(1) Mason JHN. *Mayday Hospital, Croydon, 1885–1985: A history of a century of service.* Croydon Health Authority, 1985: 16–18.

From Buxton to Lee
British anaesthesia as seen through its textbooks

D Zuck

Original presentation Reading 1986

The study of textbooks has much to offer the historian of anaesthesia. A good textbook will expound the 'state of the art'. It will describe techniques and apparatus, and explain their applications. It will indicate contemporary practices and attitudes, and will discuss the major problems of its time and the ways of tackling them. By the amount of basic science and general medicine included, it will indicate the academic standards expected of the practitioner. It may inadvertently reveal some social history in relation to the status of the anaesthetist and the structure of the specialty, and it will contain a fund of common sense and good advice from which one can still learn.

Trainees today still do most of their learning from textbooks. This was even more the case in the early part of the century, with no anaesthetic journals, virtually no societies, and certainly no organized postgraduate training. The word 'trainee' is itself inappropriate, since most anaesthetists were self-taught. So a textbook could exert a great influence on attitudes and practices; the lack of emphasis on blood pressure recording, for example, set a pattern for a whole generation. Some textbooks in their various editions were in print for more than a generation: Buxton 35 years, Hewitt 32 years, Ross (Fairlie, Minnitt and Gillies) 31 years, Lee (Atkinson, Rushman) 47 years, and of course *Recent Advances* although this is not strictly speaking a textbook.

BRITISH TEXTBOOKS

The general textbooks by British authors between 1888 and 1947 fall into two categories — major specialist texts, and practical handbooks. There were only two major texts, those of Hewitt and Blomfield, the last edition of each appearing in 1922. Of the handbooks, both Buxton and Ross were comprehensive, in some respects approaching the major works. It is remarkable that in the quarter of a century from 1922 to 1947, not one major British textbook appropriate to specialist requirements was published. This is indicative of the fact, not always recognized, that the great majority of anaesthetics were being administered by general practitioners or junior hospital doctors. Lukis's book provides a vivid picture of British anaesthesia between the wars, although Lukis herself, clearly a most formidable woman with hospital appointments in otorhinolaryngology and anaesthetics, was no ordinary general practitioner. Also apparent from Lukis, and from the second edition of Hadfield, was the revolution which took place in anaesthesia during the late 20s and early 30s. At the time this was referred to as the 'mechanization of anaesthesia', and signified the spread of anaesthetic machines in hospitals, the elaboration of techniques, and the displacement of the simpler and more portable methods.

The list I have compiled consists of those textbooks which would have been available to anaesthetists in Great Britain from about 1880 to the early 1950s. Although, as Dr Duncum has pointed out, there were no comprehensive home-produced textbooks published between Snow's and Buxton's, the first two titles on the list are American texts that were available in the UK. Lyman's of 1881 is a quite remarkable but little-known book — exceptionally comprehensive, academic and erudite. It discusses medico-legal aspects of the specialty, contains a long review of all the substances that had been used to produce anaesthesia, reproduces sphygmograph tracings of animals and man from studies of the strength of heart action from as early as 1872, and demonstrates a good knowledge of the European literature.

The third and fourth editions of Turnbull's book of 1878 are also worthy of study, containing information that we generally associate with much later periods. It includes the use of the spectroscope in blood-gas analysis, the availability of mixtures of nitrous oxide and oxygen in one cylinder, and gives the first account I have come across in a textbook, of respiratory obstruction by the epiglottis, and Clover's manoeuvre of clearing the airway by extending and raising the head. Mention must also be made of Webster, who in 1924 was described as 'professor of anaesthesiology' in the University of Manitoba. This must have been the first chair to be established in the specialty, antedating that of Waters by some years. There is a splendid photograph of Webster in Wesley Bourne's *Mysterious Waters to Guard*.

In the main, only general textbooks and some monographs have been listed, for reasons of space. Excluded are a number of books on dental anaesthesia which were published during the early years of this period, one running to 300 pages. That there were at least six titles and 15 editions indicates a trend and a need in this field. The same considerations apply to the small books on analgesia in midwifery, often aimed as much at the midwife as the doctor, of which ten titles were published in 14 editions between 1934 and 1947. Except for two or three classics, I have in general excluded books solely on regional anaesthesia, but the existence of texts such as Farr's is evidence of the dissatisfaction in the US with the quality of general anaesthesia, so vividly portrayed by Flagg. Some inclusions are subjective, notably books like Mason and Zintel, widely used by my own generation, without which the list would seem incomplete.

It will be seen that certain large American textbooks, aimed more at the specialist, were available to fill the gap during the lean years. The Year Book series from the US contained important material. British anaesthetists looked also to Hewer's *Recent Advances*, and to monographs such as Gillespie's and Rowbotham's. The main journal sources were the *Proceedings of the Society of Anaesthetists* and, after the merger, *Proceedings of the Royal Society of Medicine*, augmented from the 1920s onward by the *British Journal of Anaesthesia*.

Where ascertainable, the number of pages has been included, not for reasons of bibliographic obsessiveness, but to give an idea of the size, scope and importance of the books, and the growth of their editions. Study of the list reveals other interesting features — the trends to be picked out at certain periods, evidence of the increasing demands made by surgery advancing into new fields, the introduction of new agents and techniques, and the broadening of the ambit and responsibilities of the anaesthetist. Also worthy of note is the long association of some publishers with anaesthetic textbooks. Churchill, for example, publisher of John Snow's first textbook in 1847, survives in Churchill-Livingstone.

The books are arranged by date of first publication. The list has been checked against the actual volumes when possible, and against the catalogues of the Association of Anaesthetists, the Royal Society of Medicine, the Wellcome Institute, and the British Library, (which last catalogue has been found to be not wholly reliable). To these institutions and their staff I am indebted; and also to AJ Wright of the University of Alabama, and the magic of the Internet, for some last minute help. It will be seen that some titles changed in later editions. I would welcome corrections, or information about omissions. It is hoped to publish elsewhere a fuller analysis of anaesthetic textbooks.

A SELECTED LIST OF ANAESTHETIC TEXTBOOKS 1878–1947

Turnbull L. *(The advantages and accidents of—title of first two editions) Artificial anaesthesia: a manual of anaesthetic agents and their employment.* Philadelphia: Blakiston, 4 edns. 1878, 322 pp; 1879, 322 pp; 1890, 531 pp; 1896, 550 pp.

Lyman HM. *Artificial anaesthesia and anaesthetics.* New York: William Wood, 1881, 338 pp.

Davis H. *Guide to the administration of anaesthetics.* London: HK Lewis, 2 edns. 1887, 52 pp; 1892, 92 pp.

Buxton DW. *Anaesthetics: their uses and administration.* London: HK Lewis, 6 edns. 1888, 164 pp; 1892, 222 pp; 1900, 320 pp; 1907, 415 pp; 1914, 477 pp; 1920, 548 pp.

Hewitt FW. *Select methods in the administration of nitrous oxide and ether: a handbook for practitioners and students.* London: Baillière, Tindall and Cox, 1888, 48 pp.

Silk JFW. *Nitrous oxide anaesthesia: a manual for the use of students and general practitioners.* London: Churchill, 1888, 120 pp.

Hewitt FW. *The anaesthetic effects of nitrous oxide: when administered at ordinary atmospheric pressure.* London: John Bale, 1892, 48 pp.

Hewitt FW. (Fifth edition edited posthumously by Robinson H.) *Anaesthetics and their administration.* London: Griffin and Co, (1st edn, 2nd to 4th editions by Macmillan, 5th by Oxford Medical Publications). 5 edns. 1893, 357 pp; 1901, 528 pp; 1907, 627 pp; 1912, 676 pp; 1922, 576 pp.

Probyn-Williams RJ. *A practical guide to the administration of anaesthetics.* London: Longmans, Green & Co, 2 edns. 1901, 211 pp; 1909, 288 pp.

Lawrie E. *Chloroform—a manual for students and practitioners.* London: Churchill, 1901, 120 pp.

Blumfeld J. (4th edition, Blomfield J). *Anaesthetics—a practical handbook.* London: Baillière, Tindall and Cox, 4 edns. 1902, 109 pp; 1906, 117 pp; 1912, 134 pp; 1917, 147 pp.

Luke TD. *A pocket guide to anaesthetics for the student and general practitioner.* Edinburgh: Green, 4 edns. 1902, 148 pp; 1905, 135 pp; 1906, 136 pp; 1908, 149 pp.

Silk JFW. Anaesthesia In: Cheyne WW, Burghard FF, eds. *A manual of surgical treatment—* part 1 of 6 volumes, 4th ed. London: Longmans, 1904.

Barton GAH. *A guide to the administration of ethyl chloride.* London: HK Lewis, 2 edns. 1905, 39 pp; 1907, 54 pp.

Prenderville A de. *The anaesthetic technique for operations on the nose and throat.* London: Glaisher, 1906, 87 pp.

Boyle HEG. (Third edition co-edited by Hewer CL). *Practical anaesthetics.* London: Oxford University Press, 3 edns. 1907, 178 pp; 1911, 209 pp; 1923, 187 pp.

Bellamy Gardner H. *Surgical anaesthesia.* London: Baillière, Tindall and Cox, 2 edns. 1909, 240 pp; 1916, 220 pp.

Collum RW. *The practice of anaesthetics.* (With Gray HW. General surgical technique) Medico-chirurgical Series No 1. London: Bale and Danielsson, 1909, 382 pp.

Silk JFW. *Modern anaesthetics.* London: Edward Arnold, 2 edns. 1914, 200 pp; 1920, 191 pp.

Gwathmey JT. *Anesthesia.* New York and London: Appleton, 2 edns. 1914, 945 pp; 1924, rep. 1925, 799 pp.

Crile GW, Lower WE. *Anoci-association*. Philadelphia and London: WB Saunders, 1914, 259 pp.

Allen CW. *Local and regional anesthesia*. Philadelphia: WB Saunders, 2 edns. 1914, 625 pp; 1918, 674 pp.

Flagg PJ. *The art of anaesthesia*. Philadelphia and London: Lippincott, 7 edns. 1916, 341 pp; 1919, 367 pp; 1922, 371 pp; 1928, 384 pp; 1932, 416 pp; 1939, 491 pp; 1944, 519 pp.

Ross JS. *Handbook of anaesthetics* (continued as Ross and Fairlie, Minnitt, and ultimately as Minnitt and Gillies). Edinburgh: Livingstone, 2 edns. 1919, 214 pp; 1923, 328 pp.

Barton GAH. *Backwaters of Lethe — some anaesthetic notions*. London: HK Lewis, 1920, 151 pp.

Blomfield J. *Anaesthetics in practice and theory*. London: Heinemann, 1922, 424 pp.

Levy AG. *Chloroform anaesthesia*. London: John Bale, Sons, and Danielsson, 1922, (facsimile reprint 1986), 159 pp.

Labat G. *Regional anesthesia*. Philadelphia and London: WB Saunders, 2 edns. 1922, rep. 1923, 1924, 496 pp; 1928, 567 pp.

Hewer CL. *Anaesthesia in children*. London: HK Lewis, 1923, 111 pp.

Hadfield CF. *Practical anaesthetics for the student and general practitioner*. London: Baillière, Tindall and Cox, 2 edns. 1923, 244 pp; 1931, 336 pp.

Farr RE. *Practical local anesthesia*. Philadelphia and London: Lea and Fibiger, Kimpton, 2 edns. 1923; 1929 US, 1930 London, 611 pp.

Webster W. *The science and art of anaesthetics*. London: Kimpton, 1924, 214 pp.

Ross JS, Fairlie HP. *Handbook of anaesthetics*. (Continuation of Ross, 3rd and 4th edns, and continued as Minnitt (and Gillies)). Edinburgh: Livingstone, 2 edns. 1929, 339 pp; 1935, 299 pp.

Rood FS, Webber HN. *Anaesthesia and anaesthetics*. London: Cassell, 1930, 292 pp.

Sykes WS. *Modern treatment: anaesthesia*. London: J Cape, 1931, 128 pp.

Hewer CL. *Recent advances in anaesthesia and analgesia*. London: Churchill, 1932, 187 pp; 1937, 284 pp; 1939, 333 pp; 1943, 341 pp; 1944, rep. 1946, 343 pp; 1948, 380 pp; 1953, 440 pp; 1957, 295 pp; 1963, 358; 1967, 342 pp; and still in production.

Lukis DH. *Problems of anaesthesia in general practice*. London: Hodder and Stoughton, 1935, 158 pp.

Nosworthy MD. *The theory and practice of anaesthesia*. London: Hutchinson Scientific, 1935, rep. 1937, 223 pp.

Ashworth HK. *Practical points in anaesthesia: a clinical handbook for students and general practitioners*. London: Churchill, 1936, 160 pp.

Guedel AE. *Inhalation anesthesia — a fundamental guide*. New York: Macmillan, 2 edns. 1937, 172 pp; 1951, 143 pp.

Mason RL (2nd edn and Zintel HA) eds. *Preoperative and postoperative treatment*. Philadelphia and London: WB Saunders, 2 edns. 1937, 495 pp; 1946, 584 pp.

Rolleston H, Moncrieff AA. *Modern anaesthetic practice*. London: Eyre and Spottiswood, 2 edns. 1938, rep. 1941, 150 pp; 1946, 231 pp.

Beecher HK. *The physiology of anesthesia*. London: Oxford University Press, 1938, rep. 1940, 388 pp.

Human JU. *(The secrets of — 1st edn only) Blind intubation and the signs of anaesthesia*. London: John Bale Medical Publications (third edition by HK Lewis), 3 edns. 1938, 67 pp; 1941, 135 pp; 1947, 230 pp.

Maxson LH. *Spinal anesthesia*. Philadelphia: Lippincott, 1938, 409 pp.

Clement FW. *Nitrous oxide-oxygen anesthesia*. London: Kimpton, 3 edns. 1939, 274 pp; 1945, 288 pp; 1951, 369 pp.

Macintosh RR, Pratt (later Bannister) FB. *The essentials of general anaesthesia (: with special reference to dentistry — first two edns only)*. Oxford: Blackwell, 5 edns. 1940, 334 pp; 1941, 334 pp; 1943, 341 pp; 1947, 358 pp; 1952, 378 pp.

Minnitt RJ. *Handbook of anaesthetics* (formerly Ross and Fairlie — the fifth edition). Edinburgh: Livingstone, 1940, 364.

Robbins BH. *Cyclopropane anesthesia*. Baltimore: Williams and Wilkins, 2 edns. 1940, 175 pp; 1958, 293 pp.

Adriani J. *The pharmacology of anesthetic drugs*. Springfield, Illinois: CC Thomas, 5 edns. 1940, 46 pp; 1941, rep. 1942, 1946, 1947, 86 pp; 1952, rep. 1954, 179 pp; 1960, 232 pp; 1970, 297 pp.

Goldman V. *Aids to anaesthesia*. London: Baillière, Tindall and Cox, 2 edns. 1941, rep. 1943, 235 pp; 1948, 316 pp.

Gillespie NA. *Endotracheal anaesthesia*. Wisconsin: University of Wisconsin Press, 2 edns. 1941, 187 pp; 1948, 237 pp.

Woolmer RF. *Anaesthetics afloat*. London: HK Lewis, 1942, 120 pp.

King AC. *The principles and practice of gaseous anaesthetic apparatus*. London: Baillière, Tindall and Cox, 2 edns. 1941, 45 pp; 1946, 47 pp.

Lundy JS. *Clinical anesthesia — a manual of clinical anesthesiology*. Philadelphia and London: WB Saunders, 1942, 771 pp.

Waters RW, Rovenstine EA, Lundy JS, Beecher HK, Booth LS, Tovell RM, Wood RM. *Fundamentals of anesthesia — an outline*. Chicago: American Medical Association, 2 edns. 1942, 216 pp; 1944, 231 pp.

James NR. *Regional analgesia for intra-abdominal surgery*. London: Churchill, 1943, rep. 1944, 57 pp.

Macintosh RR, Mushin WW. *Local anaesthesia: brachial plexus*. Oxford: Blackwell, 4 edns. 1944, 56 pp; 1947, 56 pp; 1954, 62 pp; 1967, 63 pp.

Minnitt RJ, Gillies J. *Textbook of anaesthetics* (sixth and seventh editions of Ross and Fairlie). Edinburgh: Livingstone, 2 edns. 1944, rep. 1945, 489 pp; 1948, 568 pp.

Mackenzie JR. *Practical anaesthetics for students, hospital residents, and practitioners*. London: Baillière, Tindall and Cox, 2 edns. 1944, 136 pp; 1946, 172 pp.

Adams RC. *Intravenous anesthesia*. New York and London: Paul B Hoeber, 1944, 663 pp.

Rowbotham S. *Anaesthesia in operations for goitre*. Oxford: Blackwell, 1945, 104 pp.

Macintosh RR, Mushin WW (and Epstein HG, 2nd and 3rd editions; 4th edition by Mushin WW, Jones P). *Physics for the anaesthetist*. Oxford: Blackwell, 4 edns. 1946, 235 pp; 1958, 443 pp; 1963, 448 pp; 1987, 648 pp.

Parry-Price H. *A short handbook of practical anaesthetics*. Bristol: John Wright (Simpkin Marshall), 1946, 127 pp.

Adriani J. *The chemistry of anesthesia*. Oxford: Blackwell, 1946, 530 pp.

Cullen SC. *Anesthesia in general practice*. (Later *Anesthesia: a manual for students and physicians*). Chicago: Year Book Publishers, 5 edns. 1946, 260 pp; 1948, rep. 1949, 1950, 264 pp; 1951, rep. 1952, 292 pp; 1954, 312 pp; 1956, 295 pp.

Kaye G, Orton RH, Renton DG. *Anaesthetic methods*. Melbourne: Ramsey, 1946, 706 pp.

Pitkin GP, Southworth JC, Hingson RA. *Conduction anesthesia*. Philadelphia: Lippincott, 2 edns. 1946, 981 pp; 1953, 1005 pp.

Lee JA. *A synopsis of anaesthesia*. Bristol: John Wright & Son, 11 edns. 1947, 254 pp; 1950, 354 pp; 1953, rep. 1955, 1956, 1957, 483 pp; 1959, 616 pp; 1964, 774 pp; 1968, 876 pp; 1973, 991 pp; 1977, 986 pp; 1982, 962 pp; 1987, 898 pp; 1993, 994 pp. (From 5th edn. Lee JA and Atkinson RS; from 8th edn. add Rushman GB; 11th edn. *Lee's synopsis of anaesthesia*, Atkinson RS, Rushman GB, Davies JH. Butterworth-Heinemann.) Still in production.

McIntyre AR. *Curare: its history, nature, and clinical use*. Chicago: University of Chicago Press, 1947, 240 pp.

Adriani J. *Techniques and procedures of anesthesia*. Oxford: Blackwell, 2 edns. 1947, 404 pp; 1956, 568 pp.

Mushin WW. *Anaesthesia for the poor risk: and other essays*. Oxford: Blackwell, 1948, 65 pp.

Leigh MD, Belton MK. *Pediatric anesthesia*. New York: Macmillan, 1948, 240 pp.

Kemp WN. *Elementary anaesthesia*. London: Baillière, Tindall and Cox, 1948, 289 pp.

Evans FT, ed. *Modern practice in anaesthesia*. London: Butterworth, 2 edns. 1949, 606 pp; 1954, 622 pp.

Burstein CL. *Fundamental considerations in anesthesia*. New York: Macmillan, 2 edns. 1949, 153 pp; 1955, 219 pp.

Harris TAB. *The mode of action of anaesthetics*. Edinburgh: Livingstone, 1951, 768 pp.

Waters RM. ed. *Chloroform: a study after 100 years*. Wisconsin: University of Wisconsin Press, 1951, 138 pp.

Mushin WW, Rendell-Baker L. *The principles of thoracic anaesthesia: past and present*. Oxford: Blackwell Scientific Publications, 2 edns. 1953, 172 pp; 1963, 695 pp.

Ostlere G. *Trichloroethylene in anaesthesia*. Edinburgh: Livingstone, 1953, 83 pp.

Bonica J. *The management of pain*. London: Kimpton, 1953, 1533 pp.

Adriani J. *Selection of anesthesia: the physiological and pharmacological basis*. Oxford: Blackwell; Springfield, Illinois: CC Thomas; Toronto: Ryerson, 1955, 327 pp.

Dundee JW. *Thiopentone and other thiobarbiturates*. Edinburgh and London: Livingstone, 1956, 312 pp.

Keating V. *Anaesthetic accidents — the complications of general and regional anaesthesia*. London: Lloyd-Luke, 1956, 261 pp.

Mushin WW, Rendell-Baker L, Thompson PW, Mapleson WW. *Automatic ventilation of the lungs*. Oxford: Blackwell, 3 edns. 1959, 349 pp; 1969, 841 pp; 1980, 887 pp.

APPENDIX

Previously published contributions to The History of Anaesthesia Society 1986–1989

Allan LG. Clinical thermometry. Reading 1986.
Published as:
Allan LG. The history of clinical thermometry. In: Atkinson RS, Boulton TB, eds. *The history of anaesthesia. Proceedings of the Second International Symposium on the History of Anaesthesia.* London: Royal Society of Medicine Services Limited, 1989: 368–71.

Baillie TW. From Boston to Dumfries. Edinburgh 1989.
Published as:
Baillie TW. The First European trial of anaesthetic ether: the Dumfries claim. *Brit J Anaesth* 1965; **37**: 952–7
Baillie TW. *From Boston to Dumfries: the first surgical use of anaesthetic ether in the Old World,* 2nd ed. Dumfries: Dinwiddie, 1969.

Doughty A. Walter Stoeckel (1871–1961). A pioneer in regional analgesia in obstetrics. Croydon 1989.
Published as:
Doughty A. Walter Stoeckel (1871–1961). A pioneer in regional analgesia in obstetrics. *Anaesthesia* 1990; **45**: 468–71.

Howat DDC. Paul Sudeck and his inhaler. Southend 1988.
Published as:
Howat DDC. Paul Sudeck — his contribution to anaesthesia. *Anaesthesia* 1989; **44**: 847–50.

Macdonald AG. Early days in Glasgow. Edinburgh 1989.
Published as:
Macdonald AG. John Henry Hill Lewellin: the first etherist in Glasgow. *Br J Anaesth* 1993; **70**: 228–34.

O'Sullivan E. Dr Robert James Minnitt. Leicester 1988.
Published as:
O'Sullivan E. Dr Robert James Minnitt 1889–1974: a pioneer of inhalational analgesia. *J Royal Soc Med* 1989; **82**: 221–3.

Owen B. Hugh Morriston Davies 1879–1965. Southend 1988.
Published as:
Owen B. Hugh Morriston Davies 1879–1965. In: Owen B. *Meeting pioneers: Biographies of 10 pioneers in the world of medicine.* Denbigh, Clwyd: Gee and Son, 1994; 37–44.

Payne JP. On the resuscitation of the apparently dead. Croydon 1989.
Published as:
Payne JP. On the resuscitation of the apparently dead — an historical account. *Annals Royal Coll Surg* 1969; **45**: 98–107.

Rees GJ. The origin of anaesthesia for cleft palate and harelip. London 1987.
Published as:
Rees GJ. An early history of paediatric anaesthesia. *Paed Anaesth* 1991; **1**: 3–11.

Sweeney B. Franz Kuhn. London 1987.
Published as:
Sweeney B. Franz Kuhn. His contribution to anaesthesia. *Anaesthesia* 1985; **40**: 1000–1005.

Thomas TA. Self-administered inhalational analgesia in obstetrics. Reading 1986.
Published as:
Thomas TA. Self-administered inhalational analgesia in obstetrics. In: Atkinson RS, Boulton TB, eds. *The history of anaesthesia. Proceedings of the Second International Symposium on the History of Anaesthesia.* London: Royal Society of Medicine Services Limited, 1989; 295–8.

Wilkinson DJ. A sleeping giant — Dr FP de Caux. Southend 1988. Dr de Caux updated. Leicester 1988.
Published as:
Wilkinson DJ. Francis Percival de Caux (1892–1965). An anaesthetist at odds with social convention and the law. *Anaesthesia* 1991; **46**: 300–305.
Wilkinson DJ. Dr FP de Caux — the first user of curare for anaesthesia in England. *Anaesthesia* 1991; **46**: 49–51.

Zuck D. A forgotten chloroform vaporizer in its historical setting (NH Alcock). Southend 1988.
Published as:
Zuck D. The Alcock chloroform vaporizer. *Anaesthesia* 1988; **43**: 972–80.

Index